HANDBOOK
of

LOWER EXTREMITY

INFECTIONS

HANDBOOK
of
LOWER EXTREMITY
INFECTIONS

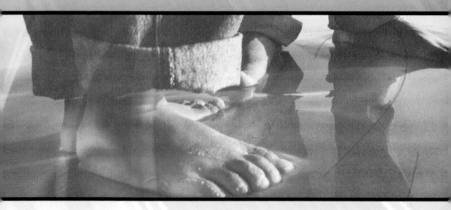

SECOND EDITION

WARREN S. JOSEPH DPM, FIDSA
Consultant, Lower Extremity Infectious Diseases

Adjunct Associate Professor
Section of Infectious Diseases
Department of Internal Medicine
Temple University School of Medicine

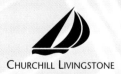

CHURCHILL LIVINGSTONE

An Imprint of Elsevier Science
New York Edinburgh London Philadelphia San Francisco

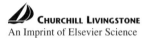 **CHURCHILL LIVINGSTONE**
An Imprint of Elsevier Science

11830 Westline Industrial Drive
St. Louis, Missouri 63146

NOTICE

Podiatry is an ever-changing field. Standard safety precautions must be
followed, but as new research and clinical experience broaden our knowledge,
changes in treatment and drug therapy may become necessary or appropriate.
Readers are advised to check the most current product information provided
by the manufacturer of each drug to be administered to verify the recommended dose, the method and duration of administration, and contraindications. It is the responsibility of the licensed prescriber, relying on experience
and knowledge of the patient, to determine dosages and the best treatment for
each individual patient. Neither the publisher nor the author assumes any
liability for any injury and/or damage to persons or property arising from this
publication.

Previous edition copyrighted 1990

International Standard Book Number 0-443-06608-6

Managing Editor: Christie M. Hart
Publishing Services Manager: Linda McKinley
Project Manager: Rich Barber
Designer: Julia Dummitt

EH-QWF

Printed in the United States

Last digit is the print number: 9 8 7 6 5 4 3 2 1

Certainly, all of the people I mentioned in the dedication of the first edition still warrant a mention in this edition. My wife, Judy, and my sons, Eric and Marc, are a constant presence in my daily thoughts and life. And, my original mentor, Jack LeFrock, MD, without whom I would have never received my initial training or inclination toward the specialty of infectious diseases.

Over the past 12 years however, I have been incredibly fortunate to have developed a second and just as important professional mentor and personal friend in Harvey Lemont, DPM. One of the truly great minds in the profession of podiatric medicine and my chairman for most of my tenure while faculty at the Temple University School of Podiatric Medicine, he allowed me to fully develop my specialty and gave direction and advice whenever needed.

Finally, I also dedicate this Handbook to all of my former students and residents who kept me on the ball and drove me to continued learning.

PREFACE

It is hard to believe that over 12 years have passed since the first edition of this Handbook was published. The response to the book has been overwhelming. Almost everywhere I lecture, someone will come up and thank me for the Handbook and relate a personal story of how helpful it was to them in board certification exam preparation or during residency interviews, or how it is the most used, dog-eared book they own. This is truly gratifying because it was my intention in writing a book of this format that it be a quick, readily usable clinical reference and not one more fancy spine up on a bookshelf.

As a testament to the ever-changing nature of infectious diseases, seemingly from shortly after the Handbook was first released, readers were asking for an update. New diagnostic testing modalities and therapeutic agents have been constantly arriving on the scene. Some of these represent relatively minor "tweaking" of older tests or drugs, whereas some changes have been truly revolutionary. The understanding of the importance of, and the ability to treat fungal infections of the lower extremity, has exploded onto our consciousness over the past decade. Barely a footnote 12 years ago, this topic now warrants a chapter of considerable length and depth.

Why did it take 12 years to publish a second edition? Basically, the time finally came when there was enough new knowledge, technology, drugs, diseases, and pathogens to justify putting out an updated book that would not be so redundant that readers of the original edition would balk at investing their hard-earned time and money to read it. To that end, although the names of the sections and chapters may appear the same, every section, chapter, and page of the original edition was carefully scrutinized and updated wherever necessary. Twelve extra years of personal patient care experience treating a wide range of lower extremity infections can significantly modify one's thinking of what was once considered dogma. Major sections have been rewritten. Updated material representing new knowledge has been added. Obsolete material was excised. Drug entries have been added, deleted, or modified based on new information. Reader comments and suggestions have been noted over the years and integrated when possible. The above-mentioned major chapter on fungal infections of the lower extremity is now included. A new appendix takes advantage of the Internet by listing sites specific for infectious diseases. And, finally, a new, useful appendix table lists pharmacokinetics parameters of every important antibiotic and provides a handy reference for information such as proper dosing (including patients with renal insufficiency).

This Handbook is not meant to be an all-encompassing text. It was designed for clinical utility and rapid reference. As such it should not be construed as a "gospel" to follow implicitly. Every case is different. The clinical judgment of the attending clinician is the most important aspect of treating a lower extremity infection. Consultation with an expert in the area of infectious diseases should be carried out whenever diagnosis or treatment is in doubt.

The treatment regimes included in this book represent opinions based on my personal experience and judgment and the current literature. As with any specialty there is more than one way to approach any clinical problem. Furthermore, knowledge about the treatment of infections and the agent to choose is changing constantly. There is no substitute for personal and independent review of the current literature and continuing education. To provide the best care possible, it behooves all clinicians to remain up to date in this dynamic area of practice.

It is my sincere hope that readers of this new edition of the Handbook of Lower Extremity Infections will continue to find it a useful adjunct to their daily clinical practices. I have tried to keep the book just as "user friendly" in layout as the original while adding all of the new material. As always, your comments are welcome.

Warren S. Joseph, DPM, FIDSA
Huntingdon Valley, PA
January, 2002

CONTENTS

PART I   **Diagnosis,** 1

    1.   Diagnosis of Lower Extremity Infections, 2

PART II   **Clinical Syndromes,** 29

    2.   Skin and Soft Tissue Infections, 30
    3.   Bone and Joint Infections, 54
    4.   Infections Following Trauma, 80
    5.   Diabetic Foot Infections, 103
    6.   Surgical Infections, 126
    7.   Fungal Infections, 147

PART III   **Antimicrobial Therapy,** 179

    8.   Principles of Antibiotic Usage, 180
    9.   Antibiotic Agents, 213

PART IV   **Microorganisms,** 277

    10.   Bacterial Microorganisms, 278

PART V   **Appendices,** 303

    Appendix 1   Oral Antibiotics and Their Usual Dosing, 303
    Appendix 2   Generic to Trade Names of Antibiotics, 305
    Appendix 3   Trade to Generic Names of Antibiotics, 307
    Appendix 4   Antibiotics against Pseudomonas Aeruginosa, 310
    Appendix 5   The Internet and Infection, 311
    Appendix 6   Drugs for Bugs, 312
    Appendix 7   Antibiotic Pharmacokinetics and Dosing, 314

PART I

Diagnosis

CHAPTER 1

Diagnosis of Lower Extremity Infections

At the beginning of a book on infectious diseases, it is important to make sure that the most basic of terms is defined to start all readers off on the proverbial "same page." Although clinicians may see infection on a daily basis, most have difficulty when asked to define the term. For this reason the following is offered.

Infection is defined as the pathologic presence of bacteria in a site or wound. This pathogenesis is evidenced by the body's response through the presence of inflammation and white blood cells.

There are some important points to take away from this definition.

1. This definition and these subsequent points are usable for any skin, skin structure, or bone and joint infection that will be covered in this book. The same may not hold true for systemic infections, pulmonary infection, urinary tract infections, or other infections.
2. The word *pathologic* is the key. Bacteria can be isolated from practically any body surface. This does not mean that the site is infected. The bacteria must be causing damage to the tissues and not just be a harmless commensal.
3. Although in rare cases there may be an altered local response to the infection, in the vast majority of cases there is almost always some identifiable response by the body. This is even true

in patients with diabetes, on systemic steroids, with vascular insufficiency and those with human immunodeficiency virus (HIV) infection.

4. Inflammation is a result of vasodilatation in the involved area, which allows greater blood flow. This causes the usual signs of redness, swelling, and heat, all of which will be discussed in detail later. Likewise, the infection will cause a chemotactic cascade that will deliver more white blood cells to the area. The combination of increased blood flow and increased white blood cells leads to two of the classic clinical findings of infection, cellulitis and pus.

Point 4 is an important point that now needs to be expanded.

Infection is a *clinical* condition and its diagnosis is made on *clinical* grounds.

CLINICAL DIAGNOSIS

■ *History*

Obtaining a complete history of the patient's chief complaint, although considered a banality in today's world of high-technology, high-cost medicine, is the important first step in the clinical diagnosis of infection. By asking the proper questions, the clinician frequently can make the diagnosis and start the patient on accurate empiric therapy before receiving laboratory results.

Etiology

Different etiologies will lead to different types of infections with various organisms. The history obtained must be detailed to properly determine the diagnosis. For example, if the patient relates lacerating the foot while swimming, it must be determined whether the water was fresh, salt, or brackish. Each of these milieus contains distinctive microbiologic flora. If a foot is punctured, the history should include the site of the wound (both anatomically on the foot and the scene of the injury), the cause of the wound, be it a nail, a piece of glass, or another object, the suspected depth of the wound, and whether shoes were worn. This history can lead to a presumptive diagnosis of osteomyelitis or soft tissue injury.

Sample Etiologies and Potential Organisms

These are just some samples of common lower extremity infections and their usually associated bacterial pathogens that can be based on just obtaining a basic history. Each will be covered in more detail in individual sections of the text.

1. Postoperative infection (no implants). By far the most common organism is *Staphylococcus aureus*. The surgical setting can also play a role. For example, if the surgery was performed in a hospital with a high incidence of methicillin-resistant staphylococcus, then that particular organism could be suspect.
2. Postoperative infection (use of implants). The most common organisms are *Staphylococcus epidermidis* or other coagulase-negative staphylococcus. This is of particular importance since a large percentage of these organisms are methicillin resistant.
3. Puncture wound osteomyelitis. *Pseudomonas aeruginosa* has been found to cause more than 90% of osteomyelitis cases following a puncture wound.
4. Cellulitis following a puncture wound. Although a common misconception is that *P. aeruginosa* is also the culprit here, as in osteomyelitis. Actually, staphylococcus and streptococcus are most common.
5. Infected ulceration in a patient with diabetes. The most common pathogens are *S. aureus* and group B streptococcus.

Clinical Signs and Symptoms

The type and severity of clinical presentation should be noted.

1. Has the patient been running a fever or feeling "feverish or flu-like"? Even if the patient has not used a thermometer, the presence of a fever has usually been recognized.
2. Has the patient experienced shaking chills, including the uncontrollable teeth chattering?
3. Has the patient awakened at night to find the bed sheets or bedclothes damp? These night sweats are a good indicator of the presence of fever.
4. Has the patient noticed lumps or stiffness behind the knees or in the groin? The patient may not relate the lumps or stiffness to the infection, and frequently it is easier to question the patient than to actually palpate the nodes. Care should be

taken in evaluating the patient's answer, however. More than one patient has confused the stiffness of arthritis with the clinician's probing about lymph nodes.

5. Has the patient noted red streaking originating at the site of infection and traveling up the leg? Patients frequently call this lymphangitis "blood poisoning."

Duration of Signs and Symptoms

Generally, the more severe the infection, the more rapidly it will spread. For example, a patient with a necrotizing, gas-forming infection of 24 hours' duration and signs of septicemia should be managed differently from a patient with a necrotizing infection related to be "brewing" for 5 days. This point may also help lead to a bacteriologic diagnosis. In the previously mentioned situation, the first patient would be treated as having a myonecrosis caused by *Clostridium perfringens*. The second patient's infection would more likely be a synergistic process containing numerous organisms. Another example is the postoperative patient in whom *S. epidermidis* may sequester in a wound for protracted periods before becoming clinically evident. *S. aureus*, on the other hand, tends to exhibit more rapid virulence.

Prior Therapy

A patient who presents with an infection may already have started a course of antibiotic therapy. This should be noted because it may affect the diagnosis and subsequent treatment. One commonly heard belief is that an antibiotic may "mask" an infection, making diagnosis difficult. There is no such thing as a masked infection, however. If an antibiotic has been given to the patient for a presumptive diagnosis of infection and the signs and symptoms disappear, this represents successful therapy, not some nefarious failure. Furthermore, if there is a true infection present and the antibiotic does not appropriately cover the organism, then the condition will surely worsen.

1. Has the patient received any antibiotics from another source, whether from another physician or an illicit source, to treat the infection? The black market for oral antibiotics is so active that it must be assumed that most intravenous drug users have already taken an antibiotic at the time of presentation. This frequent usage may be responsible for the predominance of multi-resistant infections in this population.

2. Frequently patients have partially empty bottles from past prescriptions and may begin therapy on their own.

3. Has the patient been receiving empiric therapy that has not been effective? If so, a change in that therapy, whether antibiotic or surgical, is probably indicated.

4. If the patient had been given a prior course of therapy that was seemingly ineffective, make sure that the patient actually got the prescription filled in a timely manner and had been taking the medication as ordered. If there is doubt, a call to their pharmacy or a pill count may be in order.

Medical History

Numerous underlying medical conditions have important consequences in both diagnosis and treatment of lower extremity infections.

1. The most evident preexisting condition is diabetes mellitus. Diabetic infections have unique bacteriologic and treatment considerations, which are discussed in detail in Chapter 5.

2. HIV infection will generally not have a major impact on the presentation of lower extremity bacterial infections. Most of the immune alterations in this disease involve the T cells and therefore response to fungal, viral, and parasitic infections may be altered.

3. Hypertension and its treatment may have profound effects on electrolyte balance and renal function, complicating antibiotic selection.

4. Peripheral vascular disease may affect antibiotic delivery to the site of infection, although this may be a more theoretical consideration than a real problem.

5. Venous diseases such as deep vein thrombophlebitis (DVT) may mimic infection by presenting with an acutely inflamed, painful, erythematous lower extremity. Even chronic venous congestion may present with swelling, erythema, and flaccid draining bullae that may be misdiagnosed as infectious cellulitis.

6. Other renal and hepatic dysfunctions will affect the pharmacokinetics of antibiotics.

7. Metabolic disorders, such as glucose-6-phosphate dehydrogenase deficiency, will exclude the use of sulfonamides.

8. Current medication usage may alter antibiotic selection because of the potential for drug interactions.

Allergies

Patients who relate "allergic reactions" must be questioned carefully. Many patients may have had minor gastrointestinal irritation many years ago when taking a particular antibiotic. These patients now either assume or were instructed by their physicians that they are "allergic" to the drug. In fact, most of these reactions are due to impurities in early formulations. Other allergy considerations are covered in Chapter 7.

Social History

Knowing the patient's social history can assist in both diagnosis and therapy.

1. Some patients are still reluctant to disclose that they have been diagnosed with HIV or acquired immunodeficiency syndrome (AIDS). Although it is still uncomfortable for many clinicians, even after almost 20 years of AIDS awareness, to ask about risk factors for this disease, it should still be done. If a patient discloses that he has the disease, or it is suspected but not admitted to based on the social history, be very aware of any treatment decisions. According to the Americans with Disabilities Act (ADA), it is illegal to be discriminatory in treatment based on the presence of these conditions.
2. Intravenous drug abusers will present with infections of unusual bacterial etiology regardless of the presence of AIDS. Methicillin-resistant *S. aureus* and *P. aeruginosa* infections are so common that empiric therapy of any infection in this population should include coverage of these organisms.
3. Acute alcohol abuse can affect immune defenses. Primarily, ethanol can suppress bone marrow leukopoiesis and impair neutrophil adherence. Abuse leading to cirrhosis can further impair defenses by causing lymphocyte and neutrophil dysfunction. Also, alcohol use can interfere with therapy since some antibiotics exhibit a striking disulfiram-like (Antabuse) reaction.
4. Smoking can lead to vascular disease with all of its attendant lower extremity problems.

Travel History

Indigenous organisms vary in different parts of the country and the world.

1. Travelers who have returned from indigenous areas and spent

time camping or outdoors may present with Lyme disease, which is caused by a tick-borne *Borrelia*.

2. Vacationers returning from Southern coastal areas of the United States may present with cutaneous larva migrans, which is unseen in the North.

3. Many war veterans still suffer with "jungle rot," which is seemingly untreatable with any antifungal agent. Likewise, travelers to Southeast Asia may present with unusually resistant fungal infections.

4. Mycetomas and *Mycobacterium leprae* infections, both of which directly or indirectly involve the lower extremity, still plague people from some parts of the world.

Pets

1. Pet-borne zoonosis, although rare in the foot, must also be considered.

2. Bite wounds to the lower extremity are fairly common and may lead to potentially severe infections.

■ *Physical Examination*

Performing a thorough physical examination is the second step in the clinical diagnosis of a lower extremity infection.

Overall Appearance of the Patient

Patients with a severe infection will appear "sick." They may be lethargic and slow to respond to questions. They may be diaphoretic. A man may appear unshaven and disheveled. A woman may not have applied makeup. This appearance must then be correlated with the severity of the foot infection. If the foot infection appears relatively mild yet the patient appears ill, there may be distant foci of infection. Systemic diseases that can cause this reaction in patients include subacute bacterial endocarditis (SBE) and urosepsis. SBE should be ruled out in most intravenous drug abusers presenting with infection.

Cellulitis

Cellulitis is frequently defined as an inflammatory process of the skin and connective tissues. Traditionally used to refer to infections with gram-positive organisms, in particular streptococci, the term is now applied to any inflammation having an infectious etiology. Almost any clinically important bacteria can cause this symptom. Cellulitis is usually diagnosed by the presence of the five cardinal signs of Celsus:

1. Rubor (redness)
2. Tumor (swelling)
3. Dolor (pain)
4. Calor (heat)
5. Functio laesa (loss of function)

In response to the presence of foreign bacteria, capillaries in the invaded region dilate, allowing increased blood flow to the part (rubor and calor). This dilatation causes spaces to form in the capillary wall, allowing extravasation of phagocytes and fluid into the perivascular space (tumor). The migration of phagocytes to the site of infection (chemotaxis) is mediated by organism-released chemicals known as chemotactic factors. The resulting edema causes stretching of cutaneous nerve fibers and pain (dolor). Because of this pain, the patient is unable to move easily (functio laesa).

The presence or absence of any or all of these signs is neither diagnostic nor exclusionary for infection. In the majority of cases, however, most if not all of these signs will be present. This is not a quantitative issue of how many signs equal infection. Just because the patient has three out of the five or four out of five does not mean that there is an infection present. This is because there are a number of noninfectious inflammatory conditions that can mimic infectious cellulitis.

1. Gout
2. DVT
3. Chronic indurated cellulitis (venous disease)
4. Acute Charcot's joint
5. Acute trauma
6. Early stages of wound healing
7. Postsurgical changes

As an example, take a patient 1 week postbunion surgery. The patient presents with edema of the region, pain that may limit his function, and some periincisional erythema. This patient now has four out of five signs of cellulitis; surely he must be infected! Of course, there is no infection. These are all normal changes seen postoperatively. This is an example of where the clinician's diagnostic acumen overrides any definitions written in books and papers: a prime example of the axiom that infection is a clinical diagnosis.

The extent of the cellulitis (or, as importantly, the lack thereof) should be documented. This will establish a baseline against which the resolution of the process may be compared. Some clinicians find it useful to mark the leading edge of the cellulitis in indelible ink for this purpose.

Lymphadenitis

The lymph nodes act to filter out infectious agents along the lymph channel draining the acute site. In the presence of these organisms, the nodes can become enlarged and inflamed, causing palpable masses and pain. Infections of the foot and leg will drain proximally into the popliteal fossa and the inguinal region; however, the absence of palpable nodes in the popliteal fossa does not rule out inguinal involvement. Also, popliteal nodes are significantly more challenging to find than inguinal nodes.

Lymphangitis

Lymphangitis is an acute inflammation of the lymphatic channels draining a site of infection. It presents as red linear streaks following the course of the superficial vessels.

Fever

Fever and thermoregulation are complex topics that have warranted entire chapters in textbooks, not to mention hundreds of scientific papers. A simplistic definition of fever would be an elevation in the core temperature as part of a defensive strategy against invasion by a pathogen. "Normal" temperature, contrary to popular belief, is not necessarily 98.6° F (37° C). This value varies based on the time of day, the site from which the temperature is taken, and the individual. Normal may be as high as 100.4° F (38° C) or higher.

Pyrogens

Fever is the body's response to the presence of pyrogens. There are two types of pyrogens:

1. Exogenous pyrogen is produced by some bacteria, especially the gram-negative rods. It is not, however, responsible for all fevers,

because many common organisms are incapable of producing them.

2. Endogenous pyrogen is produced by the leukocytes, in particular the monocytes, in the presence of infection.

Exogenous pyrogen has also been shown to directly induce the cells to produce their own pyrogen. The temperature control center of the brain is located in the anterior hypothalamus. Both endogenous and exogenous pyrogens appear to have a limited direct effect on this site. They mediate their activity through the production of prostaglandins, which are more readily capable of exerting their action on the brain. This prostaglandin production helps explain the antipyretic mechanism of aspirin and other non-steroidal antiinflammatory drugs (NSAIDs), which have an inhibitory effect on prostaglandin synthesis.

These various factors cause the hypothalamus to increase the body's temperature set point. Once the set point is elevated, various physiologic responses must occur for the body to reach that new level. The most common of these is shivering and shaking chills that cause excessive muscular activity, thus warming the core to the new set point.

Fever Curves

There are a number of different fever patterns. They were once thought useful for the diagnosis of a specific type of malaria but are now mostly of historical interest. The following are the two most commonly seen in lower extremity infections:

1. Continuous fever, in which the temperature is elevated for 24 hours with only small variation. This is seen in diseases characterized by continuous seeding of bacteria into the blood (e.g., subacute bacterial endocarditis).
2. Intermittent fever, with which for more than 24 hours there are significant swings with an occasional return to baseline. It is seen with abscesses, which intermittently seed the blood, and is most common in lower extremity infections.

When evaluating fever curves, it should be remembered that most people have a normal diurnal variation, with temperature spikes occurring daily. High temperature usually occurs between 4 to 6 PM and possibly as late as 8 PM. The low point for fever usually occurs around 8 AM.

Antipyretic Therapy

Fever seems to have a physiologic purpose. More and more studies are showing that fever helps the body to fight off a metabolic toll, mostly those with underlying cardiac or pulmonary disease and frail older adults. The other population in which fever should be suppressed is the very young to prevent febrile seizures.

A fever curve is also useful in assessing the progress of a treatment regimen. With adequate therapy, the curve should show a definite downward trend over a few days. The usefulness of this parameter can be masked by the use of antipyretic agents.

Therefore as a general rule, unless there is imminent danger of seizures or metabolic derangement in the case of extremely high fever, antipyretics should be used sparingly and carefully. Standing antipyretic orders should be avoided. Even in cases where the antipyretic is being used for patient comfort, there is a risk-benefit ratio to consider. Although the patient may be temporarily more comfortable, the drug may increase the severity and duration of the condition.

Nosocomial Fever

Frequently, hospitalized patients will develop fever in the face of an apparently improved wound infection or no obvious infection at all. This is referred to as *nosocomial fever*. There can be many causes of this condition, and many different mnemonics have been tried to make them easy to remember.

1. A few of the commonly involved sites that should be examined include:
   a. Lungs. Examine for atelectasis, pneumonia, and pulmonary emboli.
   b. Genitourinary tract. Order urinalysis for urinary tract infection, which is common in women but very unusual in men without an underlying predisposing factor such as catheterization, blockage, or malignancy.
   c. Indwelling catheters. This includes all intravenous and feeding tubes. Check for signs of drainage or cellulitis around the ingress (line sepsis). If found, the lines should be removed and replaced.
   d. Veins. Examine for thrombophlebitis.
   e. Blood. Blood cultures, repeated two or three times, should be performed to rule out bacteremia from any of the above or from SBE.

2. Many drugs can cause fever. This so-called drug fever is thought to be an allergic reaction. Common drugs capable of causing fever include NSAIDs, phenytoin, phenobarbital, penicillin, aspirin, and antihistamines.
3. For some patients, most commonly those with malignancies, there will be no explanation for their fever. The cause is believed to be secondary to alterations in the thermoregulatory center of the brain. This is referred to as *central fever*.

Fever of Unknown Origin

To determine the etiology of a fever when no obvious wound infection is present, a systematic approach, such as the one listed subsequently, is used to examine the previously mentioned possibilities.

1. Stop all antibiotics.
2. Stop all other drugs (if possible).
3. Observe patient for 2 to 3 days.
4. Reculture fully the wound, urine, sputum, and blood.
5. Consider the use of imaging techniques such as computed tomography (CT) scanning or nuclear scans.

If the cause of the fever cannot be determined after 2 to 3 weeks of clinical and laboratory workup, the patient is classified as having a fever of unknown origin (FUO).

Sepsis

Sepsis is the clinical and physiologic response of the body to microorganisms or their by-products in the bloodstream. It should be differentiated from bacteremia, which is simply the presence of these organisms in the blood, or septicemia, which is generally considered to be the same as bacteremia yet more severe. Sepsis causes the peripheral circulation to collapse, leading to inadequate perfusion of tissues. This is known as *septic shock*.

Clinical signs and symptoms of sepsis include fever; tachycardia; tachypnea; changes in mental status; and hematologic abnormalities, including eosinopenia, hyperglycemia, and leukocytosis. In more severe cases paradoxical hypothermia and leukopenia can result. Other manifestations of severe sepsis include adult respiratory distress syndrome and disseminated intravascular coagulopathy. In 1992 the American College of Chest Physicians and the Society of Critical Care Medicine developed criteria for the diagnosis of sepsis.

To diagnose sepsis, there must be clinical evidence of infection plus evidence of a systemic response to infection. This systemic response is manifested by two or more of the following:

1. Temperature >38° C or <36° C
2. Heart rate >90 beats/min
3. Respiratory rate >20 breaths/min
4. White blood count >12,000 cells/mm³, <4000 cells/mm³, or >10% immature (band) forms

This brief discussion of sepsis appears in this chapter instead of as a separate clinical entity because recognition of sepsis is paramount in its treatment. Along with antimicrobial therapy directed at the specific causative organism, medical management of the previously mentioned manifestations is the proper approach to therapy.

LABORATORY DIAGNOSIS

It bears repeating that the diagnosis of a lower extremity infection is first and foremost a clinical judgment. Once a history has been obtained and the physical examination completed, if it is suspected that an infection exists, then the laboratory may be an adjunct in the confirmation of that infection and may assist in determining the causative organisms and proper therapy. Laboratory testing not only can be helpful in the confirmation of a diagnosis of an infection but can also be used to follow the course of therapy.

■ *Complete Blood Count with Differential*

Probably the single most useful test for both diagnosing and following the course of therapy in an infection is the complete blood count (CBC) with differential.

White Blood Cell Count

In an acute infectious process, the body responds by increasing the number of polymorphonuclear leukocytes (PMNs) (or "polys" or "segs") produced. Therefore the first index of importance is the white blood cell count (WBC). An absolute leukocytosis is highly suggestive of infection. However, in localized foot infections, the

WBC count may be within normal limits. Also, the WBC can be elevated for many reasons other than infection. Therefore WBC testing by itself will not confirm or rule out the diagnosis of infection.

In an acute process the PMN: lymphocyte ratio will favor the PMNs. This may reverse in more chronic disease. Patients with infections caused by parasitic organisms may present with an increase in the eosinophil count. Eosinophilia can also be useful in detecting the presence of allergic reaction to an antibiotic.

Left Shift

When bone marrow production of PMNs becomes overwhelmed, immature forms, or band forms, will be released into the peripheral bloodstream. The presence of these band forms constitutes the second index of importance in evaluating the CBC, the left shift. Unfortunately, as previously mentioned, because of the localized nature of many foot infections, the left shift may also remain normal or equivocal. Interestingly, the left shift gained its name because standard pictorial drawings of the morphologic development of white blood cells always began with the most immature cells on the left of the page with the progressively more mature cell drawings being added on from left to right until the fully mature cell was on the right side of the chart. Therefore the more immature cells, the more types represented by drawings on the left side of the page.

Once appropriate therapy is begun, both the leukocytosis and the left shift will return to normal fairly rapidly. If there is no trend toward normalization following 2 to 3 days of treatment, the therapy should be reconsidered.

Absolute Neutrophil Count

In patients who are leukopenic as a result of underlying disease, chemotherapy, or antibiotic side effect, the absolute neutrophil count (ANC) can be employed to determine the level of the patient's host defenses. The ANC is calculated by adding the percentage of PMNs and the percentage of band forms and multiplying the total by the WBC. For example, a WBC of 10,000 cells/mm^3 with 65% PMNs and 5% band forms yields an ANC of 7000 cells/mm^3. If the ANC falls below 1000 cells/mm^3, reverse isolation precautions may become necessary to prevent patient exposure to exogenous infection. Patients with below 500 cells/mm^3 are at the greatest risk.

■ Erythrocyte Sedimentation Rate

The erythrocyte sedimentation rate (ESR) is determined by measuring the distance in millimeters that a column of erythrocytes falls in 1 hour. The cells fall when formed into rouleaux, which only occurs when the natural tendency for red cells to repel one another is overcome by the presence of acute phase reactants. These reactants are present when a patient has an underlying infection, malignancy, or inflammation. Because the ESR may be elevated in any of the previously mentioned conditions, elevation may be too nonspecific to be diagnostic for infection. However, if the ESR is elevated and it is believed that the elevation is because of infection, it can be useful as a baseline value to monitor the effectiveness of therapy.

■ C-Reactive Protein

One of the acute phase reactants discussed above is C-reactive protein (CRP). Although not as widely used as the ESR, in the presence of infection the CRP is found to be positive almost immediately and is generally a more sensitive indicator of infection or inflammation. The difficulty with this test is twofold. First, as with the ESR, it is relatively nonspecific. Second, to use this index appropriately, a quantitative assay should be performed. This test is difficult, expensive, and unavailable at many laboratories.

■ Antistreptolysin O Titer

Used almost exclusively in the diagnosis of acute rheumatic fever, the usefulness of antistreptolysin O (ASO) titer in the diagnosis of skin and skin structure infections has not been well documented. Theoretically, in the presence of a streptococcal organism in an infection, the ASO titer should be positive. The only potential indication for its use is in cases in which standard culture techniques cannot be employed (e.g., cellulitis with no specimen to culture) or for suspected streptococcal skin infections. The test is rarely used.

■ Teichoic Acid Antibodies

Teichoic acid is a polymer present on the cell walls of gram-positive organisms. Because it acts as a potent antigen, antibodies will be formed to it that can be assayed through immunologic tests such as the enzyme-linked immunosorbent assay (ELISA). The usefulness of this assay in diagnosing staphylococcal skin and skin structure infections has not been demonstrated. There has been some work in the area of osteomyelitis, but most of the studies are retrospective and success rates vary widely from 30% to 70%.

■ *Blood Chemistry*

Most laboratories run computerized panels consisting of 6 to 24 different chemistries. The following includes only those with direct relevance to the diagnosis and treatment of lower extremity infections.

Serum Creatinine

The serum creatinine level is the single most important chemistry. The test should be run on every patient receiving parenteral antibiotics. With only a few exceptions, all antibiotics are excreted to some extent by the kidneys. The serum creatinine level is the best hematologic index of renal function and therefore of antibiotic excretion. Dosage and dose interval of many agents may be calculated based on the renal function. Although dosing nomograms may be calculated from the results of the creatinine clearance test, the test is time consuming, requiring a 24-hour urine collection. Creatinine clearance can be calculated from the serum creatinine level by using the equation of Cockcroft and Gault:

$$C_{cr} \text{ (ml/min)} = (140 - age) \times weight \: / \: Cr \times 72 \times 0.85 \text{ (for females)}$$

Blood Urea Nitrogen

Less specific for renal function than the creatinine level, the blood urea nitrogen (BUN) level is affected more readily by the hydration state of the patient. It is used more as a secondary test to support renal function data garnered by serum creatinine testing.

Electrolytes

Sodium and potassium levels are particularly necessary for determining antibiotic therapy. A number of antibiotics contain fairly high sodium loads at therapeutic dosage. Their use may cause hypernatremia with resultant hypokalemia. The electrolytes are also useful adjuncts in determining renal function. Hypertension with concomitant diuretic use will have a major effect on the test.

Glucose

The stress of an infection will cause serum glucose levels to rise. Diabetics will often present with elevated glucose levels between 400 and 1200 mg/dl. Even patients with mild glucose intolerance may present with hyperglycemia. Furthermore, heretofore-undiagnosed diabetics will present with severity of infection out of line with the etiology. Hyperglycemia in these patients may be the only clue to their occult diabetes mellitus.

Liver Function Tests

Some antibiotics, most notably clindamycin and erythromycin, are metabolized in the liver. If these agents are to be used, then the liver function tests (LFTs) should be examined. The most common tests determine levels of bilirubin, serum proteins, serum glutamic oxaloacetic transaminase, and serum glutamic pyruvic transaminase. LFTs have also gained major importance with the availability of the newer-generation oral antifungal medications used for onychomycosis.

BACTERIOLOGIC DIAGNOSIS

■ *Gram Stain*

The Gram stain is an easy, inexpensive, and rapid in-office procedure that yields a wealth of information concerning the etiology of infection. All that is required to perform this test is a set of commercially available reagents and a microscope with a 100X oil-immersion objective. Exact timing of application for each reagent is unnecessary. The time needed to put down one bottle and reach for the next is usually sufficient to allow adequate staining. Despite this, most clinicians are not performing this test in the office and instead depend on the same commercial laboratory to which they send their cultures. For this reason, often the Gram stain result is not seen until the final culture report is received. Despite this delay, the information can still be useful.

Gram Stain Technique

1. Make a thin smear of drainage on a glass slide. Do not take the specimen with a cotton-tipped applicator, because this may absorb some of the material. Use the wooden end of the applicator or a metal probe.

2. "Heat fixing" by running the slide under a flame is not necessary. Allowing the slide to air dry for 5 minutes is sufficient.

3. While holding the slide (there is no need to put the slide on a rack, just keep it tilted away from the fingers to avoid inadvertent staining) apply the Gram crystal violet and let it sit for 5 to 10 seconds.

4. Rinse the slide with tap water. This step applies between each of the following applications. Some believe that even this is unnecessary and that immediate application of the next reagent is sufficient "rinsing."

5. Apply Gram iodine. The residual blue stain will turn black almost immediately.

6. Holding the slide at a steep angle to allow immediate drainage, apply the decolorizer until the runoff is almost clear and most visible signs of stain are removed from the slide. Rinse immediately to halt the process. This is the most critical step to successful staining. Too long an application over-decolorizes, causing all the organisms to appear gram negative. Insufficient time causes everything to appear gram positive.

7. Apply the Safranin counterstain. Because this is a fairly light color, leave the stain on the slide for at least 10 seconds.

8. Rinse. Blot dry.

9. Examine microscopically using the 100X oil-immersion objective. The organisms are too small to visualize at any lower power.

Evaluation of the Slide

The slide is properly Gram stained if the PMNs have light pink cytoplasm with darker pink-mauve nuclei. Organisms can also be used to evaluate the stain technique. If cocci appear gram negative, the stain was probably overdecolorized. Most pathogenic cocci in the lower extremity are expected to be gram positive, except in the rare case in which gonococci are suspected (e.g., in septic arthritis).

Information Obtainable from the Gram Stain

Organism Morphology

Most organisms have distinctive morphology upon examination that allows immediate identification and empiric therapy. Staphylococci appear as gram-positive cocci in "grapelike" clusters.

Streptococci appear as gram-positive cocci in chains. Table 1-1 lists Gram stain morphologies for various organisms.

Contamination Versus Infection

This is probably the most useful information that can be garnered from Gram stains received at the same time as final culture results. Many wounds and body sites are heavily colonized with microorganisms in the absence of clinical infection. Gram staining of these areas reveals large numbers of bacteria usually accompanied by an amorphous background material consisting of erythrocytes and fibrin. An infected site will usually contain not only the organisms but also a large number of white cells, predominantly PMNs. The presence of these cells points to the body's response to a pathogenic process, as referenced in the definition of infection discussed earlier in this chapter. Without these PMNs being present in the smear, there is an excellent possibility that the isolated organisms may just be colonizers of the area and not infecting organisms.

TABLE 1-1

Gram Stain Appearance of Common Organisms*

ORGANISM	MORPHOLOGY
Gram Positive (Blue)	
Staphylococcus	Cocci in "grape-like" clusters
Streptococcus	Cocci in chains
Corynebacterium	Rods in "Chinese characters"
Clostridium	Rods with a "racquet shape" caused by spore
Gram Negative (Red)†	
Gonococcus	Diplococcus within the white blood cell count (WBC)
Klebsiella	Diplococcoid bacillus may show a heavy capsule
Pseudomonas	Slightly curved rod

*Slide check: The cytoplasm of the WBC is light pink; the nucleus of the WBC is dark pink-mauve; cocci are dark blue-purple, unless gonococci are suspected.
†It is difficult to identify most other gram-negative rods on the basis of stain only.

Suspicion of Anaerobes

If the Gram stain reveals a large number of organisms of differing morphology and the culture report isolates only a few, the presence of anaerobes should be suspected. Anaerobic bacteria are technically difficult to isolate in the laboratory. Their presence may be missed on culture. If anaerobes are suspected clinically, and the organisms seen on the stain do not coincide with those reported by the laboratory, they may be assumed to be anaerobic.

■ *Culture and Sensitivity*

One of the greatest misconceptions in the approach to infectious diseases is that a culture is used to diagnose an infection. This is untrue. As repeated on a number of occasions in this chapter, diagnosis is clinical. The laboratory is just used to help confirm the diagnosis or give assistance in selections of therapies. Specifically, a culture and sensitivity are to be used once the clinical diagnosis of infection is made to determine which organisms are causing the infection that was clinically diagnosed. Therefore cultures should not be performed on clinically noninfected sites, because this may lead to false-positive results and inappropriate antibiotic therapy.

Culture Technique
Site of Culture

The site from which the culture is taken must be representative of the infection. Sinus tract cultures of osteomyelitis are notoriously unreliable in predicting the causative organism in bone. Wound swabs of heavily contaminated areas will lead to falsely cultured nonpathogenic organisms. This is particularly true of clinically noninfected but certainly colonized ulcerations in patients with diabetes.

Asepsis

If a potentially contaminated site must be entered for retrieval of material for culture, the possibility of specimen contamination should be minimized. If skin is being penetrated, the application of a topical antiseptic will prevent contamination with potential skin flora. This will not guarantee a clean "catch," however, and the culture result must be interpreted in that light. Removing tissue specimens from the base of an ulceration should only be accomplished following aggressive debridement or curettage of the ulcer base to remove superficial contamination.

Method of Collection

As previously discussed, the use of commercially available swabs is the easiest, if not the best, method of collection. Pus itself is not always the best material to culture but may be the most readily available. The organisms found in the pus may already be dead or phagocytized. The specimen should be from a deep site, if feasible. Actual pieces of tissue from the wound or material from curettage of the base of the lesion are excellent sources of culture, but obtaining them is more invasive and therefore carries a potential risk. Aspiration of an abscess can yield a large amount of purulent material for culture, although frank surgical incision and drainage, if indicated, will accomplish not only the gathering of specimen but will also be therapeutic. The long-outdated practice of applying a rubber stopper to the aspiration needle should be avoided, however, because this may lead to inadvertent needle-stick injury.

Quantitative Bacteriology and Amount of Specimen

An adequate amount of specimen must be sent to the laboratory to allow Gram stain, aerobic and anaerobic culture and sensitivity, and any special studies to be performed. Some laboratories are capable of performing quantitative Gram stain and culture, in which a tissue biopsy is homogenized and stained or cultured, allowing actual numbers of organisms to be determined per gram of tissue. This technique is known as *quantitative bacteriology*. A count of more than 10^5 organisms per gram is highly correlated with the development of wound infection if the open wound is primarily closed. This technique is frequently discussed at meetings and in papers as being a "gold standard." Unfortunately, because of the technical difficulty and time consumption involved, most laboratories are not prepared to perform this test. Therefore from a practical standpoint this is really only of academic interest and is not commonly performed by the vast majority of clinicians.

Special Studies

In addition to the usual aerobic and anaerobic bacteria, there are infecting organisms that will not fall into either of these two broad categories. If there is a high index of suspicion for an unusual pathogen based on clinical grounds or previously negative cultures, a potassium hydroxide (KOH) preparation, fungal cultures, and acid-fast smears for mycobacteria can be ordered.

Although the KOH preparation and acid-fast smear can be performed and interpreted quickly, cultures for these organisms may take many weeks to grow. There are also special immunologic studies that may be performed for particularly fastidious, difficult-to-grow organisms.

Transport to the Laboratory
Expedient delivery of culture material to the bacteriology laboratory is paramount in the recovery of some organisms, particularly anaerobes. Although modern collection containers will have appropriate media for each type of specimen, there is no guarantee that the organism will remain viable indefinitely. In the hospital setting, ideally, the specimen should be personally carried to the laboratory rather than using orderlies to transport the material. In the office, the clinical laboratory service should be called for immediate pickup rather than waiting for the standard daily run.

Antibiotic Therapy
Specimens should be collected before any antibiotic therapy. If the patient is already taking antibiotics, these should be stopped for at least 48 hours, if possible.

Culturing in the Absence of Exudate
Most lower extremity infections are purulent in nature, affording plenty of culturable material. In some infections, the most common of which is superficial cellulitis, no such luxury exists. If there is no drainage and no open wound, a culture is not useful. In these cases it may not be possible to recover an organism, and treatment must be based on empiric knowledge. Aspiration of the leading edge of cellulitis is a common method of diagnosing the causative organism. Studies have concluded that the success rate of this procedure is less than 10%. Since this is an invasive procedure, the potential risks must be weighed against these minimal results. A question that remains unanswered is whether seeding deep tissues occurs with bacteria when a needle is inserted through an area of superficial cellulitis. Although theoretically possible, there are no data to prove or disprove this theory.

Order of Specimens
As a general rule, upon opening an abscess, the anaerobic culture is the first taken, because any prolonged exposure to air may be

sufficient to inhibit their growth. The aerobic specimen is taken next, and finally, the Gram stain material.

Blood Cultures and Bacteremia

Blood cultures are used to diagnose bacteremia, which is the presence of bacteria in the blood. There are three types of bacteremia: transient, intermittent, and continuous.

Transient Bacteremia

Occurring in most patients on a daily basis, transient bacteremia develops when brushing teeth, eating hard foods, or any other manipulation of a well-vascularized, heavily contaminated area. Transient bacteremia may also occur with the surgical manipulation of an infected area such as an abscess. In most healthy patients there is little clinical significance to this event. However, in patients with compromised heart valves secondary to rheumatic fever or previous valvular surgery, the bacteria may seed the valve, causing endocarditis.

Intermittent Bacteremia

Intermittent bacteremia is most frequently found when there is a septic foci seeding the blood with bacteria. Abscess and urinary tract infection (UTI) are two of the most common causes. This bacteremia has the most clinical significance for infections in the lower extremity.

Continuous Bacteremia

Continuous bacteremia is considered diagnostic of bacterial endocarditis unless proven otherwise.

Protocol for Drawing Blood Cultures

1. There should be a high index of suspicion for bacteremia. On clinical observation the patient appears "septic," is suggested to have hematogenous osteomyelitis, or has an FUO. Blood cultures should not be routinely ordered on all lower extremity infections, because they are expensive and unnecessary. Cultures should be taken as soon as possible after the onset of fever or chills.
2. Because contamination by skin flora poses a diagnostic dilemma, aseptic technique is employed when drawing cultures. This includes the use of a topical antiseptic and sterile gloves

and avoidance of the site with ungloved fingers after skin preparation.

3. Two or three sets of cultures are drawn within a 24-hour period.

4. Cultures are drawn from rotating sites 20 to 30 minutes apart.

5. Twenty milliliters of blood are drawn each time. Bacteremias are usually of low magnitude, and drawing larger volumes of blood will improve recovery as well as provide adequate volume for aerobic and anaerobic culturing. Remember that any amount of blood from one venipuncture, no matter how many bottles it fills, is only *one* culture.

6. Usually three cultures are sufficient to detect any clinically significant bacteremia. If after five or six cultures over 2 days no organisms have been recovered, no further cultures are indicated.

7. Blood cultures cannot be considered negative until after at least 2 weeks of incubation owing to the possible presence of fastidious, slow-growing organisms.

Interpretation of blood cultures can be difficult if only a few tubes become positive or the cultures become positive only after long incubation. The presence of common contaminants such as *Corynebacterium* or *S. epidermidis* may also lend to the confusion, because these may in some cases actually be pathogenic.

■ Immunologic Diagnosis

The presence of some slow-growing, fastidious organisms is not easily demonstrated by traditional microbiologic methods of culture and sensitivity. In these cases specific antibodies against the organism can be detected. This antibody detection is usually accomplished through the use of immunofluorescence, agglutination, or immunoassay. Examples of a few of the bacteria detected in this manner include *Brucella, Legionella, Treponema,* and *Mycoplasma.* These techniques are most useful in the diagnosis of viral and fungal diseases. As most of these organisms have limited involvement in infections of the lower extremity, it is out of the scope of this chapter to cover these tests in detail.

■ Common Organisms for Common Infections

The final step in determining the bacterial etiology of the infection is to employ what amounts to an educated guess. Many common lower extremity infections have a well-documented association of certain organisms. For example, osteomyelitis following a puncture wound is caused by *P. aeruginosa* in about 90% of cases. Consequently, a patient presenting following a puncture wound with clinical, radiographic, and laboratory indications consistent with osteomyelitis can be empirically begun on antipseudomonal antibiotics pending the results of the culture and sensitivity.

HOSPITALIZATION OF THE INFECTED PATIENT

The decision to hospitalize a patient rather than to use aggressive outpatient therapy must frequently be made. The choice has become more difficult to make because of a number of factors:

1. The availability of oral antibiotics with efficacy equal to that of some of the parenteral agents, which makes the need for hospitalization to administer these agents less important.
2. The advent of home health care infusion teams, which allow parenteral antibiotics to be given in an outpatient setting. These teams can also perform any laboratory test required to monitor the infection or therapy, negating the need for a hospital laboratory.
3. Probably the biggest factor that determines outpatient versus inpatient therapy is the presence of hospital utilization review. Many hospitals require patients to meet specific guidelines before allowing admission for an infection. These may include "significantly" elevated WBC, fever, or the presence of a large, draining, open wound. Hospitals can lose much money on infection admissions. These admissions receive relatively short diagnosis-related group length of stay allowances, which are frequently exceeded.

■ *Guidelines for Hospitalization*

1. Severe infection, identified by:
   a. High fever (above 101° F)
   b. High WBC (above 13,000 cells/mm³)
   c. Systemic spread, as evidenced by signs of sepsis
   d. Infection that overcomes local defenses (proximal spread)
2. Failure to respond to aggressive outpatient therapy

3. Causative organism only susceptible to a parenteral agent
4. Need for aggressive surgical debridement requiring general anesthesia
5. Underlying systemic disease (e.g., uncontrolled diabetes)
6. Need for complete bed rest. No matter what patients promise, they won't stay in bed at home. By itself, this probably will not be acceptable to the hospital. It must be combined with one of the guidelines just mentioned.

■ Following the Course of the Infection

Assuming adequate surgical drainage is performed and antibiotic therapy is initiated, there will be a marked change in the clinical signs and symptoms of the infection. The two most important parameters to follow are:

1. The fever curve, which with appropriate therapy, should proceed remarkably downward. Nocturnal spikes will diminish over time until the patient remains afebrile throughout a 24-hour period.
2. The WBC, which should normalize within 2 to 3 days.

Continued fever spikes and a persistently elevated WBC should be considered as pathognomonic for a continuing infectious process or the presence of an undiagnosed abscess requiring surgical drainage.

There are a few clinical hints that suggest the resolution of the infection.

1. A decrease in the amount and "anger" of the cellulitis
2. The presence of skin wrinkles seen with decreased edema
3. The appearance of a band of peeling skin, similar to that seen following a sunburn, centered around the original area of cellulitis
4. Postinflammatory hyperpigmentation presenting as a violaceous discoloration in the previous site of the cellulitis. It may be confused with cellulitis in some patients, although unlike cellulitis it is not warm to the touch. In black patients it appears either dark brown or black. Patients should be reassured that this is not "gangrene," as some fear. It may be present for more than a year.

SUGGESTED READINGS

American College of Chest Physicians/Society of Critical Care Medicine Consensus Conference Committee: Definitions for sepsis and organ failure and guidelines for the use of innovative therapies in sepsis, *Crit Care Med* 20:864, 1992.

Armstrong DG et al: Value of white blood cell count with differential in the acute diabetic foot infection, *J Am Podiatr Med Assoc* 86(5):224, 1996.

Covey DC, Albright JA: Clinical significance of the erythrocyte sedimentation rate in orthopaedic surgery, *J Bone Joint Surg* 69A:148, 1987.

Epperly TD: The value of needle aspiration in the management of cellulites, *J Fam Pract* 23:337, 1986.

Mackowiak PA, Jones SR, Smith JW: Diagnostic value of sinus-tract cultures in chronic osteomyelitis, *JAMA* 239:2772, 1978.

Mackowiak PA: Temperature regulation and the pathogenesis of fever. In Mandell GL, Bennett JE, and Dolin R, editors: *Principles and practice of infectious diseases*, ed 5, Philadelphia, 2000, Churchill Livingstone.

Stumacher RJ: *Clinical infectious diseases*, Philadelphia, 1987, WB Saunders.

White A, Wheat LJ, Kohler RB: Diagnostic and therapeutic significance of staphylococcal teichoic acid antibodies, *Scand J Infect Dis* (suppl) 41:105, 1983.

PART II

Clinical Syndromes

CHAPTER 2

Skin and Soft Tissue Infections

SUPERFICIAL INFECTIONS

■ Cellulitis

Along with being a catch phrase for any localized reaction to infection, the term *cellulitis* also implies a specific clinical syndrome. Cellulitis is an acute spreading infection of the skin and connective tissues. The initial etiology is usually a trauma that violates the skin's defenses. The trauma can be severe or relatively minor (e.g., a gun shot wound, laceration, puncture wound, ulceration, bullae, surgery, or insect bite).

Clinical Presentation
The patient presents with an edematous, erythematous hot limb. Constitutional signs may be present. Boundaries are not clearly demarcated, and superficial topography is lost because of swelling. Lymphangiopathy and lymphadenopathy with proximal spread are present. There may be a lack of drainage or an open sinus. These signs may appear from a few hours to a few days after the inciting trauma. Other, noninfectious inflammatory processes, such as acute venous occlusions or acute gouty arthritis, are often misdiagnosed as cellulitis because the clinical presentation is similar.

Laboratory Findings
The cell white blood count (WBC) may be elevated with a left shift. Blood cultures should be considered because of the result-

ant bacteremia. Material for culture will not be present unless there is an open lesion around the initial site or superficial skin necrosis. These sites are often superficially colonized and therefore cannot be used to form an accurate diagnosis. Aspiration of the leading edge of the cellulitis results in poor recovery of an organism and has the potential to cause deep spread of the infection; therefore a bacteriologic diagnosis is not always possible or necessary.

Bacterial Etiology

Group A streptococcus and *Staphylococcus aureus* are the most frequently implicated causative organisms.

Treatment

Surgical drainage is rarely indicated unless abscess formation is suspected. Because bacteriologic diagnosis may be difficult, cellulitis should be treated empirically with therapy directed against the most common causative organisms, staphylococcus and streptococcus. Selection of oral versus parenteral therapy is based on the severity of the disease and extent of systemic involvement.

Oral Alternatives
1. Cephalosporin (cephalexin, cefuroxime axetil, cefdinir)
2. Penicillinase-resistant penicillin (cloxacillin, dicloxacillin)
3. Clindamycin
4. Macrolide (azithromycin, clarithromycin)
5. Penicillin V (if the organism is known to be a streptococcus)

Parenteral Alternatives
1. First-generation cephalosporin (cefazolin)
2. Penicillinase-resistant penicillin (nafcillin, oxacillin)
3. Clindamycin
4. Vancomycin
5. Aqueous penicillin (if the organism is known to be a streptococcus)

■ *Donor-Leg Cellulitis Following Saphenous Phlebectomy*

A large percentage of podiatric patients present with lower extremity vascular disease. These patients frequently undergo vascular reconstruction, which requires the harvesting of a saphenous vein graft. At any time following that operation, an acute cellulitis may occur along the donor site. The etiology is believed to be an acute interdigital tinea pedis that allows organisms access to deep tissues.

Clinical Presentation

The clinical presentation is similar to that of regular cellulitis. Differentiation should be made from acute thrombophlebitis, which mimics this disease with calf tenderness and a positive Homan's sign. This is accomplished by noninvasive vascular testing and venography.

Laboratory Findings

Laboratory findings are the same as those for regular cellulitis.

Bacterial Etiology

Group A streptococcus is the causative organism.

Treatment

Antibiotic treatment is the same as that for cellulitis, discussed previously. If only a streptococcal organism is isolated, oral or parenteral penicillin is the drug of choice. In addition, treatment should be directed at curing the tinea pedis, without which recurrence of the cellulitis is possible.

■ *Paronychia*

More commonly referred to as an "infected ingrown toenail," paronychia is technically defined as inflammation around the nail borders. A portion of the toenail, through trauma or inappropriate cutting, forms a spicule. As the nail grows the spicule may implant itself into the soft tissue of the nail border or groove. The nail then acts as a foreign body and causes an inflammatory response. Secondary bacterial infection may then ensue, although the process may remain strictly inflammatory without infection.

Clinical Presentation

The patient presents with edema, erythema, heat, and pain along the affected nail border. Proximal spread of this cellulitis into the foot is rare but may occur. A moderate amount of purulent drainage is often seen. In more chronic cases exuberant granulation tissue is formed, and there may also be a decrease in pain. The potential for osteomyelitis should be explored in chronic cases.

Laboratory Findings

Because this is a local process and there is rarely systemic involvement, routine blood testing is not indicated. The erythrocyte sedimentation rate (ESR) may be obtained if osteomyelitis is suspected. Culture and sensitivity testing of the drainage is helpful in establishing a bacterial etiology but is of questionable value in the treatment. Most paronychias are cleared before culture and sensitivity results are returned. Radiography should be considered to rule out osteomyelitis in chronic cases or in cases in which deep tracts are noted. Care should be exercised in interpretation of the radiographs, however, as chronic inflammation may cause rarefaction in bone that mimics osteomyelitis. Bone scintigraphy is rarely helpful as it is too nonspecific. Magnetic resonance imaging (MRI) may be the most useful test for diagnosing osteomyelitis in these cases.

Bacterial Etiology

Staphylococci, streptococci, *Proteus mirablis*, and, rarely, *Candida* are the suspected organisms.

Treatment

The hallmark of treatment of paronychia is removal of the offending portion of nail. Many physicians will attempt treatment with antibiotics and soaks alone with poor results. Following complete removal of the nail spicule, 75% silver nitrate may be applied to any granulation tissue present. Soaking of the involved border or the use of wet-to-dry dressings may improve drainage. The use of systemic antibiotics is not indicated, except in cases of extensive cellulitis, systemic involvement, underlying osteomyelitis, immunocompromise, and poor response to the previously mentioned therapy.

Postavulsion Complications

The vast majority of nail avulsions performed for the treatment of a paronychia heal uneventfully. There are, however, some special situations that should be discussed.

1. Phenol and alcohol procedure (P&A). This is probably the most frequently performed permanent nail removal technique (matricectomy). The question frequently arises as to whether it is appropriate to perform this procedure at the same time that the patient presents with an acute paronychia. It is believed that

by performing the definitive procedure, recurrence of the deformity will be prevented and the patient will not have to undergo a separate procedure at a future time. Although no formal studies have looked at this issue, it is performed at the same time as the therapeutic nail avulsion by many clinicians with good success. Phenol (carbolic acid) was once considered the "universal disinfectant"; therefore it should have potent activity against any infecting organisms in the site. If a P&A is to be performed, it should be remembered and the patient should be informed that prolonged drainage and inflammation is a common reaction to the chemical and not usually indicative of an ongoing infectious process.

2. Scintigraphy following nail avulsion. Often, days to weeks after an avulsion is performed, especially for a chronic paronychia, there may be recalcitrant inflammation and drainage. Clinicians, in their zeal to make a definitive diagnosis, may suspect an osteomyelitis and order scintigraphy, such as a technetium bone scan. The result is a false-positive scan secondary to direct trauma to the distal phalanx caused by the instrumentation used during the avulsion. This is an unreliable study in trying to make the diagnosis of an osteomyelitis.

3. Laser procedures. There are still a number of clinicians who will use laser or radio frequency techniques for the performance of a matricectomy. These techniques both essentially work by causing dry burns to the matrix tissue and should be treated as such. Infections with common burn wound organisms such as *Pseudomonas aeruginosa* should be considered if complications arise.

4. Patients with poor circulation. The clinical situation may arise when a patient presents with both a paronychia and clinical findings of significant circulatory compromise. The clinician is then faced with a dilemma. The patient may not have enough circulation to heal the avulsion procedure necessary to excise and drain the paronychia, *but*, if the ingrown nail and resultant abscess is not excised and drained, the patient will surely develop necrosis from the chronic process. In a case such as this, the nail avulsion and drainage should probably be performed in as atraumatic a way as possible regardless of the potential for complications. If not performed, it is nearly certain that the patient will worsen and that the toe will necrose. The procedure at least gives the toe some chance.

■ *Erythrasma*

Because of their similar presentations, tinea pedis and erythrasma are often confused.

Clinical Presentation

The patient presents with slowly spreading interdigital maceration and pruritus. Cellulitis may be present over the distal foot. Wood's lamp examination reveals a "coral red" fluorescence.

Laboratory Findings

Gram stain reveals gram-positive bacilli. Culture and sensitivity testing for both fungi and bacteria should be done.

Bacterial Etiology

Corynebacterium minutissimum is implicated.

Treatment

Oral erythromycin 1 g/day for 1 week is the classic treatment. Alternative therapies include other oral macrolides such as azithromycin or clarithromycin or topical treatment with clindamycin solution.

■ *Folliculitis and "Hot Tub Dermatitis"*

Infection within a hair follicle is rare in the foot but may occur on the dorsum as well as on toes and legs. In patients who recently used a hot tub, a whirlpool, or a Jacuzzi, any area that is weight bearing upon sitting may be involved.

Clinical Presentation

The patient presents with a small red papule that may progress to a draining pustule. If allowed to progress further, a deeper furuncle or carbuncle may develop. The disease is usually self-limiting.

Laboratory Findings

Culture and sensitivity testing is necessary when drainage is present.

Bacterial Etiology

Staphylococcus aureus, and *P. aeruginosa* in the case of hot tub dermatitis, are the causative organisms.

Treatment

Local care includes applications of warm compresses. Topical antibiotics such as mupirocin may be useful in staphylococcal disease but would be ineffective against *Pseudomonas*. Systemic antibiotics are rarely indicated. In recurrent cases, low-dose oral clindamycin may prove useful.

■ *Furuncles and Carbuncles*

Folliculitis that is permitted to progress unchecked my lead to deeper subcutaneous abscesses known as furuncles or commonly known as boils. These lesions tend to drain spontaneously and seldom need specific treatment other than warm compresses. However, in some cases they may progress to form large groups of furuncles known as carbuncles. These are quite deep, often extending into the subcutaneous fat layers and most often require surgical drainage, excision, and antistaphylococcal antibiotic therapy. Failure to aggressively treat the carbuncles may lead to bacteremia as the staphylococcus is released into the circulation. Fortunately, although folliculitis and furuncles may be found in the foot and leg, the more severe carbuncles rarely occur there.

■ *Staphylococcal Scalded Skin Syndrome*

Although uncommon as a primary disease in the lower extremity, staphylococcal scalded skin syndrome may occur following lower extremity surgery. There is usually an antecedent staphylococcal skin infection.

Clinical Presentation

This disease is most commonly seen in children. Fever and tenderness of the skin are early signs. Large, flaccid bullae form and rupture, exposing underlying areas of red, scalded-appearing skin. Septicemia may result, but it is rarely fatal and has limited morbidity. This is a different condition from toxic epidermal necrolysis (TEN), which usually occurs in adults, is more commonly secondary to a drug reaction than infection, is a deeper process, and is often fatal.

Laboratory Findings

Blood cultures are required. Other standard blood testing may show typical signs of severe infection.

Bacterial Etiology
S. aureus, phage type II, is commonly found.

Treatment
Fluid maintenance and parenteral antibiotic therapy directed against staphylococci, including nafcillin, cefazolin, and vancomycin, is therapeutic.

■ *Impetigo*

Usually described in children and limited to the upper extremity and the face, impetigo can also occur in adults on the foot and leg. This is a very superficial infection, but it is highly contagious.

Clinical Presentation
Classic honey-gold crusts that begin as vesicles are found. Yellow, creamy drainage develops under crusts. Rare cellulitic response is seen around lesions. Systemic involvement is rare, although it may occur in children.

Laboratory Findings
Culture and sensitivity testing are required. Gram stain reveals gram-positive cocci in chains and clusters. Rarely, gram-negative rods are seen.

Bacterial Etiology
Group A streptococci was classically described as the major cause. Now, however, *S. aureus* is found at least as frequently if not even more frequently than streptococcus.

Treatment
Topical antibiotic therapy with mupirocin is therapeutic. This drug has been shown to be as effective as oral therapy and probably more effective than other topical agents. Oral antibiotic therapy with penicillin (for streptococcus specific cases) and cephalosporins, dicloxacillin, erythromycin, or clindamycin in mixed cases may also be tried.

■ *Ecthyma*

Unlike impetigo, ecthyma more frequently occurs on the lower extremity. It is a deeper lesion than impetigo, extending down into the dermis and may therefore lead to scarring. These lesions frequently present in the lower extremity, especially in children and in the elderly.

Clinical Presentation
Punched out, crusted lesions with greenish-yellow crusts are found. Surrounding erythema may also be seen.

Laboratory Findings
The laboratory findings are the same as those for impetigo, but blood cultures are also necessary to rule out metastatic spread from a bacteremia.

Bacterial Etiology
Streptococci and, in the case of ecthyma gangrenosum resulting from pseudomonal bacteremia, *P. aeruginosa* are the implicated organisms.

Treatment
For streptococcal disease the treatment is similar to that for impetigo. In the case of ecthyma gangrenosum, appropriate, aggressive therapy of the underlying pseudomonal bacteremia is warranted.

■ *Injection Site Ulcerations/Abscess*

This is found in intravenous (IV) drug users that have "skin popped" because of a lack of open veins, missed the vein on injection, or injected contaminated, caustic drugs.

Clinical Presentation
Usually a round, punched out, ulcerated area overlaying a normal vein course, between the toes, or under the nail plate. If not yet opened and draining, they present as a localized fluctuant area with surrounding cellulitis.

Laboratory Findings
Findings are usually unremarkable since this problem tends to be very localized.

Bacterial Etiology
S. aureus is most frequent; however, there is a high incidence of

methicillin resistance in the IV drug using population, theoretically because of frequent, nonprescribed antibiotic usage. If the patient is using saliva on the needle ("greasing the needle"), mouth flora include streptococcus and anaerobes needs to be considered. *P. aeruginosa* is also common in this population.

Treatment

Treatment is dependent on the organism isolated. Empiric therapy should probably be directed against both methicillin-resistant staphylococcus and *P. aeruginosa*, i.e., vancomycin plus ciprofloxacin. If anaerobes are suspected, the addition of clindamycin or metronidazole to the just-mentioned treatment or the use of piperacillin/tazobactam with or without vancomycin should be considered.

■ *Erysipelas*

This is a form of cellulitis that involves lymphatic blockage and most frequently occurs on the face. More recently, however, the lower extremities have become a common location.

Clinical Presentation

Cellulitis with sharply demarcated, "geographic" advancing borders is found. The leading edge presents with a raised border. Fever and pain are common.

Laboratory Findings

Leukocytosis is usually present. Culture material may not be readily available.

Bacterial Etiology

Group A streptococcus is the causative organism.

Treatment

Parenteral or oral penicillin, depending on the severity of the disease, is therapeutic.

SUBCUTANEOUS AND NECROTIZING INFECTIONS

The classification of the necrotizing infections is difficult. The distinctions between the different "textbook" types blur when presented clinically. The depth of the involved tissues and the organisms present may be difficult to determine initially. Appropriate medical and surgical therapy must be initiated promptly and empirically, usually before determining the exact diagnosis, in order to salvage the limb. These diseases all have in common massive tissue necrosis and rapid progression. Even with early intervention, the rate of amputation and mortality is high, approaching 50% for each.

Most patients presenting with one of these infections have some underlying predisposition, commonly tissue devitalization and hypoxemia or a compromised immune system. Trauma, surgery, burns, malignancy, diabetes, and peripheral vascular disease are frequently coexistent.

These infections subsequently are described individually, beginning with the more superficial and continuing to the deeper processes. Many of these conditions sound and appear similar to others. In fact, different names have sometimes been given to nearly identical diseases. Wherever possible, this redundancy is eliminated for brevity and ease of discussion. Furthermore, only conditions that are highly prevalent in the lower extremity are included.

▤ *Clostridial Cellulitis*

Clostridial cellulitis is an infection of devitalized subcutaneous tissue. Involvement of fascia and muscle is uncommon. The pathogenesis is frequently trauma or surgery that has become contaminated with clostridia as a result of insufficient debridement or fecal contamination.

Clinical Presentation
Onset is gradual. Systemic toxicity is minimal. Signs are mostly local and include extensive gas, a dark, thin, foul-smelling exudate, and only mild pain. Progression can be rapid, although not as rapid as in deeper forms.

Laboratory Findings
Gram stain reveals a thick, gram-positive rod with blunting on one end characteristic of clostridia. X-rays demonstrate extensive superficial tissue gas.

Bacterial Etiology

Clostridium perfringens and, less frequently, other clostridial species are implicated.

Treatment

Treatment is by aggressive surgical debridement and high-dose parenteral antibiotic therapy directed against *C. perfringens*, including:

1. Penicillin, up to 24 million U/day
2. Imipenem/cilastatin, 1.5 to 2 g/day

■ *Nonclostridial Anaerobic (Crepitant) Cellulitis*

Nonclostridial anaerobic (crepitant) cellulitis is very similar in presentation to clostridial cellulitis except for its causative pathogens. The pathogenesis is less dependent on trauma or surgery. Diabetes is a common underlying factor.

■ *Clinical Presentation*

As stated, the presentation is similar to clostridial cellulitis, although there may be more systemic toxicity, and the exudate is less watery and more pus-like.

Laboratory Findings

Gram stain may show polymicrobial flora. Gram-positive and gram-negative organisms may be present.

Bacterial Etiology

Etiology is characterized by mixed flora: anaerobes, including *Bacteroides, Peptococcus,* and *Peptostreptococcus,* and facultative bacteria, including Enterobacteriaceae, streptococci, and staphylococci.

Treatment

Surgical intervention is the same as that for clostridial cellulitis. Antibiotics must be directed against organisms found on Gram stain and modified once cultures are returned. Empiric choices for mixed aerobic/anaerobic infections include:

1. Imipenem/cilastatin, 1.5 to 2 g/day
2. Ticarcillin/clavulanic acid, 3.1 g q6h to q8h
3. Ampicillin/sulbactam, 3 g q6h

4. Piperacillin/tazobactam, 3.375 g q6h or 4.5 g q8h
5. Various combinations including clindamycin or metronidazole for anaerobic coverage, plus a quinolone, third-generation cephalosporin, or aztreonam for aerobic, gram-negative activity.

■ *Necrotizing Fasciitis Including Streptococcal Fasciitis*

An acute, severe, rapidly progressive disease that predominantly affects the lower extremities, necrotizing fasciitis is differentiated from the cellulitis described previously by the involvement of the superficial and sometimes deep fascia. The diagnosis is made at the time of debridement by the ease with which a finger or blunt probe can be passed along the fascial planes. The pathogenesis is usually trauma. Even insignificant events, such as a minor laceration, may be sufficient to cause this infection. There have been a number of cases reported of streptococcal fasciitis following lower extremity surgery. Since this condition will progress rapidly, it may initially be relatively mild in appearance but can lead to sepsis and death. Clinicians need to be aware of this possibility, although it is extremely rare.

Clinical Presentation
There is very rapid onset. The patient may complain of pain within a few hours of surgery or even have minor trauma. The initial clinical presentation can be rather benign with minimal clinical signs of infection being found. This lack of symptoms can then progress to extensive cellulitis in a short period. Early pain and erythema may progress to anesthesia and necrosis as the superficial vessels are thrombosed and the nerves destroyed. Tissue gas and a foul-smelling exudate may be present. Systemic toxicity is prominent and the patient becomes septic. There is a high mortality rate.

Laboratory Findings
Gram stain reveals a mix of organisms. Leukocytosis is common. Blood cultures are frequently positive. Late in the process the patient may develop laboratory evidence of sepsis and multi-organ failure.

Bacterial Etiology
Mixed aerobic and anaerobic flora is found in general cases of necrotizing fasciitis. Streptococcal fasciitis is caused by group A, ß-hemolytic streptococcus.

Treatment

Radical surgical debridement is the hallmark of treatment. Debridement is considered adequate when subcutaneous tissue can no longer be easily separated from the fascia. Antibiotic therapy should be based on Gram stain results before return of cultures. Possible empiric antibiotic choices are the same as those listed for nonclostridial cellulitis. Total-body hyperbaric oxygen may be a useful adjunct in the therapy.

■ *Synergistic Necrotizing Cellulitis*

Closely related to necrotizing fasciitis, synergistic necrotizing cellulitis differs in its involvement of underlying muscle. This disease is also found predominantly in the lower extremity. The pathogenesis is related to diabetes and obesity.

Clinical Presentation

Onset is acute, with marked systemic toxicity. Severe pain and edema are present. Tissue gas may be present. Skin changes occur late and present as gangrenous ulcerations with a watery, red-brown, foul-smelling exudate often referred to as "dishwater" pus. Entire muscle compartments may be necrotic.

Laboratory Findings

Blood cultures are positive in 50% of patients. Leukocytosis is present. Gram stain reveals mixed gram-positive and gram-negative flora.

Bacterial Etiology

This is a mixed aerobic/anaerobic infection. *Bacteroides* or *Peptococcus,* along with facultative gram-negative bacteria, are the most common combinations.

Treatment

Treatment is by surgical debridement of involved tissue, including muscle. Amputation may be required. Empiric antibiotic therapy is similar to that described for necrotizing cellulitis. Despite aggressive surgery and antibiotics, the prognosis is poor.

■ *Clostridial Myonecrosis (Gas Gangrene)*

The term *gas gangrene* is often incorrectly used to describe any condition in which soft tissue gas or crepitus appears. True gas gangrene is synonymous with clostridial myonecrosis. This is a rapidly progressive, deadly disease that traditionally follows muscle injury, burns, penetrating trauma, or bowel surgery. However, gas gangrene may also have no obvious traumatic etiology.

Clinical Presentation
Acute onset, between 6 hours and 3 days after injury, pain that rapidly increases in intensity, and toxemia are hallmarks of the disease. The patient appears lethargic, diaphoretic, and apathetic. Fever is frequently present, as well as hypotension and tachycardia. Early local signs include a tense swelling that blanches the skin. Later, large, tense bullae may form, along with necrosis of the skin. A foul-smelling, brown-red drainage containing gas bubbles may be seen. Gas and crepitus may be present but are more common in clostridial cellulitis. The muscles undergo necrosis and develop a red-purple discoloration. They do not bleed when incised.

Laboratory Findings
Leukocytosis is present. Positive blood cultures occur in some patients, but not commonly. The hematocrit is generally reduced. Gram stain reveals large, gram-positive bacilli but few polymorphonuclear leukocytes. Radiographs show massive dissection along muscle groups and fascial planes with distinct outlines of the muscles.

Bacterial Etiology
C. perfringens and, rarely, other clostridial species are found.

Treatment
Massive surgical incision, drainage, and debridement are therapeutic. Decompression of fascial compartments is required. Amputation may be necessary in many cases. The use of hyperbaric oxygen is controversial but may be helpful. Medical supportive therapy for the septicemia is important. The antibiotic of choice for *C. perfringens* has traditionally been penicillin G in high doses of up to 24 million U/day (2 million U q2h). Other traditional anaerobic agents, such as clindamycin and metronidazole, may be less effective. Chloramphenicol has been advocated in penicillin-allergic patients and for cases in which gram-negative organisms are seen on the initial stain. Imipenem/cilastatin has an excellent anaerobic spectrum and may be useful as empiric therapy in these cases.

■ *Nonclostridial Myonecrosis*

There are a number of similar infections that can all be grouped under this category. The main difference between each is the causative pathogen. As a group, these infections are less acute and have a lower mortality than their clostridial counterparts. Usually progression is slower with much less marked tissue necrosis.

Clinical Presentation

Systemic toxicity and local pain are less marked than in gas gangrene but may progress if not treated adequately. Tissue gas may be present but will not spread as quickly. The exudate will vary depending on the causative organism, but is usually foul smelling. Muscles can be necrotic, but less so than in gas gangrene.

Laboratory Findings

Systemic response is less marked than in clostridial myonecrosis. Gram stain results will vary depending on the causative organism. Gas will usually be present on the radiograph.

Bacterial Etiology

Given the proper set of circumstances, many different organisms may cause myonecrosis. Each bacterial cause of nonclostridial myonecrosis has been given the name of a unique disease entity. When anaerobic streptococcus is isolated, the disease is known as anaerobic streptococcal myonecrosis. When a mix of anaerobes and facultative organisms are seen, it becomes synergistic non-clostridial anaerobic myonecrosis. Unusual organisms reported to cause myonecrosis include *Aeromonas hydrophilia* and vibrio following marine injuries.

Treatment

As with the necrotizing infections discussed earlier, surgical intervention with complete debridement is the key to therapy. Antibiotic therapy should be directed against the isolated organism, with empiric therapy as outlined for nonclostridial cellulitis. One drug in particular, imipenem/cilastatin, looks extremely promising in the early treatment of these infections.

■ *Infected Vascular Gangrene*

A unique type of necrotizing infection that occurs almost exclusively in the foot, infected vascular gangrene is associated with peripheral vascular disease. It is most commonly seen in patients with diabetes mellitus.

Clinical Presentation
Unlike gas gangrene, the onset and progression are relatively slow. There is little systemic toxicity. Pain is usually nonexistent because of the peripheral neuropathy in the patient with diabetes. Local changes include frank gangrene with full-thickness necrosis of skin and muscle. Gas may be present. Exudate will have a foul odor.

Laboratory Findings
Hyperglycemia may be present, and there will be some leukocytosis. Gram stain reveals gram-positive and gram-negative organisms. Localized tissue gas is seen on x-rays.

Bacterial Etiology
Mixed aerobic/anaerobic flora are the causative organisms. *Bacteroides fragilis* and other bacteroides are common. Anaerobic gram-positive cocci are also isolated. Group B streptococci are found frequently along with other streptococci. Staphylococci and Enterobacteriaceae may also be isolated.

Treatment
Treatment is by surgical debridement of ischemic and necrotic tissue. Antibiotics are directed at the organisms cultured. Empiric choices include the following:

1. Piperacillin/tazobactam, 3.375 g q6h or 4.5 g q8h
2. Ticarcillin/clavulanic acid, 3.1 g q6h to q8h
3. Ampicillin/sulbactam, 3 g q6h
4. Imipenem/cilastatin, 500 mg q6h to q8h
5. Clindamycin combined with an appropriate anti–gram-negative agent (i.e., quinolone, aztreonam, or third-generation cephalosporin)

■ *Pyomyositis*

As its name implies, pyomyositis refers to pus in the skeletal muscle. Traditionally described in the tropics or in patients who have traveled to a tropical region, it has also been seen in patients without this history. One of the more common locations is the calf muscles. The pathophysiology of the disease is not well understood, although hematogenous spread appears an unlikely route. Most likely it develops in muscles that were previously traumatized or by contiguous focus of infection.

Clinical Presentation
An early stage presents with subacute onset of localized muscle pain and fever. There is some swelling of the area. Pus is usually not found on aspiration. A later phase presents increased pain, erythema, edema, and flocculence. Aspiration reveals pus. If not treated, septicemia may result.

Laboratory Findings
Leukocytosis with a slight left shift may be seen. The ESR will be elevated. Gram stain reveals gram-positive cocci.

Bacterial Etiology
S. aureus is found in the majority of cases. Streptococci or a mix of other organisms may also be found.

Treatment
Surgical drainage of purulence is therapeutic. Parenteral antibiotic therapy directed by the culture results. Since staphylococci causes the majority of cases, treatment can include the following:

1. Cefazolin, 1 g q8h
2. Nafcillin, 2 g q4h to q6h
3. Clindamycin, 600 to 900 mg q8h
4. Vancomycin, 500 mg q6h to q8h

LYME DISEASE AND COINFECTING TICK-BORNE ZOONOSES

■ *Lyme Disease*

Lyme disease (previously called Lyme arthritis and now frequently known as Lyme borreliosis) was first discovered in 1975, when an unusual outbreak of arthritis occurred in children living in and around the town of Lyme, Connecticut. In 1982 Burgdorfer et al. first identified the etiologic agent that now bears his name: *Borrelia burgdorferi*, a gram-negative spirochete. The disease is now the most common vector-borne disease in the United States. It can also be found in many other parts of the world. Lyme disease is transmitted by its principal vector, the deer tick *Ixodes scapularis* (formerly *I. dammini*), although other ixodid ticks have also been implicated. Most transmission occurs when the tick is in the nymph stage and occurs in spring and early summer, although transmission has been reported during other times of the year and during other stages of tick development. Interestingly, the tick does not act as a reservoir for the organism. The most important reservoir is the white-footed mouse, or deer mouse. White-tailed deer, although a host for the adult ticks, is also not considered an important reservoir for the bacteria.

It is very important to note that there seems to be a direct correlation between the amount of time the tick is attached to a human and the potential for developing clinical disease. A minimum of 24 to 48 hours of attachment may be required to transmit the disease.

Clinical Presentation
The disease is usually broken down into three stages.

1. Stage 1 or "localized infection" is an early stage marked by the presence of erythema migrans (EM), which presents as an expanding annular ring of erythema centered around the initial bite site. Although the presence of EM is reported in more than 90% of patients who develop the disease, actual tick bites are rarely reported. This is primarily due to the small size of the infecting tick and the painless bite. The lesion starts as a small papule and slowly expands over time. Central clearing, giving a "target" appearance, is common.
2. Stage 2 is the "disseminated stage" of the infection. Secondary rings of EM may begin to appear at distant site from the original bite. This usually occurs days to weeks after the initial presentation. The most reliable and persistent symptoms of this stage are lethargy and fatigue. Other symptoms include transient neurologic symptoms, such as Bell's palsy, and rheumatologic and cardiac involvement.
3. Stage 3 or "persistent infection" usually occurs months to years later. It is marked by migratory arthritis and chronic neurologic symptoms. The arthritis most commonly affects the large joints of the lower extremity, although the hands and shoulders can also be involved.

Laboratory Findings

Much of the diagnosis of Lyme borreliosis is clinical. Diagnosis of the disease in the laboratory presents several difficulties.

1. Observation of the spirochete using special stains is diagnostic but difficult. Skin biopsy from the outer edge of the erythema migrans will have the highest concentration of organisms along with fluid from joints, cerebrospinal fluid (CSF), or blood. More recently, polymerase chain reaction (PCR) detection of the spirochete DNA has assisted in the identification of the organism, especially from synovial fluid.
2. Ideally, the organism should be grown on culture for definitive diagnosis. Unfortunately, the organism is fastidious and difficult to grow, and the required media are expensive.
3. Serologic testing with the enzyme-linked immunosorbent assay (ELISA) or through immunofluorescence is fraught with both false-positive and false-negative results. Furthermore, confirmation of positive and equivocal tests are necessary with Western blot techniques.
4. Serodiagnosis is further complicated by the fact that the immune response can develop very slowly.

Bacterial Etiology

The spirochete *B. burgdorferi* is causative.

Treatment

The causative organism is usually susceptible to numerous antibiotics, including penicillins, second- and third-generation cephalosporins, tetracyclines, and macrolides.

1. Stage 1 and early stage 2. Oral doxycycline 200 mg/day for 20 to 30 days is the drug of choice, but should be avoided in children. Amoxicillin 500 mg tid is an alternative, as are erythromycin, azithromycin, and cefuroxime axetil. All should be continued for about 3 weeks.
2. Late stage 2 and stage 3. Both stages can be treated with similar agents for prolonged periods. For cases of arthritis and Bell's palsy, little difference has been shown between oral and parenteral therapy. In severe cases especially in neurological and cardiac cases, parenteral therapy with the third-generation cephalosporin ceftriaxone at 2 g/day for 3 weeks may prove effective.

Prophylaxis

As with many diseases, prevention is the best course. Avoiding high-risk areas, wearing long pants tucked into socks, wearing light-colored clothing, and using insecticides containing DEET all help to prevent tick bites. As for the use of routine prophylactic antibiotics following a tick bite, the risk of contracting Lyme disease is so small that recommendations call for not using antibiotics. Nevertheless, when faced with a demanding patient, many physicians will use a 10-day course of either doxycycline or amoxicillin.

■ *Coinfecting Zoonoses*

Recently there has been an increased awareness of other tick-borne illnesses that often are cotransmitted to humans along with Lyme disease. These organisms, when acting either alone or in combination with the Lyme spirochete, cause disease states that can be significantly more severe than Lyme disease alone.

Babesiosis

Caused by the malaria-like protozoan *Babesia microti,* this disease is transmitted by the same ticks that transmit Lyme disease. This is primarily a flulike disease that can mimic many other conditions including a viral infection, although serious and fatal variants are known. It is generally self-limiting and complications are few, although relapse can occur. Treatment is usually by a combination of oral clindamycin plus quinine for 7 to 10 days.

Ehrlichioses

Human granulocytic ehrlichiosis (HGE) is caused by a small gram-negative cocci closely related to *Ehrlichia equi,* a horse pathogen. It was first described in the United States in 1994. As with babesiosis, the vector is the same Ixodes group of ticks that transmits Lyme disease. The disease itself is more severe than the others, causing a serious febrile illness that frequently requires hospitalization. Blood dyscrasias including leukopenia and thrombocytopenia are common. Fortunately, the same treatment that is effective for Lyme disease, especially doxycycline, is also the treatment of choice for HGE.

The bottom line with both of these diseases is that once a patient is suspected of contracting Lyme borreliosis, it may be worthwhile to also consider these other infections so that effective treatment can begin promptly.

"HIGHER BACTERIA" AND PARASITIC INFECTIONS

■ *Madura Foot*

Madura foot, also known as mycetoma or maduromycosis, is a chronic, deforming infection that most frequently involves the foot. It was first described in the Madura district of India, from which it gained its name. It is now seen mostly in underdeveloped tropical and subtropical countries. Although most cases in the United States are reported from the South, more cases are now being seen in other regions because of immigration from endemic areas.

The etiology of Madura foot is generally insignificant trauma that allows the organism to enter the body. Once in the foot, the organisms spread along tissue planes and deep to bone.

Clinical Presentation
It is predominant in males. It starts as a small papule on the foot, and massive edema of the foot and leg is seen. Large focal granulomas form on the foot, and multiple sinuses drain "grains" of organism. These grains may have a distinctive color or odor depending on the causative pathogen. These sinuses periodically open and close, causing scarring. With deep involvement, destruction of bone occurs. Secondary bacterial infection may ensue with classic signs and symptoms.

Laboratory Findings
Because the diagnosis of Madura foot is basically made on clinical grounds, the laboratory offers little help. Exact diagnosis of the causative organism can be made on special staining and culturing.

Bacterial Etiology
Madura foot can be categorized according to the causative agent as either eumycetoma, caused by true fungi, or actinomycetoma, caused by the "higher bacteria" or Actinomycetes. Usual species include *Nocardia brasiliensis* and *Actinomadura madurae*.

Treatment
Traditionally the cure of mycetoma has tended to be surgical. Depending on the depth of penetration, amputation was often the only cure. More recently, limited surgery along with combinations of various drugs, based on the identification of the causative organisms, is the preferred approach.

■ *Cutaneous Larve Migrans*

Commonly known as "creeping eruption," cutaneous larve migrans (CLM) is a relatively rare parasitic skin infection usually found in warm tropical environments, including the Southeastern United States, or in travelers returning from tropical beach environments. The majority of cases occur on the foot, although other parts of the body that had direct contact with ground or sand, including the legs and buttocks, can also be involved.

Clinical Presentation

CLM presents as an intensely pruritic, serpiginous, elevated, reddened skin lesion. It begins in an area of the foot that has been in contact with contaminated soil or sand. The lesion progresses around the foot, tracing the track that the organism has migrated throughout the tissue. The actual organism is usually 1 to 2 cm ahead of the visible track. The diagnosis is based on clinical findings.

Laboratory Findings

This remains an essentially local process, so laboratory diagnosis is generally not indicated. Occasionally, eosinophilia has been reported. Also, biopsy from an area ahead of the lesion may reveal the parasite.

Etiology

CLM is caused by the larval form of a dog hookworm, *Ancylosoma brazilienses*. Other canine and feline parasites have also been less frequently implicated. Essentially these organisms are found in egg form in the feces of local animals. Once the eggs are released into sandy areas, they develop into larvae and can invade the foot.

Treatment

Traditionally, treatment has been with topical thiabendazole topical (10% solution four times/day, making sure that the topical therapy is placed ahead of the lesion, where the living parasite is found). Also, oral thiabendazole (25mg/kg bid for 2 days) has been considered effective therapy. Alternatives include Albendazole (400 mg/day for 3 days), or, in a more recent study, Invermectin as a single dose has been shown to be very effective.

SUGGESTED READINGS

Bouchard O, Houze S, Scheimann R et al: Cutaneous larve migrans in travelers: a prospective study with assessment of therapy with invermectin, *Clin Infect Dis* 31:493, 2000.

Downey MS, Yu GV: Post-saphenous phlebectomy donor leg cellulites, *J Am Podiatr Med Assoc* 77:277, 1987.

LeFrock JL, Molavi A: Necrotizing skin and subcutaneous infections, *J Antimicrob Chemother* 9(suppl A):183, 1982.

Parola P, Raoult D: Ticks and tickborne bacterial diseases in humans: an emerging infectious threat, *Clin Infect Dis* 32:897, 2001.

Rolston KVI: Infections involving the skin and soft tissues of the lower extremity, *J Foot Surg* 26:S25, 1987.

Steere A: Borrelia burgdorferi (Lyme disease, Lyme borreliosis). In Mandell GL, Bennett JE, Dolin R, editors: *Principles and practice of infectious diseases*, ed 5, p 2504, Philadelphia, 2000, Churchill Livingstone.

Swartz MN: Cellulitis and superficial infections. In Mandell GL, Bennett JE, Dolin R, editors: *Principles and practice of infectious diseases*, ed 5, p 1037, Philadelphia, 2000, Churchill Livingstone.

Thompson C, Spielman A, Krause PJ: Coinfecting deer-associated zoonoses: Lyme disease, babesiosis and ehrlichiosis, *Clin Infect Dis* 33:676, 2001.

Treatment of Lyme disease, *Med Lett* 31:57, 1989.

Veinoglou G, Sadighi P, Auerbach J: Pyomyositis: a review, *Infect Surg* 8:686, 1989.

CHAPTER 3

Bone and Joint Infections

OSTEOMYELITIS

Because of the number of bones in the foot and their proximity to the surface, osteomyelitis is fairly common. For these same reasons, diagnosis of osteomyelitis is somewhat easier in the foot compared to other parts of the body since the infected bones can frequently be seen and touched. This makes treatment more straightforward. If a small pedal bone is exposed and obviously infected, simply removing it will cure the infection. Of course, this is grossly simplifying the problem. Dilemmas that arise when trying to diagnose osteomyelitis of the foot still remain. Likewise, a clinician cannot always simply remove a bone, because this may not be practical. Antibiotic therapy, either alone, or in combination with some debridement surgery, may then be required.

■ *Classification*

The literature is replete with attempts to classify a particular disease, which indicates that the process is rather complex. So it is with osteomyelitis. Traditionally, osteomyelitis has been divided into three distinct types based on etiology, all of which can occur in the lower extremity:

54

1. Hematogenous osteomyelitis
2. Direct extension, or *contiguous-focus* osteomyelitis
3. Osteomyelitis secondary to vascular insufficiency

These types can be subdivided based on the length of time the process has been present. Unfortunately, the exact definition of these distinctions is not always agreed upon, and lines of distinction often blur. They can also be used in combination (i.e., initial acute or recurrent chronic):

1. Chronic
2. Acute
3. Initial
4. Recurrent

This system, popularized by Francis Waldvogel over 30 years ago and based on the etiology of the infection, is still useful today.

Another classification system, first described by George Cierny and Jon Mader in 1985, has been widely adopted by many in the infectious diseases and orthopedic communities. Instead of dwelling on the etiology of the process, this system combines the anatomical location of the infection in the bone and pairs that to a specific "host" type. A complicated algorithm is then specified for each combination of stage and type to direct physicians in their treatment approach. This system offers many important points that need to be understood.

Anatomic stages

1. Medullary—Involvement of only the medullary canal. This is actually a "true" osteomyelitis because the dictionary defines the word roughly as "infection of the medullary bone and contiguous structures." This occurs most commonly in a hematogenous osteomyelitis.
2. Superficial—Involvement of only the outer cortex. This could actually be considered an infectious periosteitis because the cortical bone is involved with no medullary involvement.
3. Localized—This involves at least one cortex through and through into the medullary canal. The hallmark of this type is that the structure of the bone is still stable.
4. Diffuse—More than one cortex is involved plus the medullary bone. The infected bone that results is unstable because of the involvement of multiple cortices.

Physiologic Class

1. A-Host: A host with an intact immune system. An otherwise normal patient.
2. B-Host: A compromised host. This class is further divided into B_L, a locally compromised patient (i.e., vascular blockage to an extremity), and B_S, a systemically compromised host.
3. C-Host: A unique class, in which the treatment is worse than the disease. This type of patient requires only suppressive therapy or no therapy at all. Many of the patients seen with pedal osteomyelitis fall into this category. They may be elderly, debilitated, or have a systemic disease process that precludes either surgery or prolonged antibiotic therapy. The existence of this class is an admission that not all patients need to be "cured." Many individuals will go to their graves with an osteomyelitis in the foot that had *nothing* to do with their death. Clinicians using this approach must thoroughly document the reasons and explanations provided to the patient.

■ *Principles of Diagnosis*

History and Physical Examination

As with any infection, the first step in diagnosing osteomyelitis is to obtain a history and perform a physical examination. In fact, the actual diagnosis can often be made solely on the basis of these two steps. Details on questions to include in the patient history and general physical findings are found in Chapter 1. If osteomyelitis is suspected, however, the following specific questions become especially pertinent.

1. What was the etiology? An ulceration? A puncture? A bite? Different causes will have potentially different infecting organisms.
2. How deeply did the puncture or bite penetrate? Just because the patient sustained a puncture does not mean it affected the bone. It may only be a soft tissue injury.
3. How long ago did the initial signs and symptoms begin? What has been the course of those symptoms? Many patients will come to an office after being incompletely treated elsewhere. They will relate a cyclic course of exacerbations and remissions. This may be evidence that the soft tissue infection was treated but the bone could still be harboring organisms.

4. Has there ever been an opening of the skin? If so, did it drain pus? Did it close and then reopen at a later time? Sinus tracts have been known to spontaneously heal and then reopen months to years later. This may be evidence of a chronic osteomyelitis.
5. Can the area of pain be pinpointed?
6. Has there been limitation of movement?
7. If the patient is a child, has there been a change in personality, disposition, or eating habits? Very young children, of course, are unable to say what is bothering them. Therefore, things like failure to thrive or guarding a painful area may be clues to a deeper infection.
8. Have any antibiotics, prescribed or not, oral or parenteral, been taken? For how long? What effect did they have? If an antibiotic was taken and seemed to have a positive effect, it may have been an appropriate drug but was not used for a long enough period of time. This can be helpful in determining the causative organism even if bone cultures were impossible to harvest.

After the history, the patient should be examined for the following clinical signs of osteomyelitis:

1. Any evidence of exposed bone. Bone that can be freely observed or palpated with a probe, especially in a highly contaminated wound, should be considered infected. In 1995, Grayson et al objectively showed that so-called "probing to bone" has a high positive predictive value for osteomyelitis.
2. The presence of dysvascular, necrotic, soft, or "mushy" bone that easily crumbles and yields to probing upon debridement. Another clinical sign is the presence of frank purulence within a bone.
3. Pinpoint pain, swelling, or redness over a specific bone in the absence of an open ulcer of the sinus tract. This is especially prevalent in hematogenous osteomyelitis.
4. The presence of a sinus tract. However, be specific with this term. Some clinicians use it to describe any opening in the body. With osteomyelitis, it refers to a direct communication from the outside to the bone.
5. Scars over the area in question. In the absence of an active sinus tract, scars may indicate a previously closed sinus.

Laboratory Findings
Along with standard laboratory diagnostic tests (see Chapter 1), there are a few that can specifically aid in the diagnosis of

osteomyelitis. Unfortunately, because of the localized nature of many lower extremity osteomyelitis cases, all these tests may be either completely normal or only minimally elevated.

Erythrocyte Sedimentation Rate

The erythrocyte sedimentation rate (ESR) is one of the most commonly used indices for the diagnosis of osteomyelitis and the monitoring of therapy. Because the ESR is elevated in many inflammatory conditions, it is not specific enough for the actual diagnosis. However, if the ESR is elevated, and there is no other apparent reason, osteomyelitis is the most likely reason for the rise. If this assumption is made, then decreases in the ESR with osteomyelitis therapy might demonstrate efficacy of the treatment. At least one small retrospective study by Kaleta et al demonstrated a high positive predictive value for osteomyelitis in the diabetic patient with a clinical suspicion for osteomyelitis and an ESR greater than 70.

C-Reactive Protein

C-Reactive (CRP) protein is an acute phase reactant that becomes elevated in the presence of an inflammatory process. Some believe it to be a more sensitive indicator of a septic process than the ESR. To take advantage of this sensitivity, however, the laboratory must be able to perform a *quantitative* assay. Furthermore, like ESR, the CRP is too nonspecific to be of much diagnostic help but may be useful in following the course of treatment.

Teichoic Acid Antibodies

Teichoic acid antibodies can be found circulating in the patient's serum if the infection is caused by a staphylococcal organism. This test, although not specific for osteomyelitis, is useful in determining the causative organism once osteomyelitis is diagnosed. Despite its potential usefulness, it is rarely performed for osteomyelitis.

Blood Culture

Blood cultures should be drawn on every patient suspected of having hematogenous osteomyelitis. Because the organism in the bone is usually metastatic from a distant focus of infection, blood culture is the most reliable method of determining the bacterial etiology without actually culturing the bone. This procedure can yield results in approximately 50% of cases, thus minimizing the need to actually culture the bone itself.

Bone Pathology

Bone biopsy with subsequent pathologic examination may be useful in the diagnosis of osteomyelitis. Histologically, the bone presents with suppurative necrosis and destruction. Osteoblastic new bone can also be seen. The pathologist should be made aware of any previous surgery, other coexistent inflammatory processes of bone, or the presence of potential Charcot changes in the foot. In some instances, changes noted in these cases may mimic osteomyelitis, making it more difficult for the pathologist to make a definitive diagnosis. For this reason, bone pathology cannot necessarily be considered definitive.

Bone Culture

Although technically a laboratory study, bone culture is discussed separately from the previously mentioned tests because of its importance. Bone culture is the definitive method used to diagnose osteomyelitis. Basically, if bacteria are cultured from the bone, the diagnosis is made. It is important to perform this test by harvesting bone properly; otherwise, a soft tissue organism that found its way onto the bone may be grown and interpreted as a positive "bone culture." This complicates the decision to treat.

Bone for culture can be harvested in two ways:

1. The open surgical technique, in which the affected bone is visualized and inspected and multiple samples are taken from different sites. This may be an independent procedure or part of a definitive surgical debridement.
2. The percutaneous technique, in which, using any one of a number of biopsy needles, large-gauge hypodermic needles, or bone trephines, the bone is sampled through punctures in the skin. Care must be taken to ensure that the needle is in fact in the infected bone. For this reason, multiple samples should be taken, and radiographic control of the placement is warranted.

Regardless of which of these techniques is used, a few basic principles should be followed:

1. The patient should stop taking antibiotics for as long as possible and at least 48 hours before the culture. Although scientific evidence to support this practice is hard to find, it has become widely held that the presence of any antibiotic in the serum or bone will alter culture results.

2. The culture should be harvested through a *clean* site. No attempt should be made to remove bone for culture through an ulceration or sinus tract. These sites are notorious for being contaminated with multiple bacteria that have little or no bearing on the actual infecting organism.

3. Multiple specimens should be harvested. The location from which each was sampled should be clearly identified on the laboratory report. This technique allows a determination of the extent of involvement.

4. Sufficient amounts of bone should be sampled. Osteomyelitis, especially chronic forms, can have a relatively low bacterial inoculum. This can make recovery in the laboratory difficult.

5. Send separate specimens for culture and biopsy. Although this sounds like a basic rule, many well-intentioned practitioners mistakenly place culture specimens in formalin or another pathologic fixative. Culture specimens should be sent dry, in a bacterial holding solution, or in saline. The microbiology laboratory should be consulted for their preferred technique.

6. A sample of bone of sufficient size for Gram stain, aerobic culture, anaerobic culture, should be sent. Special studies for fungal infection and acid-fast examination for mycobacteria are not always necessary as a first line approach unless there is some reason to suspect these organisms. Consider these studies in special cases where other cultures are negative despite appropriate harvesting, the patient is failing to respond to traditional therapy, or in cases when these organisms may be found (i.e., infection in the site of a corticosteroid injection).

Imaging

Within the last few years there have been major advances in the techniques used for osteomyelitis imaging. Some of the more promising modalities will be listed here. Many are not in general clinical practice but may be in the near future. It will be necessary to keep up to date with the imaging department of the local hospital or center to determine which particular study they are able to perform. Despite the advent of new imaging agents, some basic principles still hold true.

1. Plain film radiography is still the first line test. Despite its relative lack of sensitivity, it is widely available in almost any office; practically noninvasive; inexpensive; and if positive, fairly diagnostic.

2. Nuclear imaging is extremely sensitive, and its specificity varies from test to test. New tests seem to be developed monthly, are invasive, and remain moderately expensive.
3. For detecting osteomyelitis, magnetic resonance imaging (MRI) is considered the "champion." It is the most sensitive and specific; however, it is very expensive and despite its popularity, it still has false positives and is operator- and site-dependent.

Plain Radiography

The most basic of these tests are plain radiographs. Their main drawback is significant lag time before the disease can be visualized. A large percentage of the mineral content of bone must be lost before the changes are picked up on the films. Although 10 to 14 days is considered the standard minimum delay before changes are seen, the delay can be shorter in more aggressive cases. Changes seen on radiographs include the following:

1. Cortical breaking
2. Periosteal elevation, which is thought to be caused by pus breaking through the cortex and lifting the periosteum from the bone
3. Lysis of bone
4. Sequestrum, a radiodense area of bone that is separated or "broken away" from the main body of bone
5. Involucrum, periosteal new bone that forms a sclerotic-appearing "tube" around the old bone. When involucrum formation becomes hyperactive, a form of chronic osteomyelitis known as *Garre's sclerosing osteomyelitis* develops.
6. Brodie's abscess, a discrete radiolucent area believed to be found in chronic osteomyelitis.

Nuclear Scintigraphy

Nuclear scintigraphy plays a role in the diagnosis of osteomyelitis. Unlike plain radiographs, changes can be seen on scintigraphic studies within hours of onset. The main drawback to these studies is their lack of specificity for infection. Many different clinical trials have dealt with these scans individually or in combination against one another to determine issues such as sensitivity, specificity, and positive predictive value. Because each study reaches different conclusions and quotes different statistics, specific values for each are not practical.

Technetium 99 MDP Bone Scans

Technetium 99 MDP scans are the true "bone scan." The technetium isotope is specific for the hydroxyapatite matrix of bone. Any metabolic activity of bone will therefore cause uptake of this isotope, with a resultant positive scan. This metabolic activity can be seen in a number of conditions:

1. Infection
2. Fractures and other trauma
3. Surgical osteotomy or ostectomy
4. Tumors
5. Diabetic neuroarthropathy (Charcot joint)
6. Gout or almost any other arthritic condition (they all cause bone metabolism)

These scans are usually ordered in three phases:

1. Flow: taken immediately
2. Blood pool: taken after 5 to 10 minutes
3. Bone: taken after about 4 hours

Occasionally, a fourth scan is added after 24 hours.

Because of its lack of specificity, the clinical usefulness of technetium bone scanning is limited in lower extremity infections. Knowing the limitations of these scans is as important as knowing their indications. Despite all the problems with these scans, they are still frequently ordered by clinicians, seemingly by rote, without any thought about the drawbacks and implications of falsely positive scans:

1. They should not be used for the diagnosis of postoperative osteomyelitis when any bone surgery was performed. A radiologist will frequently read a scan as being "positive" for osteomyelitis without even knowing that a previous surgical procedure was performed on the bone, thereby causing the increased uptake.
2. They cannot be used to differentiate osteomyelitis from changes found in diabetic osteolysis or Charcot. It is not uncommon for a radiologist to report "osteomyelitis" of an obvious Charcot midtarsus when the clinician was concerned about an infected toe. *Be specific as to location and underlying conditions in your orders!*
3. They cannot determine the "extent of involvement" of an infected bone. Remember, the scan only shows the metabolic

activity, not infection. If the extent of involvement is of interest, then MRI or even plain films would be a better choice.
4. If plain radiographs already show evidence of osteomyelitis, bone scans are an expensive, unnecessary redundancy.

The following are indications for technetium bone scans in the diagnosis of lower extremity infections:

1. To rule out osteomyelitis. If the area is well vascularized, a negative scan will rule out the disease. Of course, as previously mentioned, a positive scan will *not* diagnose it.
2. Acute hematogenous osteomyelitis.
3. Early osteomyelitis following a puncture wound.
4. In conjunction with gallium scans for the differentiation of osteomyelitis from deep abscesses.

Gallium Scans

Gallium scans are more specific for soft tissue than bone. Some practitioners will combine the two studies and compare the results. If the uptake is greater in the gallium study and fades in the third phase of the technetium study, bone infection is ruled out. If uptake is intensely focal in both, then osteomyelitis is assumed. When compared with some of the newer modalities, however, the Gallium scan is of limited usefulness for diagnosing lower extremity osteomyelitis. Many centers have substituted other white cell scans for this one.

Indium Scans

Indium 111 white blood cell scans were the first of the newer generation of white cell labeled scans. The concept behind these is that white blood cells will target sites of inflammation and infection. When paired with a bone-seeking isotope, there should be not only good sensitivity, but also more specificity than with the standard bone scans. These scans are a definite improvement over both the technetium bone scan and the gallium scan. However, they are far from perfect and even newer tests are more sensitive and specific.

Drawbacks to this test include the fact that it is expensive to perform, it takes over 24 hours to run, and it is technically difficult. Perhaps its major drawback is that it is difficult to find a center that runs the test. It has been replaced in many centers by some of the newer modalities.

99mTc-hexamethylpropylene amine oxime (HMPAO) Scans

The HMPAO scan (Ceretec) has become the most accepted white cell scan for the diagnosis of osteomyelitis. It is easier to run than the indium scan and has a superior outcome. The HMPAO scan is basically a labeled white blood cell scan using the well-known bone tracer technetium as the isotope. It has excellent sensitivity, specificity, and accuracy and may show promise in the differentiation of osteomyelitis from Charcot.

Because of this promise, there have been many attempts to improve on the concept of a technetium labeled white cell scan. Some of the more interesting and promising of these include a Tc99 labeled ciprofloxacin scan. Experts believe that ciprofloxacin, as an antibiotic, will concentrate in the site of infection. Another interesting and promising scan is the use of a Tc99 labeled anti-granulocyte monoclonal antibody fragment Fab' scan. It remains to be seen if either of these, or any other newer modality, gain acceptance in the United States.

Magnetic Resonance Imaging

Most people agree that MRI has become the gold standard for the imaging diagnosis of osteomyelitis. MRI can demonstrate changes in bone marrow composition in infected bone very early in the course of the disease. Since a specific amount of marrow involvement can be seen, MRI has been successfully used in planning surgical debridement by helping to demarcate the involved bone. Although direct visualization of the cortex is not really accomplished, this has had little effect on this test's usefulness. An added benefit is that soft tissue abscesses that may be invasive to adjacent bone are also visualized early and clearly, as are sinus tracts and even cellulitis. In addition, a negative scan will rule out osteomyelitis. Techniques (e.g., spin, fat saturation, use of enhancement) are constantly evolving and each specialist has his or her own idea of how to image an osteomyelitis. However, on a T_1-weighted image the inflammatory fluid in the marrow will be dark (decreased signal intensity) compared to the usually bright fatty marrow tissue. On a T_2 image, the reverse will be true with the infected area showing up brightly against the darker normal marrow.

No test, not even MRI, is perfect. It is expensive. It is highly dependent on technique and equipment, especially when one is looking for fine detail in the foot. Another concern is that MRI may still be ineffective in differentiating osteomyelitis from diabetic osteolysis. Furthermore, other inflammatory processes, such as acute gouty arthritis, neoplasm, and possibly trauma, may be misinterpreted as an osteomyelitis, which will lead to false positives. Finally, any metallic implant in the area will produce artifacts that make the test difficult to evaluate.

Computed Tomography

In the diagnosis of infection, computed tomography (CT) has a less clearly defined role than MRI. It has been used successfully to determine the presence, location, and size of abscesses and gas in tissue. It is probably most useful for determining the size and location of sequestrum or necrotic bone before surgical intervention or in bones not easily visualized on plain radiography. It is not regularly used for diagnosis of foot osteomyelitis but may be more helpful in cases involving the leg and thigh.

Bottom line

The bottom line when it comes to imaging for osteomyelitis is that a staged approach is probably most effective.

1. The first step is to take plain film radiographs. If these are positive, there is rarely any reason to go further. Exceptions may be the use of MRI for surgical planning of a larger bone — don't waste it for a toe.
2. If the plain films are negative but there is still significant clinical concern, consider using a nuclear technique. Tc99 bone scans are useful to rule out the disease. If the scan is negative, there is probably no osteomyelitis. A white cell scan, such as an HMPAO, can rule out the process if negative and indicates osteomyelitis if it is positive. Of course, this specificity comes at greater expense.
3. If plain films are negative, the third option is to proceed directly to an MRI. This will come at an even greater expense than an HMPAO; however, some would argue this test will eventually be performed anyway, so it is best to perform it early on.

■ *Principles of Treatment*

Some physicians believe that osteomyelitis can never really be cured. Instead, these practitioners prefer to use terms such as *arrest, quiesce,* or *sequester* when referring to the apparent successful treatment of osteomyelitis. Their reticence is understandable. Osteomyelitis is a difficult disease to manage. The literature is difficult to interpret. Success rates vary widely based on numerous factors that are difficult, if not impossible, to standardize. One school of thought calls for the use of surgical debridement with no antibiotics.

Another discounts the importance of the surgery. It is probably safe to say, however, that in most cases, the successful management of osteomyelitis calls for a combination of antibiotics, surgical debridement, and skillful postoperative management, but there are always exceptions to the rule. In the unique anatomy of the foot, infected bones can be easily resected, resulting in an easy cure. Likewise, in patients who do not require surgery, excellent results have been achieved with prolonged courses of oral antibiotics.

The discussion about the Type C Host found in the Classification section is also important. There are some patients in which treatment is not feasible. The risks of prolonged antibiotics or surgical intervention are too great compared to the risks presented by the disease itself. It is perfectly acceptable in these patients to take a "watchful waiting" approach and treat only acute symptoms as they occur.

Antibiotic Treatment

It has been traditionally taught that except in cases of hematogenous osteomyelitis, antibiotics alone are probably insufficient therapy for osteomyelitis. Clinical experience has borne out a different reality. Although surgical excision of infected bone is clearly definitive, antibiotics alone can be successful in patients who either cannot or will not undergo surgery. Even in cases where surgery is performed, antibiotics are an important adjunct in the treatment. The selection of an appropriate agent should be based on the following principles:

1. The selection should be based on appropriate bone culture results whenever possible. *The selection should not be based on sinus tract or ulcer culture swabs!* Empiric usage without supportive cultures may subject the patient to a prolonged exposure of potentially toxic, expensive, or inappropriate therapy.
2. The selected agent should be bactericidal against the causative organism. Because infected bone may be dysvascular and the organisms sequestered, the patient's immune system cannot be considered reliable.
3. The minimal inhibitory concentration (MIC) of the antibiotic for the infecting organism should be low enough that achievable tissue levels will exceed the MIC many times over. (Note that no specific number of times is given. The data are too variable for any definitive conclusion.)
4. Antibiotic treatment must last for a sufficient period of time. Approximately 4 to 6 weeks of parenteral or equivalent therapy,

following definitive debridement, is considered by many to be the standard of care for most cases of non-hematogenous osteomyelitis. Equivalent therapy is defined as the use of a drug whose pharmacokinetics allows similar bioavailability in both oral and parenteral forms. Follow-up therapy with prolonged courses of oral antibiotics is common but not necessary.

5. Despite the previous comment about follow-up therapy, keeping a patient on a parenteral drug, or equivalent, for a prolonged period of time is unrealistic. Insurance coverage, hospitalization times, drug sensitivities (both for the patient and the organism) may severely limit treatment options. In some cases it may only be feasible or practical to keep the patient on a course of a standard oral antibiotic for a prolonged period of time. Although probably not optimal, this has been accomplished successfully for years. Unfortunately, there are not enough data to definitively single out one drug or how long it should be administered.

6. If oral therapy is chosen, monitoring patient compliance is helpful. Periodic blood tests to ensure the maintenance of a serum bactericidal titer of at least 1:8 is one method. Another is pill counting. However, neither of these methods is commonly used.

7. *Bone penetration* studies offer little reliable information to the practitioner. They tend to be sponsored by pharmaceutical companies and inevitably favor their products. Until the methods and results are standardized and universally accepted, they cannot be relied on. *It can be assumed that all the antibiotics commonly used in lower extremity infections will penetrate into bone in sufficient quantity to be efficacious.* Clindamycin is the one drug that has been studied most completely and scientifically in this regard. This drug is known to have excellent bone penetration and has been comparatively very effective against staphylococcal osteomyelitis.

9. There is little evidence to support the often stated belief that antibiotics are useless in a patient with poor circulation to the lower extremity. Some mistakenly contend that if blood is not effectively circulating to the lower extremity, the antibiotic won't either. As long as the tissue is still marginally viable, the antibiotic will reach the bone. Because most antibiotics concentrate in bone, therapeutic levels should still be possible.

Surgical Treatment

Meticulous debridement of all necrotic, infected bone is the hallmark of osteomyelitis treatment. In the foot, this debridement is simplified by the normal anatomic boundaries of the numerous small bones and joints. This becomes more difficult when dealing with the long bones in the foot and leg. Some general guidelines include the following:

1. Once an entire infected bone (e.g., a phalanx) is removed and there is no evidence of proximal or distal spread, the disease can be considered cured.
2. If the infection remains superficial, on the outer surface of the cortical bone, saucerization of the area is usually sufficient.
3. Once the infection has entered the cancellous portion of the bone, the entire bone should be considered infected because the organisms have gained access to the haversian system and can migrate throughout. This is especially true if purulence is revealed under compression in the area. As previously discussed, MRI may be useful in differentiating areas of frank medullary infection.
4. If debridement of the entire bone is not feasible, then removal of frankly necrotic bone should be followed by aggressive antibiotic therapy and meticulous postoperative technique. This occurs commonly in the metatarsals, tibia, fibula, and os calcis.
5. Because of underlying health concerns, surgical intervention is not warranted in some cases. For these patients, *chronic suppressive therapy* with long-term antibiotics alone may be perfectly acceptable. The patient must be made aware that this may not cure the disease but will put it into remission. In addition, the patient must be informed that an exacerbation can occur at any time.

Dead Space Management Techniques

Following surgical debridement, there is usually a significant dead space from where the necrotic bone and soft tissue have been removed. If this area is not managed properly, a buildup of wound fluid and bacteria can cause a relapse of the osteomyelitis.

Local Wound Care with Periodic Debridement

Wound care with periodic debridement is probably the most straightforward and common approach to the dead space following debridement surgery of bone. This technique calls for the use of daily dressing changes, bedside debridement as needed, packing, and occasional surgery for further complete debridement. When the wound is clean, it is closed by delayed primary closure.

Antibiotic-Impregnated Beads

One of the more well-documented techniques for dead space management is the implantation of antibiotic-impregnated beads or fillers. They are traditionally made of polymethylmethacrylate (PMMA) and mixed with gentamicin. An incredible amount of research has been published on many different types of material and antibiotics. Some of the newer studies have used biodegradable materials such as hydroxyapatite cement or polylactic acid (PLA) as the carrier for the antibiotic. Even autogenous blood clots have been discussed as a medium into which to mix the drug. The antibiotics studied most often include gentamicin, tobramycin, vancomycin, and a number of other drugs. Supporters point to these high local levels of antibiotic with virtually no systemic complications. In fact, in Europe the impregnated beads have been used in place of systemic antibiotics. Previous detractions have mostly been silenced by the overwhelmingly positive clinical experience now reported throughout the rest of the world. Probably the greatest drawback at this time is the continued lack of an FDA-approved product for use in the United States. As a result, most surgeons continue to have to "roll their own" at the time of surgery.

Myocutaneous Flaps

The use of myocutaneous flaps operates on the principle of increased blood flow or oxygenation to the affected area to treat the osteomyelitis. Following debridement of bone, the resultant bony cavity is filled with a vascularized myocutaneous flap. These flaps are either rotated from adjacent areas or are harvested as "free flaps" from a distant site. This vascularized tissue increases blood flow to the site and thus increases oxygen delivery. This technique also has the advantage of providing dead space management.

Cancellous Bone Grafts

Another technique to control the resultant dead space following debridement is the application of cancellous bone grafts, which is commonly referred to as *Papineau grafting*. These grafts not only fill the void left by surgery but also provide a framework or scaffold onto which granulation tissue can form. Once the wound is adequately filled with granulation, a skin graft is applied to the site for coverage.

Ingress-Egress Drainage Systems

Ingress-egress drainage systems have been installed in some patients with osteomyelitis. These systems provide a continuous instillation of an antibiotic, antiseptic, or normal saline into a bone cavity following debridement. Supporters of this system point to the high local levels of antibiotic or antiseptic that it achieves. The mechanical action of continuous flushing of the wound is also considered useful. Detractors claim that the systems are technically difficult to keep patent. Maceration of the tissues with subsequent superinfection is also a possibility.

Ancillary Management

External Fixation Devices

External fixation devices are applied to lend absolute stability to the bone. It is believed that this stability allows a better ingress of capillary formation across the infected site and primary wound healing. This improved blood flow gives the bone an improved ability to fight the infection.

■ *Hyperbaric Oxygen Therapy*

It is postulated that in the site of necrotic osteomyelitic bone there is a marked reduction in oxygen tension. This relative hypoxia will lead to diminished microbial killing activity of the leukocytes. The use of hyperbaric oxygen may help overcome this deficiency. Hyperbaric oxygen therapy should not be confused with localized topical application of oxygen. In true hyperbaric oxygen therapy, the patient is totally enclosed in a chamber and breathes pure oxygen at a pressure of 2 to 3 atmospheres. Hyperbaric oxygen therapy is not a substitute for adequate antibiotic and surgical debridement. Even though the data are equivocal, it may be helpful in severe or chronic and refractory cases of osteomyelitis.

CLINICAL SYNDROMES

■ *Acute Hematogenous Osteomyelitis*

Acute hematogenous osteomyelitis (AHO) is most commonly seen in three groups of patients:

1. Very young patients (those with immature bone)
2. Older adults
3. Intravenous drug users

Of these three groups, young patients are seen most commonly with AHO of the lower extremity. In these patients, there is sludging of blood flow in the metaphyseal region of long bones and the apophyseal region of flat bones. If bacteremia is present because of a concomitant distant site infection, the bacteria may precipitate out of the blood and into the bone at these sites. Commonly affected bones include the metatarsals, the tibia, the fibula, the femur, the calcaneus, and the cuboid. Although the pathogenesis is similar in the other types of patients, the vertebrae are the bones most frequently involved.

Clinical Presentation
The following are all possible symptoms of AHO:

1. Severe pain with ambulation is reported. In preverbal children, guarding of the area may be noted.
2. Pinpoint tenderness and swelling is found over the involved bone.
3. Constitutional symptoms, including fever, chills, and malaise, are frequently present. The patient may appear septic.
4. Open draining sinus tracts are uncommon.
5. Radionuclide studies may be helpful in establishing an early diagnosis.

Laboratory Findings
1. An elevated white blood count (WBC) is frequently found.
2. Blood cultures may be positive and are one of the best ways to determine bacterial etiology.
3. The ESR will usually be elevated.

Bacterial Etiology and Special Populations
All patient groups with AHO share in common this factor: the infection in the bone is secondary to a bacteremia. The initial source of the bacteremia will help lead to a microbial diagnosis.

1. AHO is usually caused by a single organism.
2. *Staphylococcus aureus* is by far the most common cause of the disease in young people because the original infection site is usually an upper respiratory infection or distant skin and skin structure infection.
3. *Haemophilus influenzae* is less commonly seen but can be found in patients less than 1 year old. Again, this is because in this

age group, upper respiratory infections are the most common original infection site.

4. In elderly patients the gram-negative rods are the most commonly found organisms. These organisms usually arise from a bacteriuria (bacteria in the urine) secondary to a urinary tract infection.

5. Although hematogenous extra-pulmonary tuberculosis (TB) infections caused by *Mycobacterium tuberculosis* are usually found in the spine, it is possible to find them in the foot. Patients almost always have a history of primary pulmonary TB. This disease is an indolent, slowly progressing process that over time can cause massive destruction of the bony structure of the foot. Chronic pain is the most common initial presentation. Diagnosis is usually made on bone culture and pathologic examination looking for granuloma formation and examination for the organism using acid-fast staining.

6. *S. aureus*, including methicillin-resistant strains and *Pseudomonas aeruginosa* are frequently found in intravenous drug users. For patients "greasing the needle," mouth flora including anaerobes can also be found.

7. A large percentage of patients with a history of *sickle cell disease* will eventually develop osteomyelitis, frequently of the lower extremity. The vast majority of these cases will be caused by Salmonella species, with *S. aureus* also being common. The most common explanation given for the predominance of Salmonella is that the sickle cell disease causes bowel infarctions and gangrene, which allows this organism to leave the gut and circulate throughout the bloodstream. Micro-infarcts of the long bones then give the circulating organism a place to "land." Therapy for these patients should be empirically directed against Salmonella but should also include staphylococcus coverage.

8. Another group prone to hematogenous osteomyelitis is patients undergoing hemodialysis. Because of the need for frequent access by use of an indwelling catheter, both *S. aureus* (including frequent methicillin resistant strains) and *S. epidermidis* are common isolates, although a number of others have also been reported. Infection in the lower extremity can occur, but it is rare.

Treatment

1. AHO is the only form of osteomyelitis traditionally thought to respond favorably to antibiotic therapy without surgical debridement.

2. Therapy is usually begun with intravenous antibiotics for about 2 weeks and then changed to oral therapy. The oral antibiotics are continued for 2 to 3 months.
3. More recent data show that oral antibiotics alone for a number of months may be just as effective as the combination of intravenous antibiotics followed by oral ones.

■ *Osteomyelitis Secondary to a Contiguous Focus or Direct Extension*

The most common type of osteomyelitis seen in the lower extremity is contiguous focus osteomyelitis (CFO). Examples of CFO include:

1. Most postoperative infections, including pin-tract infections and prosthetic joint infections
2. Post–puncture-wound osteomyelitis
3. Osteomyelitis underlying diabetic neuropathic ulceration
4. Bite-wound osteomyelitis
5. A septic arthritis that destroys the joint and invades the bone
6. Osteomyelitis following an open fracture

Because of the wide variation of etiologies, CFO is often the most difficult to diagnose and treat. The one congruency is that all these processes are caused by an inoculation of bacteria from a heavily contaminated or infected site into a previously noninfected site.

Clinical Presentation

Because of the variety of etiologies, only general statements are made here about the disease. Specific discussions of each type can be found in the chapters dealing with each specific process.

1. Localized signs, including erythema, edema, and heat, are frequently present.
2. Fever may be present, depending on the severity of the process.
3. Draining sinus tracts are often seen. Bone is frequently exposed or easily probed, thereby simplifying the diagnosis.
4. Radiographs show the classic signs of osteomyelitis.
5. Bone scans are rarely helpful because of the antecedent trauma.

Laboratory Findings

1. The WBC is frequently normal or only slightly elevated.
2. The same can be said for the ESR. Elevations are usually related

to the extent of bony involvement. Other causes for an elevated ESR must be ruled out.

3. Blood cultures and sinus tract cultures are rarely helpful.
4. Definitive diagnosis is based on bone cultures harvested using the proper technique, which was described earlier.

Bacterial Etiology

The bacterial etiology depends widely on the type of CFO. Specifics are discussed in separate chapters.

Treatment

Although many other regimens have been successful, the three treatment steps outlined here have withstood the greatest test of time and trial. Together they have become generally accepted as the standard of care. This does not mean that they will always work. Each case is an individual challenge. It is the ultimate responsibility of the treating physician to decide what will work best for the patient. The following three treatment steps are recommended:

1. Surgical debridement of all infected or necrotic-looking bone
2. Parenteral antibiotics (or equivalent), directed by reliable bone cultures, for a period of 4 to 6 weeks following the definitive debridement
3. Postoperative adjunctive technique as needed

■ *Osteomyelitis Secondary to Vascular Insufficiency*

This type of osteomyelitis is found almost exclusively in the lower extremity. It occurs when bone becomes infected in the face of ischemic soft tissue. The three major causes are:

1. Arteriosclerosis
2. Diabetes mellitus with arterial disease (not neuropathic diabetic ulcers)
3. Frostbite

Clinical Presentation

1. Osteomyelitis secondary to vascular insufficiency is generally a local process. Minimal systemic signs of infection are found. Local signs of infection may be muted or absent because of the

body's inability to respond with typical vascular changes seen in cellulitis. These tend to progress very slowly and are often stable for long periods of time.

2. Pregangrenous changes of skin to frank gangrene are sometimes present in the most severely dysvascular cases.

3. Ulcerations occur predominately at the distal tips of the digits, subungually, under a heel decubitus ulceration, or along the first metatarsal prominence. These ulcerations have visible bone exposed in the base.

4. Severe local pain, specifically ischemic pain at rest, is present.

Laboratory Findings

1. Because this is a local process, most blood results are unremarkable.

2. Noninvasive vascular studies will show decreased perfusion of the foot.

Bacterial Etiology

1. It is classically described as polymicrobial in nature.

2. Gram-negative and gram-positive aerobes are found.

3. Anaerobes are common when frank skin necrosis is found.

Treatment

1. From a therapeutic standpoint, this is not generally an infectious problem. As noted previously, these lesions remain stable for long periods of time, and antibiotic therapy will have little effect. The ischemia must be addressed first. This may mean vascular consultation and possible reconstruction before surgical debridement.

2. If gangrenous tissue or bone is present, surgical removal is indicated. In some localized cases, such as a single toe, auto-amputation may ensue.

3. Antibiotics will not reach frankly gangrenous tissue, but they will prevent the spread of organisms to adjacent viable structures.

4. These are the patients who most often fit into the Cienry/Mader Class "C" host category in which the treatment can be worse than the disease. Frequently, no treatment is just as warranted as any sort of active approach. Since these tend to be slowly progressing, indolent processes, there is little danger to the patient.

SEPTIC ARTHRITIS

Septic arthritis (SA) is an acute disease. Immediate diagnosis and prompt aggressive treatment is necessary to prevent joint-- threatening sequelae. The pathophysiology of SA is not unlike that of osteomyelitis. SA can be divided into two types:

1. Hematogenous. Unlike osteomyelitis, hematogenous seeding of a joint is the most common etiology of SA. Due to the rich vascular supply of the joint capsule, bacteremia caused by a distant focus of infection may allow organisms to settle into the joint. Predisposing factors to hematogenous seeding of a joint include:
   a. Rheumatoid arthritis, possibly because of the previous damage to the joint
   b. Systemic corticosteroid use or immunosuppression
   c. Previous trauma to the joint
   d. Living in a Lyme endemic area
2. Direct extension, which is frequently seen in lower extremity joints following:
   a. Surgery
   b. Puncture wounds
   c. Animal bites
   d. Intraarticular injections—particularly of steroids
   e. Adjacent osteomyelitis that breaks through the cartilaginous plate

Clinical Presentation
1. Marked increase in local temperature, edema, and erythema is found. The vast majority of cases only occur in one joint (monarticular).
2. Significant guarding of the joint with limited and painful range of motion is seen.
3. Constitutional signs and symptoms may be present. One form of disseminated gonococcemia presents with high fever, chills, malaise, and SA.
4. Joint effusions are present.
5. Radiographs show increased soft tissue edema with joint swelling. Bone changes are only seen if the SA is caused by an adjacent osteomyelitis or vice versa.
6. MRI has become the diagnostic imaging modality of choice for SA since it can show distension of the joint space and

the location of the fluid buildup. It can also be used to show the presence or absence of periarticular bone involvement.

Differential Diagnosis

1. Gout. Probably the most common mimic of SA. Differentiation can be based on a number of factors:
   a. Joint aspiration for crystals or Gram stain.
   b. Age and sex of the patient. Gout is uncommon in young women.
   c. History of the process.
   d. Presence or absence of constitutional symptoms.
   e. Current medications the patient is currently taking. Gout is predisposed in patients taking some diuretics.
   f. Trial of colchicine therapy.
2. Trauma. Acute injury to a joint may mimic pain, inflammation, and limitation of motion seen in SA. Differentiation is mostly by history.
3. Pseudogout.
4. Acute rheumatoid arthritis and other inflammatory arthritides.
5. Seronegative spondyloarthropathies.

Laboratory Findings

1. Leukocytosis will be seen in more than 50% of patients.
2. Gram stain of the joint aspirate will also be positive in more than 50% of patients. Gram staining is more successful with gram-positive SA than with gram-negative SA.
3. Culture and sensitivity of the joint aspirate is the method of definitive diagnosis. Recovery rates of organisms are fairly high. The exception to this rule is gonococcal (GC) arthritis. In many cases of GC, recovery of the organism from the joint fluid is very difficult. In cases of suspected GC arthritis, the fluid must be plated on special agar. Also, urethral and throat cultures may be helpful in establishing the diagnosis.
4. In cases where cultures are negative, polymerase chain reaction (PCR) has been helpful in identifying organism DNA.
5. Blood cultures can be positive in cases of hematogenous SA. These cultures will assist not only in diagnosing the SA but also in providing a clue to the presence of an occult distant infection that is seeding the joint.
6. Synovial fluid analysis yields yellow purulent fluid with high numbers of polymorphonuclear leukocytes in a range from 50,000 to 200,000 WBCs/ml. Neutrophils make up >90% of the

cells. There may be low synovial glucose levels and poor mucin clot formation.

Bacterial Etiology

The age of the patient is an important factor in determining likely bacterial causes of hematogenous disease.

1. In children less than 2 years, *H. influenzae* was the most common pathogen, but because of common vaccination practices, it is now rare. *S. aureus* and group B streptococcus are now the most frequent pathogens in this age group.
2. In children age 2 years through adolescence, *S. aureus* becomes a more frequent cause.
3. In young adults *Neisseria gonorrheae* is by far the most common cause of SA. In fact, if a sexually active patient presents with a history of transient, migratory polyarthralgias followed by severe monarticular joint pain, gonococcal SA should be the major differential.
4. In elderly patients, staphylococci and the gram-negative enteric bacteria become the most frequent pathogens. This is probably because of urinary tract infections that invade the bloodstream.
5. In addition to the general trends just listed, any bacteria may cause SA, especially in high-risk patients. These may include unusual organisms such as mycobacteria, which has been reported in patients undergoing intraarticular steroid injections.
6. Nonbacterial causes include various fungi and viruses.
7. Direct-extension SA is caused by organisms different from those found in the hematogenous form. The organism that causes direct-extension SA depends on the etiology of disease. For example, following a puncture wound, *P. aeruginosa* is seen; following a cat bite, *Pasteurella multocida* may be seen. Both of these specific diseases are covered in Chapter 4.
8. In patients living in a Lyme-endemic area or with a history of erythema migrans, *B. burgdorferi* must be suspected. This is covered in more detail in Chapter 2.

Treatment

1. Repeat aspiration of the joint effusions is one hallmark of treatment for SA. Only in gonococcal arthritis is this potentially less important.
2. Open surgical drainage of joints is usually reserved for refractory cases and those joints that are difficult to access with a

needle. Arthroscopic examination and drainage of a joint has become a preferred method when surgery is needed and in joints where it is possible.

3. Systemic antibiotics should be started empirically based on age and presentation of the case. The final decision about antibiotic administration is based on the culture results.

4. Because antibiotics concentrate in the joint, there is some evidence that even oral therapy may be adequate in some cases.

5. Intraarticular injection of antibiotic is unnecessary and may cause a reactive synovitis.

6. Ingress-egress saline flush has been used by some, although there are little data to support or discredit its use.

SUGGESTED READINGS

Cierny G, Mader JT, Penninck JJ: A clinical staging system for adult osteomyelitis, *Contemp Orthop* 10:17, 1985.

Grayson ML et al: Probing to bone in infected pedal ulcers. A clinical sign of underlying osteomyelitis in diabetic patients, *JAMA* Mar 1:273(9):721, 1995.

Kaleta JL, Fleischli JW, Reilly C: The diagnosis of osteomyelitis in diabetes using erythrocyte sedimentation rate: a pilot study, *J Am Podiatr Med Assoc* 91:445, 2001.

Mader JT, Calhoun J: Osteomyelitis. In Mandell GL, Bennett JE, Dolin R, editors: *Principles and practice of infectious diseases*, ed 5, p 1182, Philadelphia, 2000, Churchill Livingstone.

Simon WH, Joseph WS: Clinical imaging with indium 111 oxine-labeled leukocyte scan: review and case report, *Clin Podiatr Med Surg* 5:329, 1988.

Smith BR, Rolston KV, LeFrock JL et al: Bone penetration of antibiotics, *Orthopedics* 6:2, 1983.

Smith GP, Kjeldsberg CR: Cerebrospinal, synovial and serous body fluids. In Henry JB, editor: *Clinical diagnosis and management by laboratory methods*, ed 19, p 457, Philadelphia, 1996, WB Saunders.

Smith JW, Hasan MS: Infectious arthritis. In Mandell GL, Bennett JE, Dolin R, editors: *Principles and practice of infectious diseases*, ed 5, p 1175, Philadelphia, 2000, Churchill Livingstone.

Waldvogel FA, Medoff G, Swartz MN: Osteomyelitis: a review of clinical features, therapeutic considerations and unusual aspects, *N Engl J Med* 282:198, 260, 316, 1970.

Waldvogel FA, Vasey H: Osteomyelitis: the past decade, *N Engl J Med* 303:360, 1980.

CHAPTER 4

Infections Following Trauma

BASIC PRINCIPLES

The lower extremity is immunocompromised in comparison to other parts of the body, in part because of decreased delivery of neutrophils to the foot and leg. For this reason, when a trauma occurs to the lower extremity, care must be taken to avoid infectious complications.

Trauma alone can lead to infection because of many factors:

1. Trauma causes an immune deficit. All three arms of the immune system are affected:
   a. Cellular immunity is decreased.
   b. Humoral immunity is decreased.
   c. Phagocyte function is decreased.
2. The immune system effects are "dose related": the greater the trauma, the greater the deficit.
3. Trauma generally leads to breaks in the integument, which is the first line of host defense.
4. Bacteria are often inoculated into the wound at the time of injury. This contamination can lead to infection depending on the amount inoculated and the presence of other predisposing factors. Common bacteria found in various types of traumatic injury are listed in Table 4-1.
5. Along with bacteria, foreign substances, such as soil, can also be inoculated into the wound. These foreign substances can potentiate the development of infection.

TABLE **4-1**

*Common Organisms Found Following Trauma**

Traumatic Injury	Common Organisms
Puncture Wounds	
Cellulitis	*Staphylococcus aureas* (>50%)
	α-Hemolytic streptococci
	Staphylococcus epidermidis
	Escherichia coli/Proteus
Osteomyelitis	*Pseudomonas aeruginosa* (90%)
Bite Wounds	
Human	*S. aureus*
	Streptococcus
	Bacteroides fragilis
	Miscellaneous mouth anaerobes
	Eikenella corrodens
	Hepatits B†
	Treponema pallidum†
Dog	*S. aureus*
	S. epidermidis
	α-Hemolytic streptococci
	Pasteurella canis
	Capnocytophaga canimorsus (formerly DF-2)
	Anaerobes including fusobacterium, bacteroides, and porphyromonas
Cat	*S. aureus*
	α-Hemolytic streptococci
	Pasteurella multocida
	Anaerobes including fusobacterium, bacteroides, and porphyromonas
	Bartonella henselae in cat scratch disease
Burn Wound	
Early	β-Hemolytic streptococci
1 to 2 days	*S. aureus*
	S. epidermidis
Late	*P. aeruginosa*
>3 days	Enterobacteriaceae
Open Fractures	*S. aureus*
	S. epidermidis
	P. aeruginosa
	Streptococcus
	Enterobacteriaceae
	B. fragilis
	Miscellaneous anaerobes

*Lists are not in level of frequency because of the wide variation of different series.
†Relatively rare, included only as a point of interest.

6. Trauma can lead to devitalization of tissue. Necrotic tissue acts as a perfect medium in which bacteria can grow.

The presence of foreign bodies and devitalized tissue in a wound will potentiate infection. The most efficient way to remove this debris is through aggressive debridement. Debridement will also reduce the bacterial load in a wound. It has been shown that a large bacterial load will cause a clinical infection whereas a smaller one may not. Inoculum of at least 10^5 bacteria is the often-quoted "magic number" needed to cause an infection.

Debridement techniques are both surgical and mechanical.

■ *Surgical Debridement*

1. All devitalized tissue and foreign bodies should be removed.
2. Devitalized skin is easy to identify because adequate demarcation occurs fairly rapidly.
3. Devitalized muscle is less apparent. The decision to debride muscle should be based on whether it bleeds, its contractibility, and its appearance.
4. Multiple surgical debridements are usually required.
5. Dead space management is needed to prevent the collection of wound fluids that may harbor bacteria.

■ *Mechanical/Chemical Debridement*

In the presence of vital structures, or following surgical debridement, various mechanical methods of debridement can be used.

1. High-pressure irrigation can be used to dislodge bacteria and necrotic tissue from a wound. This can be accomplished by the use of a pulsatile flow device that delivers 60 psi to the wound. If this device is not available, a 30-ml syringe with a 19-gauge needle is an inexpensive alternative that will yield similar pressure.
2. Excessive pressure should be avoided to prevent tissue damage from the irrigation and the potential for implanting organisms deeper in the wound.
3. The value of the addition of antibiotics to the irrigation solution is controversial. Supporters point to its efficacy in reducing bacterial counts, as demonstrated by numerous studies. Detractors point to other studies that show no benefit to adding

antibiotics and mention potential toxicities. The bottom line appears to be that, although the mechanical effect of irrigation is still the most important, the addition of antibiotics does not seem to do any harm and may be of benefit.

4. Frequent dressing changes using gauze dressing materials have a mechanical debriding effect with each dressing removal. Wound fluids and debris become entangled in the dressing and are pulled off the wound with the gauze.

5. The "surgical scrub" of a wound with povidone-iodine detergent, hexachlorophene, or any other commercially available presaturated sponge brush will aid in mechanical debridement. Care must be taken in treating granulating wounds to prevent damage to delicate tissue. Also, although not generally true of other povidone-iodine preparations, the detergent scrub may have some deleterious effects on wound healing.

6. Occlusive wound dressings should be avoided in grossly contaminated wounds. Severe infections, such as necrotizing fasciitis, may develop in these wounds under occlusion.

7. Topical debriding agents provide mixed results. Enzymes are expensive and of questionable efficacy. Solutions such as sodium hypochlorite (Dakin solution) often work well, although they are disliked by wound care specialists. There is still no solution or enzyme preparation that works as well as "cold steel" or mechanical debridement when indicated.

8. A myriad of other topical agents and solutions have been advocated as working well in reducing the bacterial count of a wound. The list is endless and truly ranges from the sublime to the ridiculous. Reported compounds include silver sulfadiazine, povidone iodine, acetic acid, honey, sugar, sugar mixed with povidone iodine, insulin, urine, and blood. This list proves that when proper debridement techniques and exemplary wound-care methods are followed, the actual agent has little to do with the outcome.

■ *Closure*

The decision to close a wound must be based on clinical criteria. Although reduction of bacterial load is the hallmark of good debridement, the success of this reduction is difficult to assess. The reliance on "three negative cultures" as a signal that it is safe to close a wound has been propagated for decades without any hard data to support it. Fairly sophisticated techniques, such as quantitative bacteriology and quantitative Gram staining, have been proven helpful but are generally not available to most clinicians.

Clinical criteria for closing a wound include the following:

1. No frank signs or symptoms of residual infection. The surrounding tissue should not be red, hot, swollen, or painful.
2. No purulent drainage noted. Serous drainage is to be expected from any wound, however, and is not a contraindication to closure. Furthermore, the presence of a discolored dressing is not a contraindication, because serous fluid may react with the dressing material to form a greenish discoloration.
3. No foul odor from the wound.
4. A granular and clean appearance to the base of the wound.
5. If wound cultures are taken, the presence of a light growth of normal contaminants such as *Staphylococcus epidermidis* and diphtheroids is not a contraindication to closure.

PEDAL PUNCTURE WOUND INFECTIONS

Puncture wounds are one of the most common traumatic injuries to the foot. Fortunately, most heal uneventfully. In fact, most patients do not even seek medical assistance unless the wound is very severe or a complication occurs. The information on, and principles of treating these wounds has not changed significantly in more than 10 years. The basics remain the same.

■ *Statistical Data*

1. Most puncture wounds occur between May and October.
2. Stepping on a nail is by far the most common cause of the pedal puncture wound. Other common objects include glass, rocks, wire, and sewing needles.
3. Only about 10% of all puncture wounds develop complications. The most common complication is cellulitis with or without abscess formation.
4. Severe complications, including osteomyelitis, are actually rare, occurring in less than 1% of cases. They seem common to the physician because patients with severe complications are the ones who seek help.
5. The most common cause of these complications is inadequate primary care.

6. Risk factors for the development of osteomyelitis include a delay in initial evaluation and debridement, forefoot injuries, and the wearing of shoes at the time of injury.

■ *Primary Care*

As just stated, the most common cause of complications following a puncture wound is inadequate primary care. Usually the patient's foot receives a cursory examination and a superficial cleansing. This is followed by a prescription for a broad-spectrum oral antibiotic and a pair of crutches, and minimal, if any, follow-up.

When a patient presents with a pedal puncture wound, the following steps should be performed:

1. A thorough history must be taken. This should include information about:
   a. The causative object
   b. How deeply it penetrated
   c. If it was removed cleanly
   d. Where the injury occurred
   e. What shoe gear was being worn
2. If the patient is presenting for the first time a few days after injury, additional information is needed:
   a. When the injury occurred
   b. Whether any initial treatment was received
   c. What the patient did to the wound following injury
   d. Whether there has been any exacerbation of symptoms
3. Physical examination should concentrate on the location of the wound and the direction of the tract. It must be determined whether penetration to a bony structure was likely given the location.
4. If the patient is presenting a few days after injury, it should be determined whether there are any cardinal signs of infection.
5. Radiographs should be taken to rule out any retained foreign bodies that may be radiodense. They will also be a useful baseline study if osteomyelitis does occur.
6. The wound should be debrided of any debris or necrotic tissue. Local or regional anesthesia may be necessary.
7. The wound should be probed to determine the depth of the tract, the presence of any deep foreign body, and the possibility of contact with bone.
8. Aggressive cleansing should be performed followed by copious irrigation with sterile saline.

9. The wound should be kept open with packing or a drain.
10. The patient should be instructed to do the following:
    a. Keep off the foot as much as possible
    b. Elevate the foot
    c. Soak the foot twice each day in a solution of sterile water and povidone iodine
    d. Monitor oral temperature daily
    e. Monitor the progress of the wound
    f. Return for a follow-up visit after 1 week
11. Tetanus prophylaxis should be administered (see Table 4-2).
12. The use of prophylactic antibiotics is controversial. There is still little evidence that the use of oral prophylactic antibiotics decreases the incidence of infection following puncture wounds to the foot. Unfortunately, their use may be dictated by the medicolegal definition of "community standard."

■ *Clinical Presentation*

Patients who present with infection following a puncture wound show a remarkably consistent pattern of symptomatology.

1. The patient usually reports a marked improvement following the primary therapy. This is made evident by a decrease in pain with a resultant increase in ambulation.
2. Within a few days to a few weeks following this improvement, there is a sudden exacerbation of pain, swelling, and redness.
3. If the patient is given oral antibiotics, there is usually a rapid remission of symptoms.
4. In cases of superficial cellulitis without abscess formation, this minimal treatment may prove sufficient. This is rare, however, because these symptoms usually indicate a deeper process.
5. Once the patient finishes the course of antibiotic therapy, there is usually a quiescent stage of a few days' duration followed by a return of symptoms.
6. This cycle of remission and exacerbation is indicative of a deep infectious process that requires extensive treatment. Osteomyelitis must be strongly considered.

■ *Laboratory Findings*

1. The white blood cell count may or may not be elevated.

TABLE 4-2

Recommendations for the Use of Tetanus Prophylaxis

History of Tetanus toxoid administration	Clean, Minor Wound		Other Wounds	
	Tetanus toxoid vaccine	**Immunoglobulin**	**Tetanus toxoid vaccine**	**Immunoglobulin**
Unknown or less than three doses	Yes, and proceed with basic immunization	No	Yes, and proceed with basic immunization	Yes (250 U of human tetanus immonoglobulin)
More than three doses	No, unless >10 years since last dose	No	No, unless >5 years since last dose	No

From Wood MJ: Toxin mediated disorders: tetanus, botulism, and diphtheria. In Armstrong D, Cohen J: *Infectious diseases*, p 2.18.1, St Louis, 1999, Mosby.

2. The erythrocyte sedimentation rate is frequently elevated, although a normal value does not rule out osteomyelitis.
3. Because this is a local process, all other laboratory parameters may remain equivocal at best.
4. Plain-film radiographs will remain essentially normal, except for soft tissue edema, for 1 to 2 weeks, after which changes consistent with osteomyelitis may be seen.
5. Technetium bone scans can be useful to detect changes in early cases that plain-film radiography would be unable to pick up. Detection of post–puncture-wound osteomyelitis is actually one of the best indications for these studies of any lower extremity infection.
6. Magnetic resonance imaging (MRI) has been found to be a cost-effective modality for determining the early presence of post–puncture-wound osteomyelitis.
7. Sequential gallium and technetium studies may help differentiate a soft tissue process from an osteomyelitis.
8. Gram stain and superficial culture of the puncture tract will be useless in determining the etiologic agent. Deep tissues and bone specimens should be harvested.

■ *Bacterial Etiology*

If an infection does follow a puncture wound, the microbiology of that infection is unique and unusual.

1. In cases in which superficial cellulitis or abscess formation occurs, the most prevalent organisms are *Staphylococcus aureus* and streptococci.
2. Osteomyelitis following cases of pedal puncture wounds is overwhelmingly caused by *Pseudomonas aeruginosa*. This has been proven many times in multiple published studies.
3. The reason for the predominance of *P. aeruginosa* is not clear. Despite many theories, including the often-quoted "sneaker osteomyelitis" work, showing high incidence of pseudomonas in sneakers, no definitive reason has been found because the organism has even been found in patients with bare feet at the time of injury.
4. As with any infection, these are guidelines for empiric therapy only. Definitive culture results following good, deep, culture-harvesting techniques should be used to guide final therapy.

■ *Treatment*

The treatment of puncture wound infections is able to be determined by whether the infection is of the soft tissues or of bone.

Soft Tissue Infection

1. The puncture tract should be reopened and explored. Any retained foreign body should be removed and any necrosis debrided.
2. If an abscess is present, surgical incision and drainage must be performed.
3. The wound should be packed open to prevent premature closure.

Empiric oral antibiotic selection should include one of the following (Note: antipseudomonal coverage is generally not indicated in these soft tissue infections):

1. Amoxicillin/clavulanic acid, 500 or 875 mg bid with food
2. Clindamycin, 300 mg tid
3. Cephalexin, 500 mg bid-qid
4. Levofloxacin, 500 mg qd (will include some antipseudomonal activity)

Empiric parenteral antibiotic selection should include one of the following:

1. Cefazolin, 1 g q8h
2. Ampicillin/sulbactam, 3 g q6h
3. Piperacillin/tazobactam, 3.375g q6h or 4.5 g q8h (will include some antipseudomonal activity)
4. Clindamycin, 600 to 900 mg q8h

Osteomyelitis

1. Necrotic bone should be surgically debrided.
2. Any coexistent soft tissue abscess should be incised and drained.
3. Antibiotic therapy should be continued for 4 to 6 weeks following definitive debridement. This time can be shortened by total excision of the infected bone (e.g., removal of an entire infected phalanx).

Empiric antibiotic selection could include one of the following:

1. Cefepime, 2 g q12h IV
2. Ceftazidime, 2 g q12h IV
3. Ciprofloxacin, 750 mg q12h PO
4. Piperacillin/tazobactam, 3.375 g q6h or 4.5 g q8h with or without an oral quinolone

■ *Puncture Wound in a Marine Environment*

Puncture wounds can occur when a patient is walking in a body of water. These wounds differ markedly in their etiologic organisms from those previously discussed. *P. aeruginosa*, a water-dwelling organism, may be found in marine injuries, but more unusual bacteria may also be seen.

Aeromonas hydrophilia

As "hydrophilia" suggests, *Aeromonas* is a "water-loving" organism. This gram-negative bacillus is found predominately in freshwater streams, lakes, and wells. The clinical manifestations of an *Aeromonas* infection are similar to those of any other type of cellulitis. Antibiotics to which it is susceptible include quinolones, imipenem (although the organism has been known to produce a carbapenemase), trimethoprim/sulfamethoxazole, the aminoglycosides (amikacin in particular), and for some, third-generation cephalosporins and tetracycline.

Vibrio Species

Some of the vibrio species have been reported to cause severe necrotizing infections in unwary bathers and fishermen. This is truly an ancient disease. In fact, Hippocrates is thought to have described a case from the fifth century BC of a severe foot infection that progressed to death. These organisms are found mostly in brackish and salt water. The clinical picture is one of necrotizing fasciitis with potential resultant septicemia. Treatment consists of surgical incision, drainage, and debridement of necrotic tissue. Antibiotic sensitivities include tetracyclines as first-line therapy, ciprofloxacin, and potentially, third-generation cephalosporins.

Mycobacterium marinum

One of the atypical mycobacteria, *Mycobacterium marinum,* is found in freshwater lakes, swimming pools, and aquaria. The organism causes infection predominately on the extremities. The clinical picture is that of isolated bluish-purple nodules that suppurate and potentially ulcerate. Antibiotic therapy includes the combination of rifampin plus ethambutol. The duration of this therapy is controversial, but it may need to be longer than 1 year. Macrolides, in particular clarithromycin, are becoming the drug of choice for many of the atypical mycobacteria. Tetracyclines, in particular minocycline and amikacin, may also be effective. Surgical excision of the nodules may be required in refractory cases.

Stingray Envenomation

Stingray spines contain a toxin that can cause a painful envenomation, although it is not a true infection. The clinical presentation includes severe local pain with swelling and ecchymosis. Because this is not an infection, antibiotic therapy is not useful. The toxin is heat labile, and immersion of the affected limb in hot water for 30 to 60 minutes is the suggested therapy.

BITE WOUND INFECTIONS

Dog bites are one of the most common causes of nonfatal injury in the United States with an estimated 5 million per year. Young males are the most frequently bitten group, with the average age being around 15 years old. The lower extremity is one of the most common sites for all animal bites. These wounds are not only common but also have significant infectious morbidity. Human bites, although less common in the lower extremity, are potentially even more dangerous. The potential for a bite to become infected is based on a number of variables:

1. The type of animal. Cat bites are more likely to become infected than dog bites because they are more commonly deep punctures. Human bites have the highest incidence of infection, although they are less frequent on the lower extremity.
2. The bacterial flora of the mouth. It is true that the human mouth is "dirtier" than an animal's.
3. The location of the wound. Bites of the extremities are more likely to become infected than if they occur in other locations. If near a joint or bone, the possibility of direct-inoculation septic arthritis and osteomyelitis must be considered.

4. The general medical condition of the patient, including the presence of diabetes, splenectomy, chronic alcohol usage, or other immunocompromising conditions.
5. The type of injury:
   a. Puncture, most common with cats, and the most dangerous.
   b. Tear.
   c. Crush.
   d. Scratch.
6. Delay in treatment for more than 12 hours on the extremities.

■ Clinical Presentation

1. Onset of localized cellulitis is rapid. This may occur as soon as 12 hours following the injury.
2. A local abscess with purulent drainage forms.
3. Systemic involvement, including fever, chills, and malaise, occurs infrequently, but may be seen in cases that present late.
4. Painful motion will be seen in cases following tooth puncture near a joint. Other signs of septic arthritis may also be noted.
5. Significant soft tissue damage and devitalized tissue are seen, especially with dog bites. Some dogs may exert up to 2000 psi of pressure on tissue.

■ Laboratory Findings

1. Because the infection is primarily a local condition, blood studies may prove noncontributory. If systemic involvement is suspected, the usual parameters for infection will be seen.
2. Gram stain of purulence will most likely reveal multiple organisms, both gram-positive and gram-negative.

■ Bacterial Etiology

A wide array of mixed aerobic and anaerobic bacterial flora are seen in bite wounds. Most of these organisms represent normal bacterial flora of the mouth. Recent studies show that the most common include *Pasteurella* species for both cats and dogs. Other common aerobes include streptococci and staphylococci. Common anaerobes include porphyromonas, fusobacterium, and bacteroides.

Although not truly a "bite wound," the previously named "cat scratch agent" is now formally known as *Bartonella henselae*. For a list of a few of the most common organisms found with each animal, see Table 4-1.

■ *Treatment*

1. A careful history should include when the bite occurred and the behavior of the animal before the attack. Most dog attacks occur by animals known to the victim, so observation of behavior is possible. Rabies vaccination is administered as indicated.
2. Tetanus prophylaxis should be administered according to the guidelines listed in Table 4-2.
3. Drainage of any purulence and debridement of necrotic wound edges should be performed. Cultures should be taken of the drainage and/or the wound. Debridement may be facilitated by cleansing the wound with a surgical scrub.
4. Copious irrigation of the wound with saline or saline with povidone iodine is performed.
5. The value of primary closure of a clinically noninfected open wound is controversial (of course, clinically infected wounds should be left open). In the head and neck it is somewhat routine. In the lower extremity, with its decreased neutrophil delivery and relative immune compromise, it may not be advisable especially in wounds more than 12 hours old. No clear-cut studies exist to address this question.
6. In cases in which the possibility for bone or joint involvement exists, baseline radiographs should be taken.
7. In patients presenting without established infection, the use of "prophylactic" antibiotics is controversial. However, because of the high bacterial inoculum and the potential for devastating infections, antibiotic therapy should probably be initiated. As with all prophylactic antibiotics, the selection is directed against common pathogens. Potentially useful oral antibiotics for this purpose include:
   a. Any of the beta-lactamase inhibitor compounds are considered drugs of first choice, including amoxicillin/clavulanic acid (oral), piperacillin/tazobactam, ticarcillin/clavulanic acid, or ampicillin/sulbactam (parenteral).
   b. Levofloxacin or one of the other newer generation quinolones, (i.e., moxifloxacin).

c. Azithromycin, strictly as an alternative.
d. Cefuroxime axetil or other later-generation cephalosporins, also as alternatives.

BURN WOUND INFECTIONS

Skin, the largest organ in the human body, has a number of important functions, not the least of which is to act as a barrier to prevent invasion by bacteria. When this layer of protection is destroyed, as occurs in a burn, there is a tremendous potential to develop systemic infection.

Systemic sepsis is the most devastating result of a burn wound. It is the leading cause of death in patients hospitalized with these injuries. The source of the sepsis is not just the local area of destroyed skin; pulmonary infections, urinary tract infections, and endocarditis can all result from burn wounds.

Along with destruction of the skin, another reason for this increased incidence of infection is the effect a burn has on the patient's immune system. As in other types of trauma, this effect is dose related. All three immune components are affected:

1. The phagocyte system: neutrophil chemotaxis and bactericidal activity is decreased.
2. The humoral system: the amount of circulating immunoglobulins immediately after a burn is markedly decreased.
3. The cellular system: diminished lymphocyte function has been observed.

A host of other factors contribute to the tendency of these wounds to become infected. A partial list of these includes weeping of protein-rich exudate, the presence of necrotic tissue in the eschar, and the lack of local blood supply.

■ *Clinical Presentation*

It is not within the scope of this chapter to discuss "normal" burn wounds or the alterations in homeostatic mechanisms that occur following a burn. However, to understand the pathophysiology of infections, a brief review is necessary. Burns are generally classified into three "degrees," depending on their clinical appearance.

1. First-degree burns: these are superficial, partial-thickness injuries. There is usually some erythema without blister formation.
2. Second-degree burns: these deeper burns are still considered only partial thickness. They can be further divided into deep and superficial second-degree injuries.
   a. Superficial burns are erythematous with some blister formation and are usually painful.
   b. Deep burns are usually dry. Blisters may be absent. They are frequently painless.
3. Third-degree burns: these are deep, full-thickness injuries involving skin and subcutaneous tissue. They are usually painless because of the destruction of cutaneous nerves. These are the type of burns that will most commonly present infectious complications.

Clinical signs that a burn wound may be becoming infected include the following:

1. Appearance of cellulitis in surrounding tissue.
2. Discoloration of the wound. This may range from marked darkening to the appearance of a green hue, which is indicative of *Pseudomonas* infection.
3. Spreading of necrosis into adjacent partial-thickness areas.
4. Liquefaction of the eschar.

■ *Laboratory Findings*

1. Full-thickness biopsy of the burn has been recommended as the definitive diagnosis for burn wound sepsis. These biopsies are graded depending on the extent of bacterial invasion into viable tissue.
2. Quantitative bacteriology of a biopsy specimen has also been used to define the presence of burn wound infection. A bacterial count of more than 10^5 cfu of organisms is consistent with clinical infection.
3. Swab cultures are usually discouraged because they capture such a small area. The use of larger area "contact plates" or petri dishes applied to the burn has been advocated.

■ *Bacterial Etiology*

1. Shortly after the burn, the wound is transiently sterile because the intense heat kills all surface bacteria.
2. Within 1 to 2 days, the streptococci and staphylococci harbored in the depth of the skin appendages become the major pathogens. Serious infection with these organisms is usually avoided by aggressive initial therapy with systemic and topical antibiotics. However, methicillin-resistant strains of staphylococcus are being seen more often at initial presentation.
3. Following initial treatment directed against the above organisms just mentioned, opportunistic infection with nosocomial, multi-resistant, gram-negative rods becomes a problem. The most notorious of these is *P. aeruginosa*, although any organism found in the hospital may invade. The source of this contamination is either endogenous, from the patient, or environmental.

■ *Treatment*

1. Prevention of burn wound infection is critically important. Many burn centers have gone to single bedrooms to avoid cross-contamination. Hubbard tanks have given way to bedside treatments. All contact with the patient is performed under wound contact precautions including gloves, gowns, and masks.
2. Much of the emphasis in the treatment of burn wounds has shifted toward the necessity to achieve rapid and complete burn wound closure to prevent infection. The use of aggressive surgical debridement and immediate closure, if possible, or the application of skin grafting at the earliest opportunity is now advocated.
3. It may be assumed that all deep burn wounds are heavily contaminated with organisms; thus initial treatment should be directed at lowering the bacterial load.
4. Debridement of necrotic tissue should be performed to promote increased local blood flow and remove the nidus for bacterial proliferation.
5. The application of topical antibacterial agents has become the cornerstone of burn wound treatment. This has two major benefits:
   a. It reduces the bacterial load already on the wound.
   b. It acts as prophylaxis to prevent further invasion.
6. The three most commonly used agents are mafenide acetate, silver sulfadiazine, and silver nitrate solution. Mupirocin

ointment has also been used effectively especially with gram-positive infections, including MRSA. All of these have advantages and disadvantages (Table 4-3).

7. The preferred method of topical treatment for burns, especially inpatient, is the "open method," where the topical is applied directly to the wound with no overlying dressings. This allows more access to the wound for treatment and observation. The "closed method" where an outer dressing is applied over the wound is more frequently used on an outpatient basis.

8. Culture results should be monitored regularly for changes in flora and the development of resistance.

9. Once an in vitro spectrum of antibacterial activity deep-seated infection is identified, aggressive systemic antibiotic therapy should be initiated and directed toward the isolated pathogens. This therapy should begin at the earliest signs of invasive infection, because burn-wound sepsis can have significant associated mortality if it is left unchecked.

OPEN FRACTURE INFECTIONS

One of the most important aspects of the treatment of open fractures is the prevention of wound infection and subsequent osteomyelitis. Depending on how and when the injury occurred, these fractures tend to be highly contaminated with bacteria. The goal of treatment is to reduce that contamination and prevent the infection. This goal is usually accomplished by the following:

1. Aggressive debridement
2. Antibiotic usage
3. Fixation

Because debridement techniques have been examined earlier in this chapter, this discussion will concentrate on the latter two regimens.

■ *Antibiotics*

It should be noted that the word *prophylaxis* was not just used. Because these wounds are so highly contaminated with bacteria,

TABLE 4-3

Effective Topical Chemotherapeutic Agents for Burn Wound Care

	Mafenide Acetate Burn Cream	Silver Sulfadiazine Burn Cream	Silver Nitrate Soaks	Mupirocin Ointment/Cream
Active component concentration	11.1%	1.0%	0.5%	2%
In vitro spectrum of antibacterial activity	Gram-negative—good Gram-positive—fair Yeast—minimal	Gram-negative-selectivity—good Gram-positive—good Yeast—good	Gram-negative—good Gram-positive—good Yeast—good	Gram-negative—fair, except poor against *Pseudomonas aeruginosa* Gram-positive—excellent, includes methicillin-resistant *Staphylococcus aureus*
Method of wound care	Open method	Open method or light closed method	Occlusive closed method	Occlusive closed method
Advantages	Penetrates eschar Wound appearance readily monitored Easily applied Joint motion unrestricted	Painless Wound appearance readily monitored when exposure method used	Painless No hypersensitivity reactions No gram-negative resistance	Excellent gram-positive activity Eschar penetration Novel structure Promotes cell growth?

No gram-negative resistance	Easily applied; joint motion unrestricted when exposure method used Greater effectiveness against yeasts Combine with mystatin for better yeast coverage	Closed methods reduce evaporative heat loss Greater effectiveness against yeasts	
Disadvantages Painful on partial-thickness burns Acidosis due to inhibition of carbonic anhydrase Hypersensitivity reactions in 7% of patients Gram-positive resistance developing	Possible neutropenia (batch-related) Hypersensitivity (infrequent) Limited eschar penetration Resistance of certain gram-negative bacteria Selection of plasmid-mediated multiple antibiotic resistance	Deficits of sodium, potassium, and calcium No eschar penetration Limitation of joint motion by closed method Methemoglobimemia (rare) Argyria (rare) Staining of environment and equipment	Few good studies Relatively expensive Polyethylene glycol base in ointment only Limited to smaller-area burns

Adapted from Pruitt, 1987, with permission.

this term is probably inappropriate. Instead, the use of antibiotics in these cases should be labeled *therapy*.

There is little hard proof that type I open fractures need to be treated with antibiotics. The infection rate appears similar with or without their usage.

The evidence is fairly convincing that types II and III open fractures should be treated with antibiotics, although even this convention has its detractors. Some, especially in Europe, believe that appropriate intraoperative antisepsis, debridement, and fixation are all that is needed.

1. The antibiotic should be effective against *S. aureus*, the most common pathogen. Gram-negative organisms have been reported as more of a problem, especially in type III fractures.
2. Extra coverage should be based on organisms isolated from cultures taken before the initial debridement.
3. Duration of treatment is from 3 to 7 days. This too is controversial. Some authors believe that only shorter periods are acceptable, whereas others will treat for a full 6 weeks or until the wound is closed.
4. The most commonly employed agent is cefazolin. This drug has a relatively long half-life, good staphylococcal activity, and will also work against some gram-negative organisms.
5. The work by Gustilo and Anderson in1976 (see Suggested Readings) discussed the need for increased gram-negative coverage, particularly for type III fractures. In their study they used cefazolin in combination with an aminoglycoside to cover the gram-negative organisms. Unfortunately, despite incredible advances in anti–gram-negative antibiotics over the past 25 years or more, many authors continue to parrot the requirement for the addition of an aminoglycoside. There is little to no evidence that a safer, just as effective class of drug (i.e., newer quinolones or extended spectrum cephalosporins) could not be used as a single-agent drug.
6. In centers with a high incidence of methicillin-resistant *S. aureus* infections, vancomycin can be substituted.

■ *Fixation*

Considered the standard care for treatment of a fracture, the use of fixation to add stability to the bone may also decrease the incidence of infection. The technique for this fixation is somewhat controversial. Supporters of rigid internal fixation suggest that, when performed properly, the insertion of these devices, even into highly contaminated areas, will decrease the incidence of osteomyelitis. Supporters of external fixation are wary about introducing what they view as a foreign body into a contaminated area. Because both sides have extensive experience and studies to back their respective opinions, the only conclusion to be drawn is that some form of rigid fixation is useful in decreasing infectious morbidity in open fractures.

SUGGESTED READINGS

Abrahamian FM: Dog bites: bacteriology, management and prevention, *Curr Infect Dis Rep* 2:446, 2000.

Baethage BA, West BC: *Vibrio vulnificus*: did Hippocrates describe a fatal case? *Rev Infect Dis* 10:614, 1988.

Barillo DJ, McManus AT: Infections in burn patients. In Armstong D, Cohen J, editors: *Infectious diseases,* p. 3.8.1, St Louis, 1999, Mosby.

Curreri PW: Burns. In Howard RJ, Simmons RL, editors: *Surgical infectious diseases,* ed 2, p. 873, East Norwalk, Conn, 1988, Appleton & Lange.

Fitzgerald R, Cowan J: Puncture wounds of the foot, *Orthop Clin* 6:965, 1975.

Goldstein EJC: Bites. In Mandell GL, Bennett JE, Dolin R, editors: *Principles and practice of infectious diseases,* ed 5, p 3202, Philadelphia, 2000, Churchill Livingstone.

Gustilo RB, Anderson JT: Prevention of infection in the treatment of one thousand and twenty five open fractures of long bones, *J Bone Joint Surg* 58A:453, 1976.

Joseph WS, LeFrock JL: Infections following puncture wounds of the foot, *J Foot Surg* 26:S30, 1987.

Joseph WS: Infections following lower extremity trauma. In Scurran B, editor: *Foot and ankle trauma,* ed 2, p 805, New York, 1996, Churchill Livingstone.

Lavery LA, Harkless LB, Ashry HR et al: Infected puncture wounds in adults with diabetes: risk factors for osteomyelitis, *J Foot Ankle Surg* 33(6):561, 1994.

Rode H, Hanslo D, DeWet PM: Efficacy of mupirocin in methacillin-resistant *Staphylococcus aureus* burn wound infections, *Antimicrob Agents Chemother* 33:1358, 1989.

Talan DA, Citron DM, Abrahamian FM et al: Bacteriologic analysis of infected dog and cat bites, *N Engl J Med* 340:85, 1999.

Wood MJ: Toxin mediated disorders: tetanus, botulism, and diphtheria. In Armstrong D, Cohen J: *Infectious diseases,* p 2.18.1, St Louis, 1999, Mosby.

CHAPTER 5

Diabetic Foot Infections

Patients with diabetes mellitus may develop infections of the foot. These infections are usually a result of an ulceration or other complications of sensory neuropathy, such as undetected trauma. Infections in patients with diabetes can progresses quickly. Despite the best of care, a simple, clean, superficial, noninfected ulceration may become a major infection, literally overnight. This does not mean that the clinician should go overboard using inappropriate culturing or nonindicated antibiotics. Good local wound care and proper off-loading are the keys to managing these lesions. Once an infection becomes established, then the treatment approach should be carefully determined and appropriately carried out. The statistics are sobering.

■ *Statistical Data*

1. The American Diabetes Association estimates that 16 million people in the United States have diabetes mellitus and at least 5 million of them are unaware of it.
2. Lower extremity complications have become the leading cause of hospitalization in patients with diabetes.
3. It is estimated that more than 80,000 nontraumatic lower extremity amputations occur each year as a result of diabetes.
4. Despite advances in the knowledge of the disease process and how to manage it, the number of amputations continues to rise.

5. Ulceration is the most common risk factor for amputation, occurring in almost 85% of the patients who undergo an amputation.
6. A patient with diabetes has a 15% to 20% lifetime risk of developing an ulceration.
7. The 5-year survival rate following a single leg amputation is only about 50%. Patients with one limb amputated have a greater than 50% chance of having the second limb amputated within 5 years. The 5-year survival rate for a bilateral amputee with diabetes is probably in the single digits.

PATHOGENESIS

The pathogenesis of the diabetic foot infection is related to an "unholy triad" of factors: neuropathy, angiopathy, and immunopathy.

■ Neuropathy

Probably the most important factor in the increased prevalence of infection is the presence of diabetic polyneuropathy. Depending on the study, more than 40% of patients with either type I or type II diabetes may develop clinically significant distal neuropathy. The etiology of this neuropathy appears to be multifactorial, including ischemic, metabolic (polyol pathway), and autoimmune components. With any of these, however, the common denominator appears to be hyperglycemia. The Diabetes Control and Complications Trial has shown that early aggressive control of hyperglycemia can significantly reduce the neurologic complications. Some early signs and symptoms may even be reversed.

With hyperglycemia the following may occur:

1. Nerve ischemia
2. Glycosylation of nerve protein
3. Decrease uptake of nerve myoinositol
4. Decreased activity of the sodium-potassium adenosine triphosphatase (ATPase) pump
5. Reduction in axonal transport

Diabetic neuropathy is frequently broken down into three categories, each with distinctive clinical features.

Sensory Neuropathy

Sensory neuropathy can manifest with either significant pain or loss of sensation. Although the painful neuropathy is of major clinical significance in the management of these patients, from an infectious disease standpoint, the lack of sensation is probably more important.

Sensory neuropathy may present with the following:

1. Decreased sharp-dull discrimination
2. Decreased vibratory sensation
3. Decreased proprioception
4. Decreased two-point discrimination
5. Decreased deep tendon reflexes
6. Stocking-glove distribution

Motor Neuropathy

Symptoms of motor neuropathy include the following:

1. Intrinsic muscle wasting
2. Imbalance of long and short flexors
3. Dorsal dislocation of toes, resulting in:
   a. Claw toe deformity
   b. Retrograde pressure on metatarsal heads
   c. Dorsal dislocation of fat pad
   d. "Pseudo-cavus" appearance

Autonomic Neuropathy

Symptoms of autonomic neuropathy include the following:

1. Impaired sweating
2. Xerosis of skin leading to fissuring and cracking
3. Sympathetic failure, which involves:
   a. Vasodilation
   b. Arteriovenous shunting on the plantar aspect leading to decreased perfusion into the nutrient capillaries in the skin
   c. Edema

Clinical Significance

1. These three types of neuropathy, when combined, lead to excessive stresses on tissue, formation of mechanical keratosis, and undetected tissue breakdown.

2. Once the skin barrier is breached, organisms can invade deeper tissues and become pathogenic. Whether an infection ensues, however, is not a *fait accompli*. Many patients can have open ulcerations for months or years without becoming clinically infected.

3. If an infection does occur, the patient, unable to feel pain, allows it to progress unchecked. Massive local or systemic involvement may result.

4. A unique syndrome that results from the presence of neuropathy is diabetic neuroarthropathy, or Charcot joint. The etiology of Charcot joint is multifactorial. There are biochemical changes that occur in the cartilage secondary to neuropathy. Furthermore, the lack of proprioception in the joints could lead to undetected stresses that have been postulated to cause microtrauma to the area. Although not an infectious condition by itself, Charcot joint can cause abnormal weight bearing, leading to tissue breakdown and subsequent infection. Furthermore, the osseous changes can mimic those of osteomyelitis. Differentiation of these two conditions is extremely difficult. The clinical presentation can be similar. Clinically speaking, if bone changes are seen and there are no open ulcerations or other portals of bacterial entry, Charcot is a more likely diagnosis than osteomyelitis. However, this does *not* imply that bone changes, even in the presence of a portal of entry, are necessarily secondary to osteomyelitis. Charcot can occur in these cases either without any bacterial invasion into the bone or with superimposed bone infection. Diagnostically, standard radiographic and nuclide studies may or may not be helpful. Labeled white cell scans such as the HMPAO scan may prove more specific for infection than traditional technetium bone scans. Magnetic resonance imaging (MRI) may also be helpful, but false positives do occur. Deep bone biopsy and culture, although invasive, might be the only true diagnostic modality.

■ *Immunopathy*

There is general agreement that prolonged periods of hyperglycemia lead to impairment of immune function. The humoral immune system is relatively spared. In fact, these patients may have increased levels of circulating immunoglobulins. The deficit is most likely in the phagocyte system and appears to be secondary to a decrease of superoxide ion production. Again, as with neuropathy, there is a direct correlation between immunopathy and glucose control. The immunopathy consists of the following:

1. A decrease in chemotaxis to the site of infection
2. A decrease in phagocytosis, which may be the primary deficit
3. Decreased intracellular killing of microorganisms
4. Any combination of the above three

Clinical Significance
Immune system dysfunction directly affects the treatment of these patients in three ways:

1. Glucose should be optimally controlled. Patients with relatively controlled diabetes may not exhibit evidence of immunopathy. They should not be considered immune deficient just because there has been a diagnosis of diabetes.
2. Once an infection is established, antibiotic selection should include drugs that are bactericidal in patients believed to be immune deficient. Bacteriostatic agents require an intact immune system to clear the organisms.
3. Because diabetics may be more prone to infection as a result of this immunopathy (including urinary tract and respiratory tract infection), they are administered frequent courses of antibiotics. This leads to colonization with resistant species of organisms.

■ *Angiopathy*

Arterial occlusive disease in individuals with diabetes differs markedly from that found in the nondiabetic population. In diabetes the occlusive disease is characterized by the following:

1. It is more widespread and multisegmental.
2. It occurs at an earlier age.
3. It is more frequent.
4. It progresses to more advanced stages.
5. It presents with more distal involvement.
6. It presents with more gangrene.
7. It tends to be bilateral.
8. It affects men and women equally.

Classically, the angiopathy of diabetes has been classified as microvascular, or small-vessel disease, or macrovascular, or large-vessel disease. There has been much controversy as to the presence and definitions of these two entities; however, it is beyond the scope of this review to clarify the points made by each camp. There does seem to be agreement on the following points:

1. There is increased thickening of the capillary basement membranes in some locations.
2. There does not appear to be any evidence of small-vessel occlusive disease.
3. There is increased blood viscosity.
4. Cell aging appears to be more rapid.
5. There is increased platelet aggregation.

These five points, in conjunction with the phagocyte defect, further decrease chemotaxis to the site of an infection.

Clinical Significance
1. Increased prevalence of gangrene will necessitate more frequent amputation.
2. Gangrenous tissue is a perfect breeding ground for bacteria, including anaerobes.
3. Decreased perfusion of tissue theoretically leads to decreased local antibiotic concentration. The true clinical implication of this has not been shown.

■ *Other Diabetic Changes*

Diabetes is a multisystem disease. Along with the systemic changes previously discussed, many other changes are found in the patient with diabetes. Complications in these other systems to varying degrees will also affect the etiology, diagnosis, and treatment of a lower extremity infection.

Visual Changes
Because of poor vision, the patient may not see early changes in the foot, allowing these problems to progress to serious infection. Once diagnosed as infected, the patient may not be able to perform proper care to the wound, including cleansing and dressing changes.

Joint Changes

Because of glycosylation of collagen, limitation of joint mobility frequently has been described in patients with diabetes. This may lead to structural abnormalities, excessive pressure points, and ulcerations. Again, hyperglycemia appears to be the major culprit.

Renal Changes

Some degree of impaired renal function is found in almost any patient with long-standing diabetes. Because most antibiotics are at least partially handled by the kidney, massive dosing alterations may be needed in these patients. Furthermore, the use of potentially nephrotoxic agents, such as the aminoglycosides, should be avoided.

Skin Changes

The skin of patients with diabetes differs from that of patients without the disease. Diabetic skin is more rigid and less pliable. It is not unlike skin in elderly patients. This is due to excessive collagen cross-linking. Diabetic skin also becomes hyperkeratotic more easily. Furthermore, as previously discussed, autonomic neuropathy may lead to arteriovenous shunting in the plantar skin, limiting perfusion to this tissue. These factors predispose the skin to tissue breakdown.

UNIQUE MICROBIOLOGY

For many years the microbiology of diabetic foot infections was assumed to be similar to that found in most any soft tissue infection. Gram-positive organisms predominated, with an occasional enteric gram-negative infection attributed to "fecal fallout." With the advent of new, more sophisticated laboratory techniques, this disease was seen in a new light. Not only were more organisms being isolated in each case, but also a great number of obligate anaerobes were being seen. Current thinking has now divided the condition of "diabetic foot infection" into at least two forms when it comes to microbiology. There are the mild or less severe diabetic infections that still have primarily gram-positive bacteria as their pathogenic flora. Where the really unique microbiology comes to play is in the more severe, limb-threatening infections. These cases are truly polymicrobial in nature, with an average of four organisms per patient commonly found. Furthermore, in these cases anaerobic bacteria are considered a major organism in terms of both numbers and pathogenicity for several reasons:

1. Ischemic and necrotic tissue, commonly found in these severe infections, by definition, have a lower oxygenation potential (eH), thereby supporting the growth of anaerobes.
2. Abscesses, frequently seen in these infections, have a lower eH.
3. Diabetic immunopathy supports the growth of facultative anaerobes. These organisms utilize any oxygen present to further decrease the eH and allow obligate anaerobes to grow.

■ *Clinical Evidence of the Presence of Anaerobes*

The presence of anaerobic bacteria can often be detected before the return of culture reports. In fact, because obligate anaerobes are difficult to isolate, the presence of these organisms is sometimes never confirmed by the microbiology laboratory. Therefore the following clinical hints will lead to the empiric diagnosis of anaerobic infection:

1. Foul odor (fetid foot)
2. The presence of necrotic tissue
3. Polymicrobial Gram stain with only one or two organisms isolated on culture
4. Gas in the tissues

■ *Tissue Gas*

It should be noted that gas in soft tissues is *not* diagnostic of the presence of *Clostridium perfringens*. It is not even diagnostic of the presence of anaerobes. The following are all potential causes of tissue gas:

1. Gram-positive anaerobes
2. Gram-negative anaerobes
3. Gram-positive aerobes
4. Facultative gram-negative organisms
5. Trauma and surgery
6. Hydrogen peroxide irrigation

■ *Common Organisms Isolated in Diabetic Foot Infections*

The specific organisms found in these infections will differ not only from patient to patient and hospital to hospital, but also from one part of the country to another. Furthermore, the severity and exact location of the infection will determine which organisms are found. For this reason, the following organisms are listed in relative importance, loosely based on a compilation of many studies of varying location and times.

Aerobes
1. *Staphylococcus aureus*
2. *Streptococcus agalactiae* (group B streptococcus)
3. Coagulase-negative staphylococci
4. *Streptococcus pyogenes* (group A streptococcus)
5. *Enterococcus*
6. *Proteus mirabilis*
7. Enterobacter, Citrobacter, Serratia group

Anaerobes
1. *Bacteroides fragilis*
2. *Bacteroides spp.*
3. *Peptococcus*
4. *Peptostreptococcus*
5. *Fusobacterium*

The first two organisms listed (*S. aureus* and group B streptococcus) are by far the most commonly found organisms in any foot infection in patients with diabetes. They are both practically ubiquitous in this disease. It should be noted that many organisms are not listed. This does not mean that they are not found or are not important. They are just found less commonly. *Any* organism can be found in the diabetic foot infection.

There are two deliberate omissions to the previous list. The omission of *Pseudomonas aeruginosa* is deliberate yet controversial. Many studies have isolated this organism from ulcerations and infections. However, it is questionable whether this isolation represents a primary pathogen in these infections or just a contaminant. Frequently, when a good, reliable, deep specimen is taken, this organism is not found. The omission of *C. perfringens* is more straightforward. Although when found, it is found most frequently in diabetic patients and is not a common isolate even in the presence of soft tissue gas (see above).

B. fragilis, along with other members of the *Bacteroides* group, has been consistently isolated as probably the most common organisms found in severely infected diabetic feet. These organisms have some interesting traits related to their pathogenicity that dictate the need to address them therapeutically:

1. They are resistant to many antibiotics. Although many anaerobes can be treated with penicillin, *Bacteroides* cannot. In fact, a multicenter, international susceptibility survey of the *Bacteroides* is performed and published on a regular basis in the microbiology and infectious diseases literature to keep everyone aware of emerging patterns of resistance.
2. *Bacteroides* can cause a synergistic infection in conjunction with other bacteria.
3. *Bacteroides* has the ability to form a glycocalyx, or slime layer, that increases its pathogenicity and resistance to therapy.

ULCERATION

Since ulceration is the leading risk factor for infection in patients with diabetes, it warrants its own section.

■ *Classification*

Depth and Severity Classification

Many attempts have been made to classify ulcerations in patients with diabetes. Classification allows all clinicians to have a similar basis for which to clinically describe, document, and treat these patients. Furthermore, classification allows facilitation of communications between treating practitioner and clinical investigators. It puts everybody on the "same page." Unfortunately, despite the recognized desire to accept one universal system, this has not been accomplished. Since the mid-1970s, the Wagner system has been the most commonly used. This system consisting of six "grades" of ulcers primarily describes the depth of the lesion (grades 0 to 4) or the extent of tissue destruction (grades 5 to 6). The primary drawback to this system is that co-morbidities such as infection or ischemia are not included. More recently, the University of Texas at San Antonio has proposed a system, which has since been clinically validated. It simplifies the Wagner system and includes the aforementioned co-morbidities (Box 5-1).

Regardless of which system the clinician uses, some general suggestions apply.

1. The use of a classification system is *not* required. It is optional but may be helpful especially in a group practice where more than one practitioner may see the patient.
2. If a system is to be used in documentation, it is important to detail *which* system is being used (e.g., "The patient presents

---

BOX **5-1**

UTSA Classification

Grade O No open lesions; may have deformity
A. without infection or ischemia
B. with infection
C. with ischemia
D. with infection and ischemia

Grade 1 Superficial Wound not involving tendon, capsule or bone
A. without infection or ischemia
B. with infection
C. with ischemia
D. with infection and ischemia

Grade 2 Wound Penetrating to tendon or capsule
A. without infection or ischemia
B. with infection
C. with ischemia
D. with infection and ischemia

Grade 3 Wound Penetrating to bone or joint
A. without infection or ischemia
B. with infection
C. with ischemia
D. with infection and ischemia

Adapted from Armstong DG et al: Validation of a diabetic wound classification system: the contribution of depth infection and ischemia to risk of amputation, *Diabetes Care* 21:855-859, 1998.

with a Wagner grade 1" or "The patient presents with a UT grade 2C"). Just documenting that "the patient has a grade 2 ulceration" can leave the note open to interpretation.
3. Note the size of the individual lesion, preferably in at least two dimensions if feasible. Three may be ideal but is seldom done.

Infection Classification

Despite all the excellent efforts that have been made to standardize the classification of the clinical size and severity of the mal perforans, none of the systems are specific for infection. Many will mention infection as a co-morbid factor or a complication and pay lip service to treatment with such comments as "use a broad-spectrum antibiotic." This does not do the topic justice. The approach to an ulceration is going to be different depending on whether it is even infected, how seriously it is infected, and what organisms can be expected. Once this is determined, suggestions can be listed for antibiotic therapy along with any adjunctive treatments. Only a few attempts have been made at classifying the infectious process in these patients. None are widely accepted at this point. As this is written, The Infectious Diseases Society of America guidelines committee on foot infections in diabetes is working on the problem.

For the purpose of this discussion, almost all infection classifications group ulcerations into three general categories:

1. Noninfected ulcerations
2. Mildly infected ulcerations
3. Moderate to severely infected (limb- and life-threatening) ulcerations

■ *Noninfected Mal Perforans Ulcerations*

Probably the most important question is, "What constitutes an infected ulceration versus one that is merely contaminated with bacteria?" The ubiquitous swab culture of any ulcer will most likely grow bacteria. Ulcers are perfect media to support bacterial growth. Does this positive culture mean that there is an infection? Do antibiotics have to be prescribed? Most assuredly the answer is *no*. Therapy is needed only when there are clinical signs and symptoms to support the diagnosis of an infection in conjunction with the ulceration.

There are some general rules of thumb, many of which have already been discussed in Chapter 1 but bear restating when dealing specifically with ulcers.

1. Cultures do not diagnose infection; they allow determination of what organism is causing the clinically diagnosed infection.
2. An ulceration need not be cultured if there are no clinical signs and symptoms of infection.
3. A positive culture is not diagnostic of infection.
4. A culture taken of a noninfected ulceration will generally grow organisms that are only contaminants. This may lead to unnecessary antibiotic therapy.
5. The use of antibiotics in a noninfected ulcer will not necessarily act as a prophylactic measure. If an ulcer is going to get infected, it still will, but possibly with an organism resistant to the antibiotic given, and possibly many others. This makes true therapeutic selection, if and when necessary, more difficult.
6. The concept of taking a culture in a noninfected ulceration for the purposes of determining a "baseline" organism(s) has no basis in science.
7. Although it is theoretically true that ulcerations may offer a "portal of entry" for bacteria into deeper tissues, this does not imply that every time a patient develops an ulcer he or she will get a deep infection. Patients can have ulcerations for months and never get infected.
8. To date, no published studies have shown that the routine use of antibiotics in noninfected ulcers increases the rate of healing.

Clinical Presentation

The noninfected mal perforans presents as a round, punched-out–appearing lesion overlying a weight-bearing prominence. The base has pink, healthy-appearing granulation tissue. There is minimal serous drainage and no odor. Before debridement, a ring of hyperkeratotic tissue may entirely surround the area and even cover the lesion. Excessive hyperkeratosis is frequently a sign of weight-bearing pressure. The skin in proximity to the ulcer shows no signs of cellulitis and minimal necrosis.

Laboratory Findings

Noninfected ulcerations are predominantly a local condition. Therefore hematology and chemistry studies would likely be unremarkable. Glucose may be elevated, but this is more a sign of poor compliance than infection. As stressed numerous times, cultures are not indicated.

Bacterial Etiology

As emphasized earlier, even noninfected ulcerations will grow organisms. These vary from patient to patient, but at least one of the following presents most commonly:

1. *S. aureus*
2. *Staphylococcus epidermidis*
3. *P. mirabilis*
4. *P. aeruginosa*

Numerous other community-acquired organisms may also be found. The mal perforans is a good environment for bacterial colonization, and that is what these essentially are—contaminants and colonizers with no pathological significance.

Treatment

The hallmark of treatment in the noninfected lesion is relief of pressure and local wound care. Relieving the excessive mechanical stresses on the ulceration allows granulation and subsequent epithelization of the wound. This can be accomplished by the following:

1. Use of pressure-relieving insole devices.
2. Healing sandals.
3. Removable short leg cast walkers.
4. Accommodative padding of the lesion.
5. Bed rest or crutches. Unfortunately, patients are not particularly compliant with either of these modalities.
6. Total contact casting. This is an excellent modality that has been proven to be extremely effective. Unfortunately, it is time- and resource-intensive and very applicator-dependent. If not performed properly, it can cause as many problems as it solves.

Local wound care consists of the following:

1. Periodic debridement of excess hyperkeratotic or necrotic tissue.
2. Daily to twice-daily dressing changes, preferably wet-to-dry, using saline solution or any number of other products (e.g., hydrogels, hydrocolloids, films, and others). This is known as *passive wound care*.

3. There have been many advances in wound care in the past few years. The advent of commercially available and FDA-approved growth factors and living skin equivalents has caused a major revolution in the field of wound healing. The term *active wound healing* is used to describe the use of these excellent, effective products. This field is changing rapidly, and there are entire journals and texts devoted to it. It is not within the scope of this book to review that information.

4. The use of topical disinfectants, such as povidone iodine (Betadine), has been commonly discredited by many in the wound care arena. Most of this opinion has been based on in vitro tissue culture studies looking at fibroblast activity. There is little convincing evidence that these solutions cause any problems with wound healing in the clinical setting. Many clinicians have had years of excellent clinical success with compounds, including povidone iodine and sodium hypochlorite (Dakin's solution).

5. Topical antibiotics such as silver sulfadiazine (Silvadene), triple antibiotic ointment (Neosporin), mupirocin (Bactroban), or gentamicin cream have been used by clinicians for years for the treatment of both infected and noninfected ulcers. Despite their wide acceptance, there are little hard data to support this usage. Although these are probably benign and may be helpful, adverse reactions such as sensitivity, excessive maceration of tissue, and superinfection are potential complications.

Antibiotic Selection

Antibiotic therapy is *not* indicated for clean, noninfected ulcerations.

■ *Mildly Infected Ulcerations*

Clinical Presentation

Ulcerations that present as clinically infected will differ significantly from those described previously. Instead of having a clean, healthy base, there may be necrosis present or a lack of granulation. This alone is not diagnostic because even noninfected ulcers may have some necrosis and eschar formation. Beyond this, however, there will be clinical signs of infection including surrounding erythema, edema, and increased heat. There may be purulent drainage. Differentiation of this type of infection from those more seriously infected is a matter of extent. The cellulitis found in these lesions usually will extend no more than 2 cm from the periphery of the wound. This is a very local process.

Laboratory Findings

As with the noninfected lesion, this is predominately a local condition. Hematologic findings may be normal including chemistries and white blood cell counts (WBCs). Serum glucose may be slightly elevated, but this may be more an issue of noncompliance rather than as a result of the infection. Cultures of curettage samples, pus, or deeper wound tissue are indicated. Swab cultures are not adequate.

Bacterial Etiology

Bacterial etiology of these mild infections tends to be overwhelmingly gram-positive aerobic organisms. The commonly held belief that all diabetic foot infections are caused by a mix of many types of organisms including aerobes and anaerobes does not necessarily refer to this type of infection. It is true for the more severe infections discussed subsequently. By far, the most ubiquitous organisms isolated from these wounds are:

1. *S. aureus*
2. Group B streptococci (*Streptococcus agalactiae*)

Treatment

General treatment principles remain constant with all of these lesions. Debridement and off-loading are of primary importance. However, unlike the clinically noninfected lesions, antibiotics are indicated for these infections.

Antibiotic Selection

Mild infections can be treated with oral antibiotics on an outpatient basis. All these selections are for empiric therapy, before a culture result is obtained.

Preferred Antibiotic Therapy
1. Amoxicillin/clavulanic acid, 500 to 875 mg q12h with food
2. Cephalexin, 500 mg q6h to q8h
3. Clindamycin, 300 mg q8h to q12h (especially for penicillin/ cephalosporin allergy)

Alternate Therapy
Levofloxacin, 500 mg q24h

One topical antibiotic of interest, Pexiganan, is a peptide class antibiotic derived from the skin of a particular frog species. This drug was studied in more than 900 patients and found to be as effective as oral ofloxacin when studied for mildly infected ulcerations. As of this writing the drug was rejected by the FDA, and it is not known if it will be resubmitted.

■ *Moderate to Severely Infected Ulcerations*

Clinical Presentation

This ulceration has an entirely different clinical appearance. The base is generally deep. A deeper tract that can be probed to bone may be present. There is evidence of liquefaction necrosis in the depths of the ulcer, giving it a soupy look. Drainage is more purulent and may have an odor. Surrounding tissue appears macerated and necrotic. Frank cellulitis, centered around the lesion, is present. This cellulitis extends well over 2 cm from the center of the periphery and may progress up the leg. Lymphangiitis and lymphadenitis can be present. Tissue gas and necrotizing fasciitis are rare but may be found in the most severe of these cases. There may be systemic toxicity, and the patient will most likely be febrile, especially later in the day.

Laboratory Findings

Although the ulceration itself may be localized to the foot, the infection may have spread more systemically. For this reason, there may be positive laboratory findings not seen with the previous types of ulcers. WBC count will likely be elevated, although some studies have shown, even in significant infections, that the elevation may be minor. Serum glucose will most likely be significantly elevated. The patient's chemistries will be altered. In particular, renal function may be diminished as demonstrated by elevated creatinine and blood urea nitrogen (BUN). Erythrocyte sedimentation rate (ESR) will likely be elevated. If sepsis is suspected, significant changes in almost all laboratory parameters will be seen. Deep wound, blood, and bone cultures may be indicated. Swab cultures are not adequate.

Bacterial Etiology

Bacterial etiology of these serious infections tends to be polymicrobial. A mix of gram-positive, gram-negative, aerobic, and anaerobic organisms can be seen. Studies have shown that as many as six different organisms may be isolated. The following are those most commonly found:

1. *S. aureus*
2. Group B streptococci
3. Gram-positive anaerobes—*Peptococcus/Peptostreptococcus*
4. Multiple gram-negative aerobes—*Escherichia coli/Proteus/Enterobacter*
5. Gram-negative anaerobes—*B. fragilis/Bacteroides species*

Treatment

Similar principles of local care and mechanical protection apply to those mal perforans that are not frankly infected. The daily care routine may need to be more aggressive, and absolute bed rest stressed more strongly. Total-contact casting is contraindicated in the grossly septic ulceration. Aggressive surgical incision and drainage is frequently necessary. Hospitalization may be required, especially in case of the following:

1. A previous course of outpatient/oral therapy has been unsuccessful in stopping the progress of the infection.
2. The patient requires aggressive surgical incision and drainage.
3. The patient requires intravenous antibiotics in a controlled setting (home parenteral or oral equivalents of parenterals are not possible).
4. There is clinical evidence of sepsis.
5. Medical or metabolic co-morbidities are present that must be handled in the inpatient setting.
6. The patient is noncompliant with off-loading. Unfortunately, few if any insurance companies consider this by itself an indication for hospitalization. It can only be achieved by using one of the previous more "medically necessary" reasons.

Antibiotic Selection

These infections are generally treated inpatient with intravenous (IV) therapy. That being said, there are instances when outpatient therapy is warranted or when the patient refuses hospitalization. Furthermore, a number of newer antibiotics, including most quinolones, have bioavailability that is equivalent both orally and parenterally. Therefore there is no reason why oral therapy should not be equivalent. Again, these are empiric selections for use before obtaining culture results.

Preferred Antibiotic Therapy

Any of the β-lactam/β-lactamase inhibitor compounds are preferred.

1. Piperacillin/tazobactam, 3.375 g q6h or 4.5 g q8h.
2. Ticarcillin/clavulanic acid, 3.1 g q6h.
3. Ampicillin/sulbactam, 3 g q6h with or without a quinolone for extended gram-negative coverage.

Other primary choices

1. Clindamycin, 600 to 900 mg q8h (if the patient is penicillin allergic).
2. Levofloxacin, 750 mg q24h with or without clindamycin. Both available PO if patient refuses hospitalization or if intravenous access is difficult.
3. Ertapenem, 1 g q24h.

Alternate therapy

1. Moxifloxacin, 400 mg q24h PO.
2. Imipenem/cilastatin, 500 mg q6h to q8h. Unless the renal function and seizure history of patient is known, treatment should be started with q8h dosing to reduce the risk of drug-induced seizure.
3. Meropenem, 1 g q8h.
4. Linezolid, 600 mg IV/PO q12h, especially if a resistant gram-positive is involved such as MRSA or enterococci. This can be used with or without gram-negative coverage (i.e., quinolone).
5. Cefoxitin, 2 g q6h.

■ *Arterial Ulcerations*

Ulcerations of the foot secondary to arterial insufficiency are rarely an infectious problem. They are included because they are frequently inappropriately grouped in with mal perforans. They require different approaches to treatment and have significantly higher morbidity.

Clinical Presentation

Unlike the mal perforans ulcerations, arterial ulcers do not necessarily occur in high-pressure regions. They are most frequently found on the distal aspect of the toes, the medial side of the first metatarsal head, the lateral side of the fifth metatarsal head, and in the posterior heel. They are usually exquisitely painful, although the pain may be dulled somewhat if profound neuropathy is present. The pain is worse at night and is relieved somewhat by dependency. Relief of pain may require narcotic analgesics. The lesions themselves have necrotic bases with extensive eschar formation. Frank gangrene may be present surrounding the area. An interesting finding, especially seen on the first or fifth metatarsal head lesions, is direct visualization of the underlying joint with the skin freely movable over the area. It is rare to find any evidence of cellulitis associated with these ulcers. These tend to remain stable for long periods of time and do not improve, or for that matter worsen, particularly quickly. Only after revascularization is a rather massive post-bypass hyperemic flush seen that is often confused with bacterial infection.

Laboratory Findings

There are no unique hematologic or chemistry laboratory changes for this condition. Only evidence of systemic vascular changes may be found. The vascular laboratory is the most useful. Noninvasive studies including pulse volume recordings, digital plethysmography, and transcutaneous oxygen tensions are used. Once these tests are completed, angiograms may be ordered. Cultures are rarely necessary because these lesions are heavily colonized but not usually infected.

Bacterial Etiology

These are *not* infectious problems. They are vascular in nature and are rarely infected.

Treatment

Treatment of these lesions centers around the diagnosis, and, hopefully, the correction of the underlying arterial insufficiency through bypass or angioplasty. "Cold steel" debridement must be carried out carefully to avoid further tissue damage and is used sparingly. Chemical debridement with topical enzymes may play a role in breaking down eschar formation. Antibiotics have a limited utility, because infection is not really an issue. The entire concept of antibiotics being useless and "unable to get down there" because of the vascular disease has never been proved.

MISCELLANEOUS INFECTIONS

▣ *Dermatophyte Infections*

Fungal infection of the skin is very common in diabetic patients. Studies have shown that patients with diabetes have a twofold to threefold higher prevalence than those without diabetes.

One major concern in the patient with diabetes is the potential for secondary bacterial infection. This is especially dangerous with interdigital tinea. The skin in the web spaces is thin. With maceration, the tissue easily breaks down, allowing bacteria growing on the moist skin to become invasive. The anatomy of the toe webs allows the organisms to spread into the foot via the numerous tendons that insert into the area. A severe plantar or dorsal space infection may result. For this reason, dermatophyte infections should be treated aggressively. This disease will be covered in detail in a separate chapter.

▣ *Plantar Space Infections*

The most severe of the diabetic foot infections is the plantar space infection. Although frequently a continuum from the moderately to severely infected ulcer previously described, the presentation is unique enough to deserve its own description. Furthermore, the condition can arise without an obvious point of entry–such as an ulcer. This is the disease that rightfully bears the pseudonym "the fetid foot." The foot is divided anatomically into multiple fascial spaces. There are at least seven distinct plantar spaces. Three are located centrally, one medially, and one laterally. Purulence will take the path of least resistance when put under pressure, as in the case of an abscess. Therefore an infection in one part of the foot will usually track proximally and distally within the involved plantar space.

Clinical Presentation

The foot and leg will be massively edematous, erythematous, and warm. The cellulitis will usually center around the space with the deep abscess formation. Occasionally, a secondary nidus of cellulitis will appear at the original source (i.e., the web space or a toe). The patient may or may not appear sick. There may be minimal pain because of the neuropathy, although palpation of the plantar arch will frequently elicit a surprisingly brisk pain response from the patient. Fever is usually present, especially if the patient is seen in the afternoon or evening. The abscess can cause localized tissue necrosis and form a draining sinus that can be distant to any original nidus or entry point. Bone is frequently involved. The drainage has an extremely foul odor. The patient generally has overall good circulation and will bleed profusely. However, because of necrosis and thrombosis caused by the infection, there may be localized areas that demonstrate no perfusion.

Laboratory Findings
Usually there is an elevated white blood cell count. The ESR may be elevated. Serum creatinine and BUN levels are usually elevated because the patient is not only renally impaired but probably also dehydrated. The glucose level is usually extremely elevated, and the patient may present in diabetic ketoacidosis. Gram stain reveals many white blood cells and many organism morphologies. Radiographs may show tissue gas. Osseous changes are usually evident to some extent.

Bacterial Etiology
As discussed previously, the microbiology of the diabetic plantar space infection is similar to that described for the severely infected ulcers. A mix of anaerobes and aerobes is usually present.

Treatment
No attempt should be made to treat these patients with antibiotics alone. The purulence must be surgically drained and the necrosis debrided. Early and aggressive incision and drainage is the key to saving these limbs.

Medical therapy is aimed at rehydration, controlling the glucose level, and supporting the septic patient. The glucose level must be controlled to allow the immune system to assist the antibiotics. Antibiotic choices are the same as listed in the section on severe infection.

■ *Dorsal Space Infections*

A variation of plantar space infections, dorsal infections differ slightly in etiology. Usually a fissure or ulceration in the dorsum of a toe or in the web space allows bacterial entrance and abscess formation around the extensor hood apparatus. The organisms then track dorsally along these tendon sheaths. Although otherwise similar to their plantar counterparts, their consequences can be more grave because the smaller amount of skin and soft tissue present on the dorsal aspect of the foot makes debridement more difficult, the chance of bone and joint involvement greater, and possibility for functional reconstruction less.

SUGGESTED READINGS

Aldridge KE, Ashcraft D, Cambre K et al: Multicenter survey of the changing in vitro antimicrobial susceptibilities of clinical isolates of Bacteroides fragilis group, Prevotella, Fusobacterium, Porphyromonas, and Peptostreptococcus species, *Antimicrob Agents Chemother* 45(4):1238, 2001.

Armstrong DG, Perales TA, Murff RT et al: Value of white blood cell count with differential in the acute diabetic foot infection, *J Am Podiatr Med Assoc* 86(5):224, 1996.

DCCT Research Group: The effect of intensive treatment of diabetes in the development and progression of long-term complications in insulin dependent diabetes mellitus, *N Engl J Med* 329:977, 1993.

Ge Y, MacDonald D, Henry MM et al: In vitro susceptibility to pexiganan of bacteria isolated from infected diabetic foot ulcers, *Diagn Microbiol Infect Dis* 35(1):45, 1999.

Greene DA, Lattimer SA, Sima AAF: Are disturbances of sorbitol, phosphoinositide, and Na+-K+–ATPase regulation involved in pathogenesis of diabetic neuropathy? *Diabetes* 37:688, 1988.

Joseph WS: Treatment of lower extremity infections in diabetics, *J Am Podiatr Med Assoc* 82(7):361, 1992.

LoGerfo FW, Coffman JD: Vascular and microvascular disease of the foot in diabetics. Implications for foot care, *N Engl J Med* 311:1615, 1984.

Sapico FL, Canawati HN, Witte JL et al: Quantitative aerobic and anaerobic bacteriology of the infected diabetic foot, *J Clin Microbiol* 6*(suppl 1)*:S171, 1980.

Tanenberg RJ, Schumer MP, Greene DA et al: Neuropathic problems of the lower extremities in diabetic patients. In Bowker JH, Pfeifer MA, editors: *Levin and O'Neal's: the diabetic foot,* ed 6, St. Louis, 2001, Mosby.

CHAPTER 6

Surgical Infections and Prophylaxis

It is hard to believe that it has been less than 150 years since the work of Pasteur, and only slightly later, Lister revolutionized the practice of medicine and surgery. Before their work with antisepsis, surgical procedures were overwhelmingly doomed to failure. Even the most basic procedure would be complicated by infection. Since antibiotics were not developed, deaths were common. With the golden age of antibiotics beginning in the 1940s, even more infections could be prevented, and lives could be saved after surgery.

Despite these incredible advances in a relatively short time, it is estimated that in the United States, approximately 500,000 surgical site infections (SSIs) still occur each year. The cost of treating these infections is thought to exceed $1.5 billion. Granted, the vast majority of these infections are *not* related to lower extremity surgery or even general orthopedic procedures. Rather, gastrointestinal, genitourinary, and posttransplant infections account for the vast majority of SSIs. Of the procedures commonly performed on the lower extremity, only limb amputation surgery has a significant rate of SSIs.

It is difficult to accurately determine the infection rate following lower extremity surgery. Studies directed exclusively at the lower extremity and of large enough proportions have not been performed. It is well accepted that the overall infection rate is quite low, with 1% to 2% the most commonly heard estimate.

Actually, it is reasonable to assume that the true infection rate is even lower, probably below 1%. The best data available on infection rates are from the National Nosocomial Infections Surveillance system (NNIS). Even the latest data collected for this study between 1992 and 1998 do not specifically single out lower extremity surgery. The closest information relating to foot and ankle surgery in this study is probably the "other musculoskeletal" category. The stated rate of infection in this group is 0.65%. Of course, this rate may not be directly applicable. This is a "nosocomial" study. Surgery performed in a physician's office, as are many foot procedures, is not included.

When infections do occur, they are costly—not only in a real dollar sense—but also in an emotional sense for the patient and surgeon. One of the major causes of medical malpractice suits is the postoperative infection.

One controversy in operative wound infections is the definition of what constitutes an infection. How can one determine whether a wound is dehisced or infected? Just because bacteria are cultured from a serous discharge or superficial swab, is an infection present? It has been recognized for decades that despite appropriate antisepsis and surgical technique, wounds will frequently become contaminated with bacteria. If the wound is frankly purulent and necrotic, the diagnosis is easy. As has been stated previously, decisions should be made on clinical grounds.

FACTORS IN SURGICAL INFECTON

When discussing surgical infections, numerous determinants are taken into consideration. This can be demonstrated as a simple formula (Figure 6-1). These determinants can then be conveniently grouped into three broader categories:

1. Surgical factors: microbial contamination and virulence, surgical technique breaches, use of prophylactic antibiotics
2. Patient factors: general and local host immunity
3. Pathogen factors: microbial contamination and virulence, resistance to antibiotics

A fourth category, environmental factors, also will be discussed, although it is not directly included in the equation.

$$\frac{\begin{array}{c} \text{Microbial} \\ \text{Contamination} \\ \text{and Virulence} \end{array} \times \begin{array}{c} \text{Surgical} \\ \text{Technique} \\ \text{Breaches} \end{array} \times \begin{array}{c} \text{Resistance to} \\ \text{Antibiotics} \end{array}}{\begin{array}{c} \text{General and Local} \\ \text{Host Immunity} \end{array} \times \begin{array}{c} \text{Prophylactic} \\ \text{Antibiotics} \end{array}} = \begin{array}{c} \text{Risk of Surgical} \\ \text{Infection} \end{array}$$

FIGURE 6-1
The contribution of various factors in the risk of surgical infection. (From Mandell GL, Bennett JE, Dolin R: *Principles and practice of infectious diseases*, ed 5, Philadelphia, 2000, Churchill Livingstone.)

■ *Surgical Factors*

Microbial Contamination and Virulence

Contamination of the surgical site can result from a number of breaks in technique. Tearing of gloves, sweating into the wound, excessive movement or talking, and inappropriate instrument handling all are potential sources of wound contamination. The clinical significance of this contamination is based on the amount and type of the contamination along with various patient factors. As early as the 1960s, an attempt was made to classify wounds by their level of contamination. When modified to apply to lower extremity surgery, the classification would traditionally consist of:

1. Clean wound—a nontraumatic wound with no inflammation and no breaks in technique
2. Clean-contaminated wound—a minor break in technique
3. Contaminated wound—a fresh traumatic wound or major breaks in technique
4. Dirty or infected wound—a wound in which acute bacterial inflammation has occurred because of the presence of devitalized tissue, foreign bodies, fecal contamination, trauma from a dirty source, delayed treatment, or the presence of frank pus.

Although this system has been used successfully for years, shows good correlation with the risk of infection, and is easy to use, it has drawbacks. The most obvious is that it does not take any patient factors into account (i.e., immune status). For example, a clean wound in an immunocompromised patient may have more risk of infection than a clean-contaminated wound in an otherwise healthy patient. Likewise, surgical factors, such as length of the procedure, are not figured into this system. More recently, organizations such as the NNIS system of the Hospital

Infections Program of the National Center for Infectious Diseases, Centers of Disease Control and Prevention, are now using a more detailed system that takes these factors into account. For instance, the American Society of Anesthesiology patient risk classification is used, as is a factor for the length of the procedure corresponding to the 75th percentile duration of surgery for any given procedure.

Microbial virulence plays another important role. It is well known that a traditionally low virulence organism such as *Staphylococcus epidermidis* can play a major role in prosthetic joint implants. These infections may not become evident until months or even years after the surgery, yet they were inoculated at the time of the procedure. Other organisms, such as group A streptococcus can produce rapidly progressive infections that can cause a limb to go necrotic in 24 hours.

Surgical Technique

Many breaches of surgical technique may play an important role in the potentiation of a postoperative wound infection. Good surgical technique is probably the most important aspect to preventing postoperative infections.

Dead Space/Hematoma

The presence of dead space in a wound leads to the accumulation of wound fluids and hematoma, which is one of the major causes of postoperative infection. Both wound fluids and blood support the growth of bacteria by supplying a nutrient medium and suppressing immune function. The iron in the red blood cells can potentiate bacterial growth while inhibiting neutrophil activity. The obliteration of this dead space must be done judiciously to minimize these factors. A further complicating factor is that a postoperative hematoma may mimic the clinical signs and symptoms of infection. Erythema, edema, and pain are often found. There is frequently drainage, although it is more likely serous, serosanguinous, or coagulated blood as opposed to purulent. In fact, this may be the most important distinguishing factor. Documentation of this finding thus becomes important. This is most often found following a surgery to remove a mass, such as a neuroma or where a significant piece of bone has been removed. Treatment consists of appropriate excavation of the hematoma and, if necessary, drain placement and hemostasis. Since there is no infection present, antibiotics would not be indicated.

Drains

The use of drains to eliminate fluid accumulation is a double-edged sword. Although effective for draining fluid, drains also provide a conduit by which external bacteria enter the wound. This is especially seen with Penrose-type drains. Sealed suction-drainage systems appear to be the safest. Drains will also cause a localized inflammatory response that may promote localized tissue damage and prevent the neutrophils from being available to attack any bacteria. Drains, like any foreign object in a wound, also act as a site for bacterial adherence and may potentiate infection in that way. For these reasons, it has been suggested that, if used, drains exit from a site different than the surgical incision. Furthermore, they should be removed as soon as possible.

Sutures

Traditionally, surgeons have been relatively secure in using monofilament sutures to close wounds. It has been demonstrated that the number of bacteria needed to cause an infection significantly decreased when braided silk sutures were used, because the braids harbor bacteria. Newer studies point to the actual chemical composition of the suture, not the physical structure, as being the most important determinant. Synthetic materials cause less infection than natural materials.

Suture Technique

All sutures, regardless of composition or structure, act as a foreign body and potentiate infection. The surgeon's technique in using the suture is probably the most important factor. Excessive suture use and strangulation of tissue, which causes necrosis, should be avoided.

Implants

The use of implants has significance similar to that of suture material. The number of organisms required to cause an infection is greater than 10,000-fold lower in cases in which a foreign body is left in the wound. For this discussion, *implant* refers to any metal or polymer joint or fixation device. A marked decrease in phagocyte activity can be demonstrated in the presence of these materials. Furthermore, bacteria can firmly adhere to the device as a result of various patient and bacterial "adherence factors." Probably the most notorious of these factors is the glycocalyx or slime that is produced by the bacteria and covers the growing colony. This capsule renders the colony resistant to most antibiotics. The use of prophylactic antibiotics or antibiotic flushes has not been shown to prevent this phenomenon.

Traditionally it was believed that eradication of infections in the face of prosthetic joint implants usually required implant removal. More recent studies have shown that when the device is not loosened and the organism is susceptible to antibiotics, so-called "debridement and retention" strategies along with long-term oral antibiotic therapy will work almost as well and will be more cost-effective than removal/replacement of the joint.

Timing of Closure

Closing a wound that may be heavily contaminated with bacteria will potentiate the development of infection. Studies have shown that the presence of greater than 10^5 bacteria present in a wound at the time of closure will lead to a greater likelihood of infection. Unfortunately, the quantitative bacteriologic testing needed to determine this number is not widely available in clinical micro labs. Therefore the ideal time to close a wound is realistically a clinical judgment. However, the old bromide about requiring "three negative cultures" before a wound can be closed is still frequently repeated. There are simply no hard data to back this assertion.

Tissue Injury

Necrotic tissue acts as a nidus for bacterial growth. The rough handling of tissues, inappropriate instrumentation, and overutilization of electrocautery or the laser will potentiate the development of necrosis.

Irrigation

Copious amounts of intraoperative irrigation may reduce the potential for infection, predominately through the mechanical loosening of bacteria and the dilution of contamination. Techniques and the controversy over antibiotic flushes are covered in Chapter 4.

Length of Operation

There is a direct correlation between length of operation and infection rate. The longer a surgical wound is kept open, the greater the potential for contamination from the operating room or the surgical personnel. The tissues are most likely being handled for greater periods of time. Prolonged procedures performed under tourniquet control may cause ischemia of tissue.

Length of Stay

Both preoperative and postoperative hospital stays can markedly increase the potential for infection. Patients can colonize quickly with multiresistant nosocomial organisms. This has become less of an issue recently because patients are generally pushed out of the hospital by insurance requirements more quickly than they used to be. Furthermore, more surgery is now done outpatient or on a very short stay (less than 24 hours).

Preoperative Preparation

Despite good hard scientific evidence to substantiate the points listed subsequently, the surgical preparation for both the patient and the surgeon seems to remain ritualized. Some surgeons are almost superstitious about changing a protocol that has worked for them in the past.

Patient

1. Showering the night before surgery with an antibacterial agent seems to reduce the infection rate.
2. Shaving of the limb before surgery may cause small lacerations or nicks. If performed more than 2 hours before surgery, bacteria will have a chance to multiply in the site and potentially cause infection. For this reason many facilities have eliminated shaving as part of the preoperative preparation. If some sort of hair removal is necessary, either a chemical depilatory or hair clippers should be used before the operation.
3. Surgical scrub of the limb on the operating table may actually increase the infection rate. Theoretically, the scrub, while cleaning superficially, may cause bacteria present in the hair follicle to rise to the surface. If a preoperative shower is taken, painting the limb with an antiseptic solution before draping is probably sufficient.

Surgeon

1. The traditional 10-minute scrub is now passé. The prolonged procedure may actually increase the number of organisms recovered from the skin via a mechanism similar to that of the patient scrub. A shorter 3- to 5-minute initial scrub is equally effective. The surgeon may scrub for subsequent surgeries for even shorter times. Some centers now eliminate the later scrubs in favor of the use of antibacterial alcohol foams. Isopropyl alcohol is an extremely effective hand disinfectant with rapid

killing and a sustained period of activity. It is considered by some to be the standard for this purpose.

2. A large percentage of surgical gloves may have defects. These defects may already exist or may occur during surgery. The clinical significance of this is unknown. With proper surgical scrub of the hands, the infection rate increases minimally, if at all. However, double gloving may be warranted, at least for especially combative cases. This concept does not appeal to some surgeons, who point to dimunition of tactile sense with the extra gloves. They believe that this dimunition may indirectly lead to even higher infection rates.

3. Epidemiologically, an outbreak of infections, usually caused by staphylococci, may be traced to one particular surgeon. Although the immediate tendency may be to question the surgical or preparation technique, potential nasal carriage of the organism must be considered. The anterior nares of the operating staff should be cultured. If an organism is recovered, it should be phage typed against the infecting pathogen and the contaminated parties treated. Combinations of oral and topical agents have been used to eliminate nasal carriage with variable, frequently temporary, results.

■ *Patient Factors*

Most organisms that cause surgical wound infections are inoculated into the wound from the patient's own bacteriologic flora.

Surgery's Effect on the Immune System
Surgery is a form of trauma; it therefore has similar effects on all three arms of the immune system:

1. The number of granulocytes decreases. Decreases also occur in phagocytosis and chemotaxis.
2. Cellular immunity decreases.
3. Antibody formation and circulating complement decreases.

Age
The infection rate increases in older adult patients for several reasons:

1. Underlying chronic medical conditions
2. Immune senescence

3. Long-term exposure to resistant pathogens, especially in nursing homes or hospitals
4. Malnutrition

Nutrition

Malnourished patients show a higher rate of wound infection. Trace elements, such as zinc, have been shown to have a beneficial effect on wound healing.

Obesity

Obese patients tend to have higher wound infection rates. The mechanism for this is not clear.

■ *Pathogen Factors*

Virulence of the Organisms

Some organisms are inherently more invasive and likely to cause infection than others. These bacteria are of concern when examining a wound and checking on culture results. For example, *Staphylococcus aureus* is known to be a notorious pathogen. *S. epidermidis*, on the other hand, had never been considered a pathogen. Now it is realized that, in the case of implant infections, this bacteria is a major problem. Furthermore, *S. epidermidis* may cause latent infections that do not become evident until months if not years after the implant is placed. This can make diagnosis difficult.

Resistance to Antibiotics

Some organisms are intrinsically more resistant to antibiotics than others. Some have the ability to develop rapid resistance to therapy. To use the example previously given, *S. epidermidis* is quite frequently resistant to methicillin (more than 80%) and therefore to all penicillins and cephalosporins. Furthermore, if a particular hospital or community has a particularly high incidence of fairly resistant organisms (this can be determined by scrutinizing a hospital antibiogram), then the chance of SSI infection by one of these pathogens may be increased.

Ability to Form a Glycocalyx

Certain organisms (*Staphylococcus, Bacteroides, Pseudomonas,* among others) are capable of elucidating a proteinaceous capsule that surrounds developing colonies. This lends significant resistance to antibiotics and the patient's immune system.

■ *Environmental Factors*

Some of the environmental factors that may play a role in the development of a surgical infection include:

1. Proper sterilization. The proper use of steam-autoclaved instruments, when appropriate, should be ensured for any invasive procedure. If instruments cannot be autoclaved, then gas or proper cold sterilization techniques, using approved solutions such as gluteraldehyde, should be used.
2. Apparel worn by personnel. Appropriate scrub suits should be worn as opposed to street clothing. These should only be used in the operating room (OR) area to prevent contamination. Impermeable gowns, shoe coverings, and masks and head coverings that cover all exposed hair, should also be worn. Interestingly enough, at least one study suggests that mask usage does not affect the infection rate, although this use still is highly recommended.
3. Operating room surfaces. All operating room surfaces need to be appropriately disinfected both between cases and, even more thoroughly, at the end of the day. Phenol-containing compounds are the most commonly used.
4. Air handling. It has been estimated that as many as 90% of wound pathogens gain access via the air in the OR. The use of laminar-air flow operating suites appears to decrease the infection rate, as does high-volume ventilation, positive pressure OR efficiency suites, and high-efficiency particulate air filtration (HEPA).
5. Hygiene of OR personnel. Although this seems basic, poor hygiene or the presence of a seemingly unrelated skin condition or infection in OR personnel can have dramatic consequences. At least one report of a series of significant postoperative infections has been traced to a nurse with seemingly inconsequential onychomycosis.

ANTIBIOTIC PROPHYLAXIS

Any discussion of the use of antibiotic prophylaxis is difficult. Every aspect, from the actual definition of *prophylaxis* to when and how to use it, is debatable. The literature is sparse at best. A Medline search of the terms *antibiotic prophylaxis* in combination with *foot surgery* or *orthopedic surgery* covering the past 15 years reveal no articles specific to prophylactic antibiotic use in lower extremity surgery. A few papers look at the incidence covering all orthopedic surgery, although most are specific for prosthetic joint implants of the hip or knee. There is one large series out of the United Kingdom, by Taylor, of almost 13,000 elective orthopedic procedures. The lower extremity procedures with the highest in-patient infection rate included ankle fusion (9.3%) and subtalar fusion (5.8%). The overall infection rate for all open elective orthopedic procedures was only 1.43%. His conclusion was that antibiotic prophylaxis may be helpful in these higher-incidence procedures, although his study did not directly look at the effect of that usage. Some pharmacokinetics papers compare one antibiotic to another. The problem is that the incidence of infection in foot and ankle surgery is so low that performing a study to show any difference would take excessively large numbers of procedures over a protracted time.

The following are questions commonly asked about the use of prophylaxis:

1. When is it indicated?
2. What agent should be used?
3. Against which organism should the agent be directed?
4. Within what time frame should it be given and for how long must prophylaxis be continued?

Some of these questions are easier to answer than others. In fact, an in-depth discussion of antibiotic prophylaxis often raises more questions than it answers. To address these questions, some basic definitions and rules are in order.

■ *Definition*

Antibiotic prophylaxis must be differentiated from therapeutic usage. Simply put, *prophylaxis is the use of antibiotics for the purpose of preventing infection*. If any infection is already present, the antibiotic becomes therapeutic, and an entirely different set of criteria for their use must be followed.

■ *Golden Rules of Prophylaxis*

Whenever prophylactic antibiotics are considered, there are two golden rules that will apply.

First Rule of Prophylaxis

There is one criterion that, if followed, will ensure the proper use of prophylactic antibiotics.

Rule 1: *The antibiotic must have achieved its maximum levels at the time of initial incision or insult.*

This is the most scientifically validated principle of all when it comes to prophylaxis. *Timing is everything.* Numerous studies, most significantly by Burke, have shown that there is a crucial time window for using antibiotics. Giving the antibiotic too soon before or even within an hour afterward will significantly increase the infection rate.

If this first rule cannot be applied to a particular case, then the use of the drug in that situation should be reevaluated. As discussed later, this rule will exclude the use of prophylaxis in many cases in which it is commonly being used. It also helps to answer important questions about the timing of administration and length of usage.

Second Rule of Prophylaxis

This rule addresses the questions of which agent should be selected and against which organism it should be directed.

Rule 2: *The antibiotic should be directed against the most common organism found if an infection were to occur in that particular situation.*

Although it seems quite obvious, obedience to this rule requires a thorough understanding of the pathophysiology, microbial etiology, and antibacterial susceptibility of a variety of infections. For example, an understanding of bacterial adherence factors helps explain the common finding of coagulase-negative staphylococci, which are often methicillin resistant, following implant surgery.

■ Indications

In the lower extremity, antibiotic prophylaxis is considered in four general situations:

1. Following wounds
2. For surgery
3. For prophylaxis against bacterial endocarditis in the surgical patient with a compromised heart valve
4. For dental patients

Wound Prophylaxis

The following are the most common types of traumatic wounds that present in the lower extremity:

1. Puncture wounds
2. Lacerations
3. Bite wounds

Frequently when these patients present to the physician immediately following injury, the question arises as whether prophylactic antibiotics need to be administered. Broad-spectrum oral drugs are most frequently prescribed. If the first rule is applied in these situations, antibiotics are not indicated. By the time the patient presents for treatment, the antibiotic prescription is filled and the drug is taken and absorbed, a significant amount of time has passed since the insult.

In the case of punctures and lacerations, most studies show that prophylactic antibiotics do not alter the incidence of infection following these injuries. Only some small series suggest a role in puncture wounds of the foot. The time interval between the injury and the presentation of the patient for therapy and the extent of local wound care is more important than whether the antibiotic was given. Antibiotics will be beneficial only in the first few hours after an injury. As for puncture wounds, there is no hard evidence to suggest that prophylaxis with an anti-pseudomonal agent, such as ciprofloxacin, decreases the incidence of pseudomonal osteomyelitis.

Animal bites present a different situation. Bite wounds are highly contaminated with numerous types of microorganisms. The physician must differentiate whether the use of antibiotics constitutes prophylaxis or actual therapy. Because of the high incidence of infection following these wounds, antibiotic therapy should be initiated along with aggressive debridement.

Surgical Prophylaxis

Although definitive studies are lacking, there is at least a theoretical basis on which recommendations can be made. Antibiotic prophylaxis should generally be considered in the following surgical cases:

1. Prolonged surgery lasting longer than 2 hours
2. Surgery on immunocompromised patients
3. Trauma surgery

4. Implant surgery
5. Any other surgery in which an infection would cause such a devastating result that any potential risk from the antibiotic is overshadowed

Prolonged Surgery

Prolonged surgery exposes the patient to a greater risk of exogenous contamination. This refers to organisms that may invade the wound from the following sources:

1. The operating room environment
2. The operating room personnel
3. The patient's own flora

Immunocompromise

Immunocompromised patients are unable to fight contaminating organisms with a properly functioning immune system, which places them at greater risk for developing an infection. Individuals with the following disorders are considered to be immunocompromised:

1. Uncontrolled diabetes mellitus.
2. Diseases requiring treatment with immunosuppressive agents, such as carcinomas.
3. Rheumatoid arthritis or other conditions requiring treatment with systemic corticosteroids.
4. Genetic or acquired immune defects. It should be noted that there is no evidence that human immunodeficiency virus (HIV) infection alters the postoperative infection rate for lower extremity surgery. HIV primarily affects the CD_4 cells of the cellular immune system. This tends to mediate infection by parasites, fungi, and viruses, but not bacteria.

Trauma

As discussed in Chapter 4, trauma has been shown to cause a significant immune defect. Furthermore, depending on the type of injury, there may be significant amounts of devitalized tissue that may potentiate infection.

Implants

Implants, either metallic or polymer, have been shown to have a significant deleterious effect on local immune responses. Furthermore, organisms may tightly adhere to the implant and form a polyglycolic "slime" around their colonies. This slime layer prevents most antibiotics from penetrating to the organism. However, most work in this area has focused on prosthetic joint implants, not necessarily metallic fixation devices.

Devastating Results

The term *devastating results* is the "wastebasket" indication that causes some surgeons to use prophylaxis in all surgery. This category is more properly applied in non–lower extremity surgery (e.g., the placement of a central nervous system shunt).

■ Selection and Administration of Agents

The selection of an antibiotic as a surgical prophylactic agent should be based on a number of factors:

1. As the second rule states, the selection should be directed against the most common organism found in the event of an infection. In most lower extremity operations, this is fairly straightforward.
   a. *S. aureus* is by far the most common postoperative pathogen.
   b. Variables with *Staphylococcus* include its susceptibility to the penicillinase-resistant penicillins (methicillin resistance) and the recently discovered tolerance to vancomycin ("vancomycin intermediate").
   c. The presence of methicillin-resistant staphylococci is usually endemic in a given hospital or community. Although traditionally thought of as a "nosocomial" pathogen, methicillin-resistant staphylococcus is now beginning to show up as a community organism.
   d. Implant infections are most frequently caused by *S. epidermidis*. This is often methicillin resistant.
2. The agent selected should have a sufficiently long half-life to provide adequate levels throughout the procedure and into the early postoperative period.
3. There is limited hard evidence to support the use of oral antibiotics for surgical prophylaxis. On the other hand, there is also limited evidence showing that, given adequate absorption and tissue levels, they would not work. This is particularly true given some of the new oral antibiotics that have similar bioavailability when given either orally or parenterally.
4. As stated in the first rule, antibiotic levels should be maximal at the time of incision. To ensure this, the following guide-

lines are recommended (it is recognized that these are "idealized" suggestions because many studies have shown that only a small percentage of patients receive their prophylaxis appropriately):

a. The intravenous infusion should be timed so that it is completed no more than a few minutes before elevation of the tourniquet or initial incision. For this reason, it has been suggested that the patient receive the antibiotic by the anesthesiologist in the OR suite as opposed to the preoperative area.

b. If the intramuscular route is used, the antibiotic should be given approximately 45 minutes to 1 hour before the start of surgery.

(1) Oral antibiotics should be given at least 1 hour before surgery.

(2) The too-often-followed practice of performing a surgery and giving the patient a postoperative prescription for a week of some oral antibiotic does not constitute appropriate prophylaxis and has no basis in science. This is commonly seen in outpatient surgicenter or in-office procedures.

5. The duration of antibiotic use is of some debate. Originally prophylactic antibiotics were given for up to 3 to 7 days following surgery. Then the recommendations were decreased to 24 hours. There is even some good evidence that that amount is excessive and that just the preoperative dose is sufficient. However, there are newer studies showing that 3 to 5 days of postoperative continuation decreases the infection rate. The bottom line is that no one is certain. Some general observations for most lower extremity surgery:

a. The initial preoperative dose is sufficient for most surgery of relatively short duration.

b. If surgery lasts more than 2 hours, a postoperative or intraoperative (for very long procedures) dose should be given.

c. Full 24 (+?) hour dosing should be used if the patient is significantly compromised or the surgery was extensive (e.g., internal fixation of a severely fractured ankle).

■ Specific Antibiotics

These antibiotics have all been used in surgical prophylaxis. Doses and specific uses are listed where indicated.

Cefazolin

Cefazolin is probably the most frequently used antibiotic for lower extremity surgical prophylaxis, and with good reason. Its half-life is longer than any other first-generation cephalosporin, allowing one- or two-dose prophylaxis with good levels throughout even the longest cases. It is relatively inexpensive. Antistaphylococcal activity is very good. It also has some gram-negative activity for coverage against the rare cases of infection caused by these organisms. Dosage is 1 to 2 g IV or IM before surgery. One extra gram should be given following longer cases.

Cefuroxime

Cefuroxime is a second-generation cephalosporin that has been used by some surgeons for prophylaxis. Most of the studies, however, have been in cardiothoracic surgery. There is some evidence that it may actually have better antistaphylococcal activity than cefazolin. It also has a fairly long half-life. Its main drawback is that its price is significantly higher than cefazolin, with only questionable returns.

Ceftriaxone

This third-generation cephalosporin has also been used for prophylaxis. Although it has the longest half-life of any cephalosporin, it has a very high price and relative lack of antistaphylococcal activity when compared to less expensive agents. Although its use has been studied in orthopedic prophylaxis, there are other less expensive, more effective drugs to use. Use of this drug is not suggested in lower extremity surgical prophylaxis.

Vancomycin

Some hospitals have now limited the use of this drug for routine prophylaxis because of the development of vancomycin-resistant or tolerant strains of gram-positive organisms. Its primary use is in patients with documented severe penicillin or cephalosporin allergy. This drug can also be considered for prophylaxis when surgery is being performed where a high level of methicillin-resistant staphylococci might be expected, such as at a hospital with a large percentage of MRSA or in implant surgery because of its activity against coagulase-negative staphylococci. Dosage is 1 g begun 1 hour before the surgery and infused slowly over that hour. Vancomycin should not be administered in a bolus. If postoperative administration is desired, 1 g can be given 12 hours following the first dose.

Clindamycin

Although not used frequently for surgical prophylaxis, clindamycin is mentioned for one special case: it has been shown to be effective at penetrating the bacterial glycocalyx. Therefore it may theoretically prove useful in prophylaxis for implant surgery. It may also prove useful as a substitute for the now more carefully regulated vancomycin in beta-lactam allergic patients. Usual dosage is 600 to 900 mg IV.

Ciprofloxacin

Since its introduction, ciprofloxacin has been used in just about every imaginable scenario. It should *not* be used in surgical prophylaxis for lower extremity surgery. The antistaphylococcal activity of this drug is quite mediocre compared to the other agents previously mentioned. Furthermore, there are no studies proving its efficacy in this situation.

Levofloxacin

This quinolone antibiotic has better activity against staphylococcus and streptococcus than ciprofloxacin. It also has the advantage of having a longer half-life, allowing less frequent dosing. As with other quinolones, its achievable levels with oral dosing are similar to that with parenteral. It may be an attractive oral alternative for prophylaxis in beta-lactam–sensitive patients. That being said, it has little to no hard data to support its use in this situation.

Teicoplanin

Although not approved for use in the United States at the time of this writing, this glycopeptide antibiotic is very similar to vancomycin in its spectrum and mode of activity. It has been studied for prophylactic usage for orthopedic surgery in a one-time dosing form.

■ *Endocarditis Prophylaxis*

The situation frequently arises in which a patient scheduled for lower extremity surgery has a history of a damaged heart valve. The valve may be damaged as a result of mitral valve prolapse, rheumatic fever, or previous endocarditis. The patient, having been instructed to take an antibiotic whenever dental work is done, wonders whether the drug is needed before surgery. The key question is whether the procedure is likely to cause a bacteremia. These circulating organisms may then stick to the damaged heart valve, leading to an endocarditis. In 1997 the American Heart Association revised its guidelines for the prevention of bacterial endocarditis. This was of major importance because for the first time specific mention was made of surgeries other than those considered traditionally high risk such as oral or gastrointestinal surgery. Finally, there were guidelines that the lower extremity surgeon could use in everyday practice.

1. Any clean elective surgery performed through surgically prepared skin is considered low risk for causing a bacteremia, and therefore prophylaxis is *not* indicated. This covers the vast majority of surgeries that would be performed.
2. Incision and drainage of an abscess, cutting through infected tissue, or any other manipulation of infected tissue has been shown to cause bacteremia. This therefore is considered high risk, and prophylaxis should be used.
3. The prophylaxis used in point No. 2 should be directed against common pathogens found in that particular infection that is being manipulated.
4. The manipulation of the oropharynx during intubation anesthesia for lower extremity surgery may place the patient at risk.

Agents for Endocarditis Prophylaxis
Unlike previous recommendations that were only directed against bacteremia caused by streptococci (high-dose amoxicillin, tetracycline), the new guidelines are very clear that the suspected organism needs to be covered. They spell out that in skin, skin structure, or bone and joint infection, *S. aureus* is the most commonly isolated pathogen. Therefore the recommendations are specific for the use of an antistaphylococcal penicillin or cephalosporin as first-line agent. Only if there is a concern about manipulation of the oropharynx should streptococcus be covered with the traditional agents.

Dental and Prosthetic Joints Patients
These two seemingly disparate groups of patients are lumped together near the discussion of endocarditis prophylaxis because all are related by concerns of blood-borne, distant-site colonization. The question can be looked at in two directions.

1. If the patient has a prosthetic joint in the foot or ankle, is it necessary for him or her to receive prophylaxis before undergoing a dental procedure? There have been a very few cases in the

literature of late prosthetic joint infection following a dental procedure. However, recent guidelines formed by consensus between the American Academy of Orthopedic Surgery and the American Dental Association seem to go against routine prophylaxis because no scientific benefit has ever been identified. Only in patients who are at high risk, such as immunocompromised patients, is prophylaxis still recommended. That being said, it is still common practice by some dentists and orthopedic surgeons. Frequently the dentist will defer to the surgeon for his or her preference. If prophylaxis is considered, then the use of cephalosporins as opposed to the frequently employed penicillins or erythromycin may be the best selection.

2. If a patient has a prosthetic joint elsewhere in the body (i.e., hip or knee), is it necessary to use prophylaxis if a foot or ankle procedure is being performed? Again, there is little real science to back up any answer to this question. It is probably safest to consider the endocarditis guidelines since the concern is creating a bacteremia that may colonize the joint just as it may the heart valve. To this end, if the procedure is clean and is being performed through surgically prepared skin then, no, it is not necessary. However, if there will be manipulation of infected tissue, then the use of a cephalosporin or antistaphylococcal penicillin may be warranted.

■ *Adverse Effects and Failures of Prophylaxis*

Prophylaxis is not innocuous. If it were, there would be no reason not to use it on everybody. Many of the adverse effects noted in Chapter 9 might be seen. Some of the sequelae of long-term therapy are avoided, but there are other potential pitfalls:

1. Multiresistant organisms may cause an infection despite the prophylaxis against more common, susceptible pathogens. This is also known as *superinfection.*
2. Money may be spent on antibiotics unnecessarily, a significant consideration in this age of cost containment.
3. Occasionally a patient may develop an infection days to weeks after the surgical procedure. This should not necessarily be considered a failure of the prophylactic antibiotic. More likely it is an infection caused by a newly inoculated organism from the environment secondary to a wound dehiscence or the noncompliance of the patient with postoperative instructions (i.e., dressing care).

SUGGESTED READINGS

Cruse PJE: Wound infections: epidemiology and clinical characteristics. In Howard RJ, Simmons RL: *Surgical infectious diseases*, ed 2, p. 319, East Norwalk, Conn., 1988, Appleton & Lange.

Dajani AS, Taubert KA, Wilson W et al: Prevention of bacterial endocarditis. Recommendations by the American Heart Association, *Circulation* 96:358, 1997. Reprinted in *J Am Podiatr Med Assoc* 88(2): 93-104, 1998.

Fisman DN, Reilly DT, Karchmer AW et al: Clinical effectiveness and cost effectiveness of two management strategies for infected total hip arthroplasty in the elderly, *Clin Infect Dis* 32:419, 2001.

Fry DE, editor: *Surgical infections,* Boston, 1995, Little, Brown & Co.

Kernodle DS, Kaiser AB: Postoperative infections and antimicrobial prophylaxis. In Mandell GL, Bennett JE, Dolin R, editors: *Principles and practice of infectious diseases,* ed 5, p. 3177, Philadelphia, 2000, Churchill Livingstone.

Lister J: On the antiseptic principle of the practice of surgery (reprinted), *Rev Infect Dis* 9:421, 1987.

Martone WJ, Nichols RL, editors: Recognition, prevention, surveillance and management of surgical site infections, *Clin Infect Dis* 33(suppl 2): S67-S106, 2001.

NcNeil SA, Nordstrom-Lerner L, Malani PN et al: Outbreak of sternal surgical site infections due to *Pseudomonas aeruginosa* traced to a scrub nurse with onychomycosis, *Clin Infect Dis* 33:317, 2001.

Nelson JP: Prevention of postoperative infection by airborne bacteria. In Gustilo RB, editor: *Orthopedic infections,* p. 75, Philadelphia, 1989, WB Saunders.

Taylor GJ, Bannister GC, Calder S: Perioperative wound infection in elective orthopedic surgery, *J Hosp Infect* 16:241, 1990.

Widmer AF: New developments in diagnosis and treatment of infection in othropedic implants, *Clin Infect Dis* 33(suppl 2): S94, 2001.

Zdeblick TA, Lederman MM, Jacobs MR et al: Preoperative use of povidone-iodine. A prospective, randomized study, *Clin Orthop* 213:211, 1986.

CHAPTER 7

Fungal Infections

When the first edition of this book was published in 1990, there was no reason to include a chapter on fungal infections of the foot. Griseofulvin was the only approved oral medication for onychomycosis, and it had been around for decades with little usage. There was a plethora of topical agents available for tinea pedis, and all of them worked to varying degrees. Frankly, nobody paid much attention to these conditions or would have cared to read about them.

In the mid-1990s, all of this changed with the introduction of oral itraconazole followed quickly by oral terbinafine for the treatment of onychomycosis. The disease nobody thought could be consistently cured was now fully treatable. The frenzy over these new drugs was fueled by the hundreds of millions of dollars spent by the pharmaceutical industry on promotion and education about the disease, the need to treat, and the products themselves. Never had any lower extremity infection received so much attention by "Big Pharma." Things heated up even more at the start of the new decade with the release of ciclopirox 8% lacquer, the first FDA-approved topical therapy for onychomycosis. The competition became fierce and maybe even a little dirty. Good information was often mixed in with bad. Lines blurred between promotion and education.

In terms of patient morbidity, lower extremity fungal infections are just as important as bacterial infections. These are true infectious diseases, not simple cosmetic problems. This chapter examines the issues in dealing with both tinea pedis and onychomycosis.

Background information, mycology, and disease classifications along with the need to treat and therapeutic options will be discussed fairly and objectively.

TINEA PEDIS

Tinea pedis is probably the most common lower extremity infection. The U.S. Department of Health and Human Services has estimated that 5% of the U.S. population has a "foot infection" each year. This definition includes athlete's foot, warts, and other fungal infections. The majority of these infections are probably some variant of tinea pedis. Other studies have actually put the prevalence of tinea pedis three times higher, at close to 15% of the population.

▨ Definition

Tinea pedis is an infection of the skin of the feet caused by the dermatophytic fungi. Synonyms include athlete's foot, ringworm, dermatophytosis, and dermatomycosis.

▨ Dermatophytes

Dermatophytes are fungal organisms that, by definition, cause infection in the skin and can invade stratum corneum and human keratin. There are three genera able to cause human disease that can be placed into this group. These are further broken down into individual species. The clinically important organisms include the following:

1. *Trichophyton*
   a. *T. rubrum*
   b. *T. mentagrophytes*
   c. *T. tonsurans*
2. *Microsporum*
   a. *M. andouinii*
3. *Epidermophyton*
   a. *E. floccosum*

These organisms are sometimes then broken down by their natural reservoirs as the following:

1. Anthrophilic—natural pathogens of humans

2. Zoophilic—natural pathogens of animals
3. Geophilic—organisms found from the soil

Of course most human disease, and all of the species just listed, are classified as anthrophilic fungi, but the other two types have also been known to cause human disease.

■ *Microbiology of Tinea Pedis*

By far the vast majority of cases of tinea pedis are caused by *T. rubrum* followed by *T. mentagrophytes* and more infrequently, *E. floccosum.* Yeasts, in particular *Candida albicans* and *Candida parapsilosis,* may also be isolated from the foot, especially the interdigital spaces. Of the two, *C. albicans* is the more likely pathogen to cause primary infection of the interdigital spaces. *C. parapsilosis,* along with other *Candida* species, may be isolated as pathogens or, more likely, contaminants.

Some of the saprophytic molds, long thought to be simple contaminants, have also been implicated in causing tinea pedis. *Scytalidium dimidiatum* (formerly *Hendersonula*) or *Scytalidium hyalinum* are the organisms most frequently cited. The argument as to whether these are true pathogens or simply isolated colonizers continues, with many authorities citing "true" cases with just these organisms.

The isolation of bacteria, most frequently from the interspaces, most likely represents colonization of tissue broken down by the fungus as opposed to primary pathogens. *Pseudomonas aeruginosa, Proteus mirablis,* and others are usually cultured from macerated interspaces; thus the concept of "gram-negative tinea." It is impossible to say with certainty, but most likely these represent bacterial colonization superimposed on a case of dermatophytosis complex.

■ *Patient Predilection*

There are many factors that may predispose a particular patient to fungal infections of the foot.

1. Genetics. Zaias has clearly shown a genetic predisposition for fungal infections, which may be passed on by an autosomal dominant trait that causes a cell-mediated deficit in the ability to fight off dermatophyte infections.
2. Environment. Patients who work in areas where their feet are constantly exposed to moisture or who wear shoes for

prolonged periods so that they cannot dry out sufficiently between wearings will become predisposed to developing infection. Moisture of the skin leads to easy access to the stratum corneum, allowing fungal invasion.

3. As previously discussed, the anatomic or physical occlusion of the interdigital spaces will predispose to a dermatophytosis complex development.

■ Clinical Presentation

There have been many descriptions of tinea pedis presentation on the plantar aspect of the foot. The following are the most common:

1. Moccasin type. This is usually caused by *T. rubrum*. It presents as dry scaling skin found in a "moccasin distribution" (i.e., on the plantar aspects of the feet and along the sides to the junction of the plantar and dorsal skin). The lesions are serpiginous with central clearing and peripheral scale, representing the advancing edge of the infection. The lesions usually are bilateral. There may be itching and burning.

2. Vesicular type. This is usually caused by *T. metagrophytes*. This is a more acute, aggressive infection because the organism is more invasive. It presents with inflammation and vesicle formation. The vesicles have a "punctate" look to the roof. On opening, they drain a clear serous fluid and show distinctive septae that run from the roof to the tissue in the base. There is frequently either pain or intense pruritus.

Moccasin tinea pedis that presents on the plantar skin but also interdigitally can be further broken down here as described by Leyden.

1. Dermatophytosis simplex. This presents as dry scaling between the toes. There may or may not be any itching or burning. Frequently the patient is not even aware of its presence. It is commonly found in patients with onychomycosis who may not have evidence of fungal infection elsewhere on their feet.

2. Dermatophytosis complex. When dermatophytosis simplex is put under occlusion, anatomically from toes that are close together, or in shoe or stockings, moisture gets trapped between the toes and a florid infection develops. Maceration, tissue breakdown, and significant inflammation occur that can spread both dorsally and plantarly. There is usually pain and

burning and frequently a foul odor. Bacterial overgrowth occurs and can be cultured even more readily than the fungus. This is an environmental condition. Correction of the environment that caused the occlusion will reverse the process back to a dermatophytosis simplex. Antibiotics are frequently prescribed because of the inflammation that mimics bacterial cellulitis. They are generally *not* indicated.

■ *Diagnosis*

The diagnosis of tinea pedis can be accomplished either clinically or mycologically.

1. Clinical diagnosis. This probably is the most commonly used technique. The lesions are somewhat classical in appearance, as is the history. Frequently the patient is not even aware of the situation, and it is found on routine examination. Treatment is begun on an empiric basis because the organisms are well defined and generally sensitive to all commonly used therapies.
2. Mycologic diagnosis. Mycologic testing is performed either in the clinician's office or through a central laboratory. Three techniques are commonly employed.
   a. KOH preparation. This test is either performed in the office or by the central laboratory. The site of harvesting is important to increase yields. Scales are scraped off the skin from the leading edge of the lesion and placed on a microscope slide with 10% to 20% potassium hydroxide. This dissolves the keratin while leaving the fungal elements intact. Frequently gentle heat or dimethyl sulfoxide (DMSO) is used to accelerate the process. Various dyes or inks may be combined with the KOH to make visualization easier. The slide is then examined under the microscope for the presence of fungal hyphae or other elements. This will not identify the genus or species of the organism, just its presence.
   b. Fungal culture. Again, this either is performed in the office or in a central laboratory. This test is more definitive because it allows identification of the exact organism that is found from the specimen. Notice that the words "causing the infection" are not used because the potential always exists for contamination as opposed to true infection. Various specific media can be used to perform the culture.

(1) Dermatophyte test media (DTM). This is the most frequently used medium in an office setting. It is basically a dermatophyte-specific growth agar along with a color indicator. The specimen is placed with the underside of the lesion or nail in contact with the agar, and the cap is loosely replaced. If the medium turns red, then the organism is most likely a dermatophyte.

(2) Sabouraud's agar. This is an all-purpose nutrient agar for growing fungi–including dermatophytes and molds.

(3) Mycosel agar. This essentially is Sabouraud's agar containing cyclohexamide and antibiotics to inhibit the growth of bacteria and molds. It is more specific for dermatophytes.

c. Wet mount. Once the organism grows in the culture, it can frequently be identified by looking at its colony morphology on the media. If this is not specific enough, then a wet mount must be performed. Basically, some fungus is teased away from the colony and mixed with lactophenol cotton blue, a stain that makes the fungi easier to visualize. This then is examined under the microscope. This must be done by a skilled mycologist schooled in the microscopic morphology of different organisms.

There is no fast and easy automated testing procedure that can produce a completed identification in a matter of hours as there is when one deals with bacteria. Fungal culture and identification is a time-consuming science that can takes weeks to physically perform and requires a skilled mycologist to individually identify each organism.

■ *Fungal Sensitivities*

Unlike bacterial culture and sensitivity testing, sensitivities for fungus are not routinely performed.

1. The National Committee on Clinical Laboratory Standards (NCCLS) has no set standards for dermatophyte sensitivity testing. There are guidelines for yeast, cryptococcus, and some molds.

2. Only a handful of specialty laboratories perform testing. The focus tends to be on in vitro testing for new antifungal drugs as opposed to regular testing of patient isolates.

3. Unlike with bacteria, there is unknown correlation between in vitro sensitivity and clinical efficacy. Many more variables come into play, so the laboratory findings are not directly relevant.

4. Unlike with bacteria, there is little fear of resistance development with the fungi. Although some resistance has been reported in some *Candida* strains, it is not clinically relevant in dealing with dermatophytes. Therefore testing of individual patient isolates is unnecessary. Antifungal activity against one specific species (i.e., *T. rubrum*) can be translated into sensitivity for all isolates of that species.

■ *Treatment*

When one considers the treatment of any infectious disease, it is necessary to consider the natural history and epidemiology of that disease. This can be broken into three components; there is a constant balancing act among them. Each one needs to be considered to successfully treat the disease. Some are more easily modified than others.

1. Host. This is by far the most difficult to modify. The genetic predisposition of these patients is not easy to change. Therefore more care must be paid to affecting the other two elements. Fortunately, this is relatively easy to accomplish in fungal disease treatment.

2. Environment. This may be one of the easiest aspects to change. By keeping the patient's feet dry, there is a good chance that the environment will not be favorable for fungal invasion. Keeping the patient in an environment that presents little opportunity for infection, such as changing shoes regularly and using fungicidal sprays and powders in the shoes, will help eliminate spores that can lead to infection. Refraining from walking barefoot in public areas, especially swimming pool decks or hotel carpets (areas known to harbor fungal organisms) can also be helpful.

3. Pathogen. This may be the easiest component to master. There are many effective topical and systemic antifungal agents available both by prescription and over the counter. These all work well against dermatophytic organisms with variable activity against yeast and nondermatophyte molds and come in different formulations including creams, gels,

solutions, sprays, and powders. They are available in forms to be used once or twice a day. They are approved anywhere from 7 days to more than 3 weeks.

Once the visible fungal infection is eliminated from the skin, a concerted effort must be made to control the environment and prevent reinfection with the pathogen. Curing one bout of tinea pedis without follow-up examination will guarantee either a return visit from a less-than-satisfied, reinfected patient, or, worse yet, a patient who will go to a different physician for definitive care.

■ *Antifungal Agents for Tinea Pedis*

Antifungal agents used for the treatment of tinea pedis fall into many different categories. The majority are either imidazole or allylamine compounds, with other groups also being represented by excellent, effective drugs. All these drugs have been shown to be effective in multiple controlled trials for the treatment of tinea pedis. Comparative trials that looked at two drugs within the same class or compared drugs of different classes all showed essentially good activity. The major differences are in the amount of time needed for treatment, frequency of application, and side benefits such as antiinflammatory activity. It should also be noted that most drugs have been tested for interdigital tinea only. Moccasin tinea, being more chronic and difficult to eradicate, is only sometimes included in the clinical trials. All these drugs are extremely safe. The only reported adverse events were occasional local skin reactions such as burning or redness.

Many of these preparations are available in various forms. These include creams, solutions, and gels.

1. Creams. This is the most common formulation and tends to be somewhat moisturizing and soothing. They usually are used for plantar involvement. If used between the toes, care should be taken to avoid heavy applications that may cause occlusion and maceration.
2. Gels. These tend to be alcohol-based preparations. They are cool upon application and dry as they evaporate. For this reason they are particularly useful for interdigital or other moist areas that would benefit from their drying action. Because of the alcohol content, care should be taken to avoid fissured or otherwise broken skin because gels can cause significant, yet temporary stinging.

3. Solutions. Solutions are essentially a compromise between creams and gels. Most are water-based, although some alcohol-based solutions are available. The water-based products are less likely to cause stinging and can also be used, but probably less effectively, to dry out interspaces. When solutions are available as sprays, large areas of skin can be covered more easily, and therefore solutions are mostly used for diseases such as tinea versicolor on the trunk.

The agents listed subsequently are all topical therapies. Oral antifungals are very useful and effective in the treatment of tinea pedis, but only one, griseofulvin, is approved for that use. All the oral agents will be included in the discussion on onychomycosis. Furthermore, there are a number of "natural" or "nontraditional" treatments for tinea pedis such as tea tree oil (*Melaleuca alternifolia*) that have been shown to be effective therapies. Their exclusion is not meant to diminish their usefulness. They are not included in the list because this chapter discusses only approved drug therapies. The following are listed alphabetically by class. See Table 7-1 for further information on dosing and duration.

Allylamines

The allylamine antifungals are fungicidal agents that work by inhibiting fungal squalene epoxidase. As a general statement, probably because of the cidal activity, these drugs tend to be required for shorter periods than the azoles to achieve a cure. All are in 1% preparations.

Butenafine (Mentax)—Indicated for interdigital tinea twice daily for 1 week or once daily for 4 weeks. This is probably one of the lesser-known agents in this class, having no particular advantage over other drugs. It is available as a cream in 15 and 30 g.

Naftifine (Naftin)—The first of the allylamines that was made available for treatment of tinea pedis. Indicated for once-daily (cream) or twice-daily (gel) treatment of tinea for up to 4 weeks. It is available as a cream in 15, 30, and 60 g and as a gel in 20-, 40-, and 60-g tubes.

Terbinafine (Lamisil AT)—Probably the best known and most used of all of the topical allylamines, this is an extremely effective drug for all cases of tinea pedis including moccasin. It is approved for twice-daily, 1-week use for interdigital tinea and twice-daily, 2-week use for moccasin. This drug went over the counter (OTC) within the last few years, making it less desirable for patients with insurance coverage for prescriptions. It tends to be the most

Topical Antifungals

TABLE 7-1

Drug	Times Per Day	Duration	Dosage Forms
Butenafine (Mentax)	Twice	1 wk	Cream
	Once	4 wk	15, 30 g
Naftifine (Naftin)	Once (cream)	Up to 4 wk	Cream: 15, 30, 60 g
	Twice (gel)		Gel: 20, 40, 60 g
Terbinafine (Lamisil AT)	Twice	1 wk—interdigital	Cream: 12, 24 g
		2 wk—moccasin	Spray: 30 ml
Clotrimazole (Lotrimin AF)	Twice	4 wk	Cream: 12 g
			Solution: 10 ml
Clotrimizole+betamethasone (Lotrisone)	Twice	Up to 4 wk	Cream: 15, 45 g
			Lotion: 30 ml
Econazole (Spectazole)	Once	Up to 4 wk	Cream: 15, 30, 85 g
Ketoconazole (Nizoral)	Once	Up to 6 wk	Cream: 15, 30, 60 g
Oxiconazole (Oxistat)	Once or twice	Up to 4 wk	Cream: 15, 30, 60 g
Sulconazole (Exelderm)	Twice	Up to 4 wk	Cream: 15, 30, 60 g
Ciclopirox (Loprox)	Twice	Up to 4 wk	Cream: 15, 30, 90 g
			Gel: 30, 45 g
			Lotion 30, 60 ml

expensive OTC. It is available as a cream in 12 and 24 g and as a spray solution in 30 ml.

Azoles

The azole antifungals are primarily considered fungistatic agents that work by inhibiting ergosterol synthesis. Because many of these are older drugs, they tend to be less expensive than the allylamines. The success and relative cost of these drugs may be dependent on the length of time they are used. All are in 1% preparations unless noted.

Clotrimazole (Lotrimin AF)—One of the venerable older azoles, which has been OTC for many years. Compared to some of the newer drugs, this is a relatively weak antifungal that needs to be used twice a day for a prolonged period, but it is inexpensive. Many patients come to the physician's office already having been on this drug. It is used twice daily for up to 4 weeks and is available OTC as a cream in 12 g and as a solution in 10 ml.

Clotrimazole and betamethasone dipropionate 0.05% (Lotrisone)—This combination of an antifungal and a relatively high-potency topical steroid seemingly offers "one-stop shopping" as a dermatologic preparation. The antifungal would take care of the infection; the steroid would take care of the inflammation and itch that may be present. For this reason it has gained wide acceptance. The problem is that there are more effective antifungals on the market, and most of the time the steroid is redundant because the symptoms resolve quickly with an effective therapy for the infection without the attendant possible risks of long-term use of the steroid. It is used twice daily for up to 4 weeks and is available as a cream in 15 and 45 g and as a lotion in 30 ml.

Econazole (Spectazole)—Probably the most popular and widely used prescription azole antifungal for tinea pedis by podiatrists and dermatologists. This is a broad-spectrum drug with activity against dermatophytes and most yeast. It also has the advantage of once-daily use; however, it needs to be applied for up to 4 weeks. It is available as a cream in 15-, 30-, and 85-g tubes.

Ketoconazole (Nizoral)—A broad-spectrum topical antifungal (also available as an oral) that works against dermatophytes and yeasts. It is indicated for once-daily treatment of tinea pedis but for a 6-week course. It is available as a 2% cream in 15-, 30-, and 60-g tubes.

Miconazole—One of the oldest azole antifungals, it is now available as an OTC product with many different brand names in many different formulations.

Oxiconazole (Oxistat)—A fairly standard azole antifungal that is indicated for once- or twice-daily dosing for 4 weeks. It is available as a cream in 15-, 30-, and 60-g tubes and as a 30-ml lotion.

Sulconazole (Exelderm)—Another standard azole antifungal that is approved for tinea pedis. It is applied twice daily for 4 weeks and comes in 15-, 30-, and 60-g tubes.

Hydroxpyridone

This unique class of antifungal does not inhibit sterol biosynthesis as do the other two. This is a fungicidal drug with a complex mechanism of activity based on the chelation of trivalent cations.

Ciclopirox (Loprox)—A broad-spectrum drug that is effective against dermatophytes, yeasts, molds, and even gram-positive and gram-negative bacteria. It is fungicidal and sporicidal. It also has the unique property of being antiinflammatory, with induced sunburn studies showing antiinflammatory activity on par with mild potency topical corticosteroids. It is prepared as a 0.77% cream, lotion, and gel and is available in 30- and 45-g gels, 15-, 30-, and 90-g creams, and 30- and 60-ml lotions.

ONYCHOMYCOSIS

Onychomycosis is one of the most common conditions seen by clinicians who treat the lower extremity. Some pertinent facts and figures:

1. Onychomycosis affects 5% to 15% of the U.S. population.
2. The incidence increases in the elderly, with almost 50% of patients more than 70 years old being infected.
3. Patients with diabetes are two to three times more likely to have onychomycosis than those without diabetes.
4. Patients with diabetes who have onychomycosis have a significantly higher incidence of foot ulceration and foot gangrene than those without onychomycosis.
5. The average podiatric physician sees approximately 160 patients per month with this condition.

6. Medicare spent almost $250 million in 1999 just on debridement of mycotic toenails.

Contrary to the beliefs of many patients, physicians, and especially insurance companies, onychomycosis is *not* a cosmetic problem. It is a real infection that has significant medical and psychosocial affects on a patient. There are many published studies that have used statistically validated quality-of-life questionnaires. Probably the most important was by Lynn Drake who found the following:

1. Forty-eight percent of patients with onychomycosis had pain.
2. Thirty-eight percent had difficulty wearing shoes.
3. Seventy-four percent were embarrassed by their nails, leading to secondary issues like fear of intimacy and fear of contagion.
4. Forty percent related pressure from their nails.
5. During a 6-month period, 1.8 medical visits per patient were required for treatment of this disease.

Any disease that causes almost one half of patients to relate pain is a significant problem that needs aggressive, appropriate therapy. Given the prevalence of this infection, the possible co-morbidities, and the effects on quality of life, the point cannot be stressed enough that this is not *just* a cosmetic condition.

■ Definitions

1. Onychomycosis. This is a general term that means any fungal infection of the nail. It is not specific for which type of fungus or yeast may be causing the infection.
2. Tinea unguium. This means specifically a fungal infection of the nail caused by the dermatophytes.

Although most of the cases of toenail infection are caused by the dermatophytes, the term *onychomycosis* is more generally used in practice and will therefore be the default terminology used in this section.

■ Microbiology of Onychomycosis

There has been great debate over the causative organisms for onychomycosis of the toenails. Various authors and lecturers have claimed that these infections are primarily dermatophyte, mixed dermatophyte and saprophytic mold, yeast, mostly saprophytic mold, and every other conceivable combination. A critical look at the literature reveals the following:

1. Most published authors agree that more than 90% of toenail onychomycosis is "caused" by dermatophytes.
2. The saprophytic molds are frequently isolated from nail cultures, but it is difficult to prove that they actually caused the infection. It is assumed that they are contaminants living off of nail previously destroyed by the dermatophytes.
3. If very strict criteria of "causation" are used (i.e., repeat isolation of a specific nondermatophyte organism, failure to culture a dermatophyte on repeat attempts), then some of the molds may be implicated in causing disease. The following molds are most frequently indicted:
    a. *Scopulariopsis brevicaulis*
    b. *Scytalidium dimidiatum*
    c. *Aspergillus* species
4. *Candida* is a relatively rare cause of toenail onychomycosis. It remains a major cause of paronychia and infection in fingernails.
5. There are bacterial infections that can mimic the changes seen in onychomycosis. In particular, *P. aeruginosa* can cause a dark green discoloration of the nail that, on superficial examination, may mimic onychomycosis.

■ *Clinical Presentation and Classification*

The classification system most widely used in describing the clinical presentation of onychomycosis was first described by Zaias. This original system has been altered and modified through the years by various authors. It is also descriptive of both toenail and fingernail onychomycosis and therefore is not directly applicable for lower extremity purposes. However, the basics still remain. There are three clinical presentations of onychomycosis generally seen in the toenail.

1. Distal subugual onychomycosis (DSO)—By far the most common presentation. The infection begins in the skin around the nail unit. Some unspecified trauma causes a break in the seal between the nail and the nail bed at the distal hypony-

chium. The fungus can then invade into the nail bed stratum corneum. As the fungus produces hyperkeratosis (the scaling that is seen on the skin), this builds up under the nail plate, lifting the plate from its attachments. As the plate is lifted from distal to proximal, the fungus can then progress into newly exposed nail bed. This is most commonly caused by *T. rubrum*. Onychomycosis, in particular DSO, is an infection of the nail bed stratum corneum. It is not actually an infection of the nail plate. Furthermore, onychomycosis does not cause long-term changes to the nail matrix, as does psoriasis. This is why treatment that addresses the fungal infection can result in a clinically normal-appearing nail. The clinical presentation is one of a progressively thickening, discolored, crumbly nail plate with significant subungual debris. At least two variations of this condition have been described.

   a. Lateral subungual onychomycosis—Basically the same condition, but instead of the invasion occurring distally, it occurs laterally.

   b. Total dystrophic onychomycosis—A condition that starts as DSO but eventually involves the entire nail plate.

2. White superficial onychomycosis (WSO)—The pathophysiology of this condition is a direct invasion of the superficial dorsal layers of the nail by *T. mentagrophytes*. This is a much more aggressive organism capable of implanting itself into the nail plate and causing direct damage to the plate. It presents as a "chalky" white appearance on the outer surface of the nail. The nail is not actually thickened as seen in DSO. Because there is no subungual invasion, there is no debris.

3. Proximal white onychomycosis. This is an infection of the proximal portion of the nail unit as opposed to the distal or superficial invasions discussed in the other two classes. It is proposed that the fungus invades under the nail from the eponychium or posterior nail fold. There has been a very specific correlation between this presentation and infection with human immunodeficiency virus (HIV). Although most commonly seen in these patients, it is not limited to only HIV-infected individuals. The most common causative organism is *T. rubrum*.

Treatment Implications of Classification

Classifying the different presentations of onychomycosis is not just an academic, intellectual exercise. There are very specific treatment implications for each of these conditions. (Complete discussions on treatment are found in a later section.)

1. Because DSO is an infection of the nail bed stratum corneum, therapy must be directed at the nail bed. Until recently, with the availability of ciclopirox lacquer, topical medications were mostly unable to penetrate through the nail to attack the fungus where it lives. Nail debridement, including thinning, or total removal, may potentiate treatment, allowing this medication to get to the stratum corneum.
2. Lateral involvement is often more difficult to treat because the nail may be detached from the bed at the lateral margins, making oral antifungal therapy less effective.
3. Totally dystrophic nails often grow in thickness as opposed to length. These nails may take much longer to cure, if they can be cured at all, because the total nail is involved and they are much thicker. Few if any antifungal clinical trials have even allowed these nails to be included because uninvolved new nail growth at the proximal portion had to be demonstrated.
4. WSO has always been the most amenable to topical therapies because the infection is in the outermost portion of the nail. Nail debridement and removal are usually unnecessary. Oral therapies tend not to be as effective.
5. Patients with proximal white onychomycosis need to be treated aggressively because there may be even more significant medical and/or psychosocial implications to their disease. Also, the underlying immunodeficiency needs to be addressed adequately.

■ *Diagnosis*

Some of the principles of diagnosis and fungal testing are the same regardless of whether the patient presents with onychomycosis or tinea pedis. The preceding statements made about KOH, fungal cultures, identification, and sensitivities hold true whether one is trying to make a mycologic diagnosis of skin or nail disease. However, the diagnosis of onychomycosis is complicated by a few other factors.

Recently issued FDA guidelines stress the need for proper laboratory evaluation of the nail specimen before beginning oral antifungal therapy.

1. Clinical diagnosis. This is an area of great debate in the literature. Some authors believe that the clinical diagnosis of onychomyco-

sis cannot be made on a reliable basis, while others believe that an experienced clinician can make a correct call the vast majority of the time. In fact, a commonly quoted "factoid" is that only 50% of nail dystrophies are caused by fungus, with the rest being caused by a plethora of other conditions. Therefore a differential diagnosis must be considered, including the following:

a. Psoriasis—complicated by the fact that a patient can have a psoriatic nail with superimposed fungus infection
b. Lichen planus
c. Pityriasis rubra pilaris
d. Darier's disease
e. Malignancy
f. Posttraumatic changes
g. Congenital conditions (i.e., pachyonychia congenita)

The fact is most of these are extremely rare conditions, while onychomycosis is extremely common. This is especially true in special populations, such as older adults and diabetics seen by most clinicians. Therefore most of the time a dystrophic nail probably will be caused by mycosis.

2. Mycologic diagnosis. To ensure that the dystrophic nail that is clinically suspected of having a fungal infection is indeed infected, it is necessary to perform a KOH and fungal culture. As mentioned earlier, these tests are the same as described previously for tinea pedis. The important difference comes in the harvesting of the specimen. Since most clinicians do not perform these tests in their offices, it is necessary to ensure that the clinical laboratory gets everything it needs to make an accurate diagnosis of the true infecting pathogen. This can be accomplished by adhering to the following guidelines.

a. Wipe the nail with alcohol before starting the culture. This simple step will decrease the possibility of skin bacteria contaminating the specimen.
b. Debride away the distal end of the nail and *discard*. The distal nail area is most likely contaminated with saprophytic molds and bacteria. Live dermatophytes are seldom found in this tissue.
c. Using a curette, harvest the specimen for culture from the *most proximal subungual debris*. Since the infection is in the nail bed stratum corneum, the debris represents the shedding, fungal-laden tissue.

d. Send as much material as possible. A common error clinicians make is sending in a few dusty flakes of material. The more material, the better the chance of recovery. Also, a lack of material may preclude the laboratory from doing all the necessary tests.

3. Histologic diagnosis. On occasion, the laboratory may not be able to recover any fungal organisms on culture or KOH. This does not mean that the dystrophic nail is not onychomycotic. Confounding factors, such as previous antifungal treatment, lack of adequate specimen, or a specimen submitted that does not contain an organism, all can contribute to this negative result. In these cases a specialty laboratory may be able to confirm the diagnosis based on a histologic sectioning of the material followed by special preparation with a stain such as periodic acid-Schiff (PAS), which may allow direct visualization of the organism. Recent studies have pointed to this technique as being a rapid and accurate test.

■ *Treatment*

For decades manual debridement with the occasional surgical permanent excision was the mainstay of therapy for these thickened, painful, unsightly, mycotic nails. Although effective in reducing the thickness and the pain, these approaches did little to address the underlying fungal infection. Patients needed to return on a regular basis for maintenance care. The refrain "if only I could invent a treatment for these nails I would be rich!" was once heard by clinician and patient alike. No effective topical antifungal therapy was available. The only oral agent approved by the FDA was griseofulvin, which, whether right or wrong, had developed such a bad reputation that few doctors or patients wanted to even try it. All of this began to change in the mid-1990s with the introduction of new oral antifungals, itraconazole and terbinafine, that could effectively and safely for the first time actually cure onychomycosis. The FDA approval of ciclopirox 8% lacquer, the first topical agent, followed, giving the clinician a choice of effective treatment modalities. Today, available approaches include manual debridement, surgical treatment, topical antifungals, oral antifungals, and various combinations of all four.

Manual Debridement

Debridement remains the mainstay of onychomycosis management for many podiatric clinicians. Podiatric physicians performed more than 7 million debridement services for Medicare patients alone in 1999. Although an invaluable aspect of onychomycosis management, debridement does not address the fungal infection that caused the problem. Essentially, "debridement is not treatment." Furthermore, because of the attempt of the clampdown by the Office of the Inspector General (OIG) to prosecute practitioners for incorrect billing of these services, one can go even further. "Debridement is not treatment, and you can't get payment!" There are pros and cons:

Pros

1. Debridement is useful in reducing the "fungal load" of the nail.
2. Debridement thins the nail, making it more comfortable because it reduces pressure from shoes.
3. Reduction in shoe pressure leads to a lower probability of nail bed ulcerations.
4. Debridement can temporarily improve the appearance of the nail.
5. Thinning of the nail allows some topical agents to penetrate better.
6. Some patients are unable to take oral medications or apply topicals. It is therefore the only available therapy.
7. It is relatively inexpensive and safe, with no concerns about adverse effects or drug interactions.

Cons

1. Debridement does nothing to "cure" the problem. It does not actually treat the fungus directly.
2. Since the fungus is not getting treated, the thickness recurs, making continual return visits, *ad infinitum*, necessary. (Some may actually consider this a bonus because it ensures a steady flow of patients into the office.)
3. Patients may get frustrated with the lack of a cure.
4. Debridement codes are coming under increased scrutiny. Unreasonable demands on diagnostic criteria and charting, not to mention the constant threat of an audit, make routine use of this procedure, while safe for the patient, risky to the clinician.

Surgical Treatment

Before the availability of the oral or topical antifungals, if a patient was tired of having routine debridement performed and wanted a permanent solution, the only answer was surgical removal of the nail plate. This could take two forms.

1. Removal of the nail followed by topical antifungal therapy. The thought was that if the nail was removed, any topical cream could be used on the nail bed to kill the fungus. This would allow new nail to grow in on a clean bed. The problem with this viewpoint was that the surgery would occasionally damage the nail bed and nail matrix, and the new nail would grow in dystrophic, although mycologically clear.
2. Nail removal with matricectomy. This permanent removal of the nail and matrix prevents a new nail from growing in. Often the patient develops some hyperkeratosis over the nail bed, which looks very much like a new nail.

Pros

1. If a patient has severe pain from an extremely dystrophic, thickened, and ingrown nail, permanent removal can be the treatment of choice.
2. It is especially effective for single nail involvement where oral antifungals may be judged to be overkill.
3. It is usually a satisfactory cosmetic result even with the nail permanently removed.
4. It is useful for a patient desiring a permanent solution but unwilling or unable to take oral antifungals or to apply daily topical therapy.

Cons

1. Invasive procedures come with all of the attendant risks, including anesthesia.
2. It is painful. Even under the best of conditions and with the best surgeons, despite claims to the contrary, this procedure may cause some significant postoperative discomfort.
3. There is a possibility of postoperative bacterial infection that could lead to osteomyelitis, the need for prolonged antibiotics, and possible surgical resection of bone. This is a remote possibility, but it happens.
4. Some patients are not comfortable with the concept of losing a nail. They think that it is necessary for everyday functioning.

Topical Antifungals

Over the years many topical products have been claimed to be effective for the treatment of onychomycosis. A number of OTC products could be found in any pharmacy, usually placed next to the cash register. Then, in the early 1990s, the FDA released a position statement that no topical antifungal agent could make claims for the treatment of nail fungus because they had never been formally studied or approved. Overnight, these OTC products were removed from the shelves, only to find their way back in a matter of weeks to months with new names and new labels. Then, instead of saying that they were effective for nail fungus, instead the product manufacturers would recommend application to the skin around the nail or would label the product as useful for the treatment of tinea pedis while showing toenails in their advertisements. The letter of the law was certainly being followed, if not the intent.

As with the previous section on tinea pedis, there are many "alternative" topical therapies for onychomycosis that have varying degrees of support in the medical literature, on the Internet, and in the press. Tea tree oil has again appeared, as has Vicks VapoRub; urine soaks; as well as numerous products with evocative names such as Pretty Nail, Compound N, Mycocide, and FungiNail. Each of these compounds enjoys its share of support. However, because this chapter's purpose is to provide medical information on approved therapies, they will not be covered.

Meanwhile, throughout Europe and other parts of the world, there are many formally approved topical therapies being used. Compounds containing antifungals in different preparations or antifungals in combination with agents used to soften nails are available. Drugs such as amorolfine, tioconazole, and bifonazole plus urea are widely used and studied. Some, most likely amorolfine, may eventually make it into the United States. In 2000 ciclopirox nail lacquer 8% became the first compound formally approved by the FDA in the United States for the topical treatment of onychomycosis. Before its approval, it had been available in 41 countries for almost 9 years.

Ciclopirox Nail Lacquer 8% (Penlac)

According to its official labeling, ciclopirox lacquer is indicated for mild to moderate onychomycosis without lunula involvement caused by dermatophytes. Two identical double blind, randomized, placebo-controlled, multicenter studies were submitted to the FDA as the pivotal trials. Entry criteria for the studies were as listed on the package insert. Efficacy evaluation criteria were unusually strict for an onychomycosis trial and included three levels: mycologic cure, almost cured (defined as less than 10% involvement at the end of the trial), and complete cure (defined as 0% involvement at the end of the trial). Percent involvement was calculated using a very exact computerized planimetry technique previously used in diabetic ulceration trials. Package insert efficacy rates are listed as a complete cure of up to 8.5% and an almost cure of up to 12%. Subsequent meta-analysis of multiple clinical trials throughout the world place the clinical success rate at a respectable approximately 68%.

Ciclopirox is available as an 8% clear lacquer in 3.3-ml and 6.6-ml bottles. It is applied once daily to affected nail(s) for 6 to 9 months, up to 48 weeks, or until the nail clears. Removal of excess buildup with alcohol or nail polish remover should be done every 7 to 10 days. Routine debridement of buildup will help penetration.

Pros
1. Ciclopirox is useful as an alternative therapy in patients who refuse to take oral antifungals or cannot take oral antifungals for medical reasons.
2. Topical application is preferred by many patients over taking pills.
3. It has practically no side effects or drug interactions.
4. Ciclopirox (see previous section on tinea pedis) is a broad-spectrum antimicrobial active against dermatophytes, yeasts, molds, and bacteria.
5. It has been shown in two studies to penetrate the nail plate to the level of the nail bed.
6. It may be useful as a prophylactic agent to prevent recurrence of infection in previously cleared nails.
7. It is less costly than oral therapy.
8. It has meta-analysis efficacy rates that approach those seen with oral antifungals.
9. In some studies the combination of ciclopirox lacquer plus an oral agent has been shown to increase the efficacy over oral therapy alone.

Cons
1. It is not as effective as oral agents in achieving cures.

2. It may not be covered by the patient's insurance plan as readily as an oral agent.
3. Daily application along with the need to remove buildup every 7 to 10 days and regular nail debridement can lead to lack of compliance in the long run.
4. Its slower results than those with the orals may discourage some patients.
5. Patients who wish to use toenail polish need to accommodate for this therapy because it cannot be applied on top of nail polish.

Oral Antifungals

Clinicians hoped that the introduction of itraconazole followed quickly by terbinafine in the mid-1990s would revolutionize the oral treatment of onychomycosis. Before these approvals, the only oral agents used in the treatment of onychomycosis were griseofulvin and ketoconazole. Because of perceived toxicities and less than stellar results with these two drugs, they received poor acceptance by most clinicians. Unfortunately, they also developed a thought paradigm in many clinicians' minds that oral antifungals were dangerous, expensive, and not terribly effective. For this reason, despite the huge amounts of promotional and educational dollars poured into the field by the pharmaceutical industry, the newer oral agents have not lived up to their potential. By all accounts these are relatively safe, very effective cures for onychomycosis. They represent the gold standard of onychomycosis treatment.

With these newer antifungals having been available on the market for more than 5 years, many common issues still arise whenever they are discussed. The questions and concerns surprisingly have not changed much from when they were introduced. Commonly heard refrains and the appropriate responses include the following:

1. "Oral antifungals are dangerous; they destroy the liver." Actually these newer oral antifungals are relatively safe drugs. There have been very few liver toxicities associated with their use. Even though recent FDA reports have cited a few cases of death and need for liver transplantation, when put in the context of the more than 20 million patients in the United States alone who have been treated, the number of complications are miniscule. Furthermore, some of these patients already had elevated liver functions that were never checked

before they started the drugs. This is not meant to minimize the issue, but rather to stress the need for proper monitoring and respect for *any* systemic drug administered to a patient.

2. "There are too many drug-drug interactions to worry about." This certainly is more true with itraconazole than with terbinafine. However, very few of these interactions are actual contraindications. They may be of little clinical importance, especially if "pulse" dosing is used. If a patient is taking many other drugs, either consider terbinafine or topical therapy. However, frequently the patient desiring treatment is on no other medications, making this a non-issue.

3. "They are too expensive, running upwards of $800/course." Yes, these drugs *are* expensive. However, their cost can be decreased by using the abundance of samples that have been distributed or by creative dosing schedules, such as pulse dosing. Furthermore, when considering that these are the most effective treatments currently available, the $800 buys 3 months of pills, but the medication is effectively in the nail for 6 to 9 months, and the price should buy a "cure" for a chronic condition the patient has lived with for years, the patient may reconsider the cost objection. Also, the cost of treating the concomitant tinea pedis will be eliminated because this disease is usually cured by oral antifungals.

4. "Insurance won't pay for them." Many insurance plans will, in fact, cover oral antifungal therapy. Some require preauthorization or an underlying medical condition such as diabetes. Some will dictate which drug you need to use or require certain confirmatory tests before giving approval. Granted, this is a major hassle for no direct financial return to the doctor. Finally, if not covered at all, it has been shown in studies that many patients are willing to pay cash for a cure. While it is never a good idea to subject a patient to "sticker shock" at the pharmacy, it is equally a bad idea to presuppose that a patient is unwilling to pay for a cure out of his or her own pocket. Refer to the previous answer.

5. "Why should the patient spend the money to treat the nails when the infection will just come back?" As is true with tinea pedis, these patients are probably genetically predisposed to develop a fungal infection. This does not mean that treatment should be withheld. A cure is still possible. This needs to be followed by long-term preventive maintenance. These patients become patients for life. Furthermore, some long-term studies

have shown maintenance of cures 3 to 5 years after stopping therapy. Thus a medication is given for only 3 months to treat a long-term problem, and 3 to 5 years later the patient is still asymptomatic.

6. "If I cure the onychomycosis, I will 'cure' away my practice." Without a doubt, this is the most short-sighted and naive objection that has ever been raised, and it is surprisingly frequent. It is the responsibility of a physician to cure the patient, if possible. Maintaining a patient in a state of "suspended animation" when an effective treatment is available for the sole purpose of individual financial gain is unethical at best and immoral at worst. Furthermore, curing these patients will not destroy a practice. As mentioned in answer 5, these patients require lifelong maintenance, and they are an excellent source of referrals because their chronic condition has been successfully treated.

7. "My patients have been told not to take them by their primary care doctor." Many primary care providers are less well versed on the issues surrounding the importance of treating onychomycosis and the safety of available agents than the foot care provider. This becomes a positive educational/communications opportunity rather than a negative.

Monitoring Therapy

Despite pharmaceutical representative claims to the contrary, it is an excellent idea to monitor liver function tests (LFTs) and white blood counts on any antifungal therapy. The single most important test is a baseline test. In FDA reports of deaths due to these drugs, frequently the patients never had any baseline testing to detect a liver abnormality before beginning the drug. Depending on the drug, most recommendations call for any one baseline LFT level of twice top level of "normal-range" to be a contraindication to beginning therapy. This was generally what was used in the various clinical trials as exclusion criteria. Some clinicians are not comfortable with levels this high, so options include:

1. Hold therapy for 1 month and recheck in 1 month. Many LFTs elevate in a transient fashion and quickly return to normal.
2. Starting the drug but monitoring more frequently than recommended for further elevations, and stopping the drug if levels continue to rise.

As long as the baseline tests were OK to start the therapy, recommendations for follow-up monitoring vary. Individual recommendations will be listed as needed. However, if LFTs begin to rise or white blood counts begin to drop, similar options present:

1. Wait until levels are twice normal to stop the drug.
2. Continue the drug but monitor more frequently.
3. Stop therapy and recheck in a few weeks.

Oral Antifungal Agents

The following drugs are listed in the order in which they became available, starting with the oldest.

Griseofulvin (Fulvicin, Gris-Peg, Grisactin)

The first of the approved treatments for onychomycosis, it is also useful for the treatment of tinea pedis. Treatment successes in onychomycosis are frequently only reported in the 20% range despite up to 18 months of therapy. At that period, the drug dosing has become prohibitively expensive even if the per-pill cost is lower than newer drugs. The drug is probably safer than it is perceived to be. Side effects include headache, photosensitivity, liver dysfunction, granulocytopenia, and hypersensitivity reactions. Griseofulvin should be avoided in patients on oral contraceptives. There also may be cross sensitivity to penicillins.

Griseofulvin is available in multiple formulations including microsize and ultramicrosize and various amounts, mostly in 250- and 500-mg tablets. Dosing usually for the ultramicrosize is up to 1 g/day given for up to 18 months for onychomycosis. Recently "reintroduced" Gris-Peg is being marketed as a useful treatment for chronic tinea pedis at a dose of 500 mg/day, divided, for 6 to 8 weeks or until the patient is clinically cured.

Pros
1. It is effective short-course therapy for refractory tinea pedis.
2. Its per-pill cost is relatively low.
3. It is probably much safer than its reputation would lead one to believe.

Cons
1. It is fungistatic, allowing organism regrowth upon cessation of therapy.
2. Its efficacy rates for onychomycosis are relatively low.

3. Its course of therapy is protracted, up to 18 months for ony-chomycosis.
4. For the protracted course of therapy, it is extremely expensive for minimal results.

Ketoconazole (Nizoral)

This drug is included solely for completeness' sake. It has been used for onychomycosis. Its official indication is for "severe recalcitrant cutaneous dermatophyte infections" without being specifically labeled for onychomycosis. Given the side effect profile, the potential for serious liver disease/failure with long-term use, and the drug interaction profile, in light of the newer, safer agents, there is *absolutely no use* for this drug in the treatment of onychomycosis.

Fluconazole (Diflucan)

This is a safe, effective oral antifungal that has been in wide use in the medical community for more than a decade. It is considered the drug of choice for many systemic fungal infections, oral thrush, and vaginal candidiasis. It also enjoyed acceptance as a treatment for onychomycosis, despite not having an FDA approval for that purpose, for many years before itraconazole and terbinafine became available. There have been studies looking at this drug for treating onychomycosis, including a pivotal trial submitted to the FDA. That study looked at once-weekly dosing of 150, 300, and 450 mg. All of the dosing forms were found to be effective and safe. Unfortunately, the FDA decided not to approve the drug, purportedly because there were too few patients in any one dosing group to make a determination. Therefore any use of fluconazole for onychomycosis would be considered "off-label." This of course, does not prevent a licensed physician from using it. It appears as efficacious as itraconazole with fewer potential drug interactions.

It is available in a number of strengths and formulations, but the recommended dosing for onychomycosis would be 300 mg once weekly for 6 months.

Pros

1. It has once-weekly dosing.
2. It has fewer adverse events and drug interactions than other azoles.
3. It has the longest track record of any oral antifungal.

Cons
1. It is not FDA-approved for onychomycosis, so usage is off-label.
2. It needs to be used for 6 or more months compared with shorter courses for other orals.

Itraconazole (Sporanox)

The first of the so-called "new" antifungals for the oral treatment of onychomycosis, this drug had almost a 1-year lead over oral terbinafine. Before receiving the onychomycosis indication, it had been available for many years for the treatment of systemic infections including histoplasmosis and blastomycosis. It also received an indication for the treatment of *Aspergillus*. It has excellent activity against *Candida*, including fluconazole-resistant strains. For these reasons the drug is considered to have broader spectrum than other agents. Like terbinafine, itraconazole demonstrates a reservoir effect. Although the pills are only given for 3 months, active levels are found in the nails for 6 to 9 months. The drug is relatively safe and effective; however, the FDA recently released new guidelines that recommend not using it in patients with a history of congestive heart failure. This, on top of its already long list of potential drug-drug interactions, has scared many clinicians away from this useful drug.

This drug's efficacy against onychomycosis is listed in the package insert as a complete cure rate of only 14%. However, as is the case with the ciclopirox lacquer, meta-analysis reveals an overall clinical success rate in the low 70% range.

It is available in 100-mg capsules. Its officially approved dosing is 100 mg twice a day taken with a fatty meal or carbonated beverage to increase absorption. However, by far the most frequent and best way to dose this drug is pulse dosing; this consists of 200 mg (two pills) twice daily (400 mg/day) for 7 days. Patients then are taken off the drug for 21 days and repeat this course for 3 months total. In other words, the drug is taken for 1 week out of each month for 3 months. The rest of the time represents a so-called drug holiday. This form, approved in fingernails but not for toenail onychomycosis, nonetheless has been shown to be the safest and most effective way to dose this drug. It is also readily available with complete instructions for the patient in a commercial "PulsePak."

Recommendations for monitoring have never been conclusive because the pulse therapy is not approved for the foot. However, after baseline, at least one subsequent level should be checked for protection of the physician and the patient.

Pros

1. Pulse dosing is preferable for many patients, especially those who do not like to take medications.
2. Pulse dosing lowers the price over more traditional daily regimens.
3. Broader spectrum against yeasts and molds may yield a perceived advantage over terbinafine, but clinical data are lacking.
4. It is a proven effective antifungal for onychomycosis.
5. Although not FDA approved, a single 1-week pulse is effective in the treatment of moccasin tinea pedis.

Cons

1. There is significant potential for drug-drug interaction because it is a potent inhibitor of Cytochrome P-450 isoenzyme 3A4. The list of drug interactions is long and ever growing with more and more being added, including some frank contraindications. These include lovasatin, simvastatin, triazolam, and midazolam.
2. New warnings against using the drug in patients with congestive heart failure or other cardiac dysfunction further limit the available patients.
3. The FDA has not approved pulse dosing for toenails. This is not a problem for any licensed practitioner; however, some clinicians still worry about this.
4. Itraconazole must be taken with food.
5. Pulse dosing can be confusing to some patients even with explanations.

Terbinafine (Lamisil)

Although the oral form of terbinafine was released many months after itraconazole, this drug had the advantage of being preceded by a topical compound of the same makeup and name. Because of the name recognition that the topical cream enjoyed, its better-perceived efficacy and safety than itraconazole, and an aggressive marketing campaign, oral terbinafine overwhelmingly became the most-used oral antifungal by podiatric physicians, while other specialties, such as dermatology and general practice, were not quite as quick to begin using it. The drug has proven safe and effective without the contraindications or drug interactions of itraconazole. However, as with any drug, there are some drawbacks. Taste disturbances, although possible with either drug, seem to be more frequent and profound with terbinafine. This limits its usefulness in patients who depend on taste for their livelihoods, such as chefs, restaurateurs, or sommeliers. Neutropenia may also be slightly more of an issue with this drug. Both are reversible in the vast majority of cases.

This drug's efficacy is listed in the package insert as a complete cure rate of 38% with meta-analysis again showing overall success rates in the low- to mid-70% range. At least one head-to-head comparison, funded by the manufacturer, showed terbinafine to be significantly more effective than pulse itraconazole, although that sort of difference has not been substantiated in other series.

The drug is available in 250-mg tablets. Usual dosing is 1 pill once daily for 90 days. Pulse regimens of 500 mg/day for 1 week out of the month have been tried, as has every other day for 6 months, with mixed results. There is no difference in taking it with food or not.

Monitoring recommendations again include the need for a baseline. Recently the previous recommendation for retesting at 6 weeks has been lifted by the FDA, so there are no formal recommendations for subsequent testing.

Pros

1. It is probably the most effective antifungal for the treatment of onychomycosis. It may have slightly better efficacy rates than itraconazole.
2. Once-daily dosing is easier for some patients to remember.
3. There are no significant contraindications or drug-drug interactions.
4. It has better activity in vitro against the dermatophytes that cause most onychomycosis.
5. Requirements for interim LFT testing no longer exist; however, CBCs are still suggested for treatment over 6 weeks.
6. Although not FDA approved, it can be used short course (2 to 4 weeks) for recalcitrant moccasin tinea pedis with excellent results.

Cons

1. It is the most expensive oral therapy for onychomycosis.
2. It has the potential for taste disturbances.

SUGGESTED READINGS

De Donker P, Gupta AK, Marynissen G et al: Itraconazole pulse therapy for onychomycosis and dermatomycosis: an overview, *J Am Acad Dermatol* 37:969, 1997.

Drake LA, Scher RK, Smith EB et al: Effect of onychomycosis on the quality of life, *J Am Acad Dermatol* 38(5):702, 1998.

Evans EGV, Sigurgeirsson B: Double blind, randomized study of continuous terbinafine compared with intermittent intraconazole in treatment of toenail onychomycosis, *Br Med J* 318:1031, 1999.

Gupta AK, Fleckman P, Baran R: Ciclopirox nail lacquer topical solution 8% in the treatment of toenail onychomycosis, *J Am Acad Dermatol* 43(4):S70, 2000.

Gupta AK, Konnikov N, MacDonald P et al: Prevalence and epidemiology of toenail onychomycosis in diabetic subjects: a multicentre survey, *Br J Dermatol* 139:665, 1998.

Rippon JW, Fromtling RA, editors: *Cutaneous antifungal agents,* New York, 1993, Marcel Dekker.

Scher RK, Breneman D, Rich P et al: Once weekly fluconazole (150, 300, or 450 mg) in the treatment of distal subungual onychomycosis of the toenail, *J Am Acad Dermatol* 38(6):S77, 1998.

Zaias N, Tosti A, Rebell G: Autosomal dominant pattern of distal subungual onychomycosis caused by *Trichophyton rubrum, J Am Acad Dermatol* 34:302, 1996.

Zaias N: Onychomycosis, *Arch Dermatol* 105:263, 1972.

PART III

Antimicrobial Therapy

CHAPTER 8

Antibiotic Usage

Principles of Antibiotic Selection

The flow of new antibiotics coming to market has slowed considerably from the heydays of the late 1980s and early 1990s. At that time it seemed like a new cephalosporin was being released on a daily basis. Now, in the ever-changing world of bacterial pathogenesis and pharmaceutical development, cephalosporins almost seem passé. Quinolones, once new and exciting panaceas for all that ails the patient, have fallen onto some hard times. A number have been pulled from the market because of adverse reactions. Various bacteria have become resistant to either individual agents or the entire class. Now exciting new classes of drugs, like the oxazolidinones, are taking the market by storm. How can a practicing physician keep abreast of all the new discoveries? How can he or she be certain of selecting the proper agent?

Despite all the hoopla, the basic principles of selection of antibiotics remains unchanged from when the earliest drugs were introduced.

■ Drug of Choice

The definition of what constitutes the drug of choice for any given infection has not changed in the almost 60 years that constitute the "antibiotic era." The drug of choice is that agent characterized by the following:

180

1. It has the narrowest spectrum against the organism(s) isolated. If the therapy is "empiric" (i.e., the organism's identity is not yet known), then using a "best guess" technique to assume the identity of the bug(s) is a legitimate method of selection. This is the "sliver bullet" approach to antibiotic selection. By using the narrowest-spectrum antibiotic, there is theoretically a better chance of hitting the infecting organisms without setting the patient up for resistance development. Also, the narrower the spectrum (generally but not always), the lower the price.

2. It is the safest selection possible. This is not as much of an issue in the treatment of lower extremity infections as it may be with some systemic conditions. The commonly used antibiotics are all fairly safe with few exceptions, such as the aminoglycosides. This class has little use in lower extremity infections for just this reason.

3. It has the lowest cost. This has to take into account the cost of the course of therapy, not just the per-pill (per-gram) cost of drug acquisition. A single pill may be expensive, but when only given once daily for a short course, it may still be less expensive than a significantly cheaper drug given three to four times per day. Furthermore, the cost of an antibiotic is not reflected in the purchase price of the drug alone. The cost of administration, monitoring of therapy, possible toxicities, and extra hospital days for those toxicities must also be figured into the overall expense.

■ *The Microbiology Laboratory*

If one were to track a bacterial culture from the hospital floor or office to the microbiology laboratory to a final result, the procedure would be something like this:

1. Culture material is gathered on a swab, the paperwork is filled out, and a microbiology order is placed for a gram stain, culture, and sensitivity. This is actually the most vital part of the process. The lab needs a good specimen. Collect as much material as possible. Tissue biopsies or samples, bone, and aspirates of purulence will all increase the bacterial yield.

2. The swab is picked up and transported to the lab.

3. The specimen is logged in and given an accession number.

4. The swab is then plated and then smeared onto a number of different solid media (primary plates) to spread out the speci-

men and try to find individual colonies of different types of bacteria. This is then incubated.

5. Anything left on the swab is then placed onto a microscope slide for gram staining.

6. The mostly "spent" culture swab is placed into a tube of a liquid media (broth subculture) that will tend to grow out anything that may be left on it. This is what is meant when a report is returned claiming an organism was found "from broth subculture only."

7. After about 24 hours, the primary plate is examined and individual colonies with unique morphologies are identified and subcultured either onto other plates or placed into the automated identification/susceptibility device. At this point, a trained microbiologist could have a good idea of the identity of the organism just by looking at colony morphology, color, odor, and presence or absence of hemolysis around the colony. If the primary plates are negative, the broth subculture is examined for turbidity. If found to be turbid, it is then subcultured onto a plate. A preliminary report may be produced at this time.

8. Identification is performed as subsequently described.

9. Antibiotic sensitivity of the identified organism is performed through either of the techniques that will be described.

10. The final report is relayed to the clinician.

■ *Identity of the Organism*

The identity of the infecting organism can be ascertained through a number of clinical and laboratory methods:

1. Gram stain
2. Culture and sensitivity
3. Special immunologic techniques including enzyme-linked immounsorbent assay (ELISA) or western blotting
4. Molecular assays such as polymerase chain reaction (PCR)
5. An educated guess as to what might be causing the infection

Some of these more common methods are described in detail in Chapter 1. The bacterial organism must be identified once it is isolated in the laboratory. Most laboratories use automated devices that can biochemically identify an organism and report antibiotic sensitivities within a few hours. Some smaller hospitals and laboratories may still rely on the older methods described here. These more labor-intensive techniques are still used to determine the identity and susceptibility of organisms that may not have been picked up by the automated device or on special request of the clinician. Identification is frequently performed in two steps—a preliminary and a final identification.

Preliminary identification, which is usually available within 12 to 18 hours of initial plating, is performed by a number of methods:

1. Looking at how the organism affects the media (e.g., noting the presence of hemolysis: ß-hemolysis is complete clearing of the blood around the colony; α-hemolysis is a partial clearing that leads to a green discoloration; and γ-hemolysis is no change).
2. Examining colony morphology, including shape, size, color, and odor.
3. Simple biochemical reactions (e.g., the slide coagulase test for staphylococci).

Final identification requires performance of a chain of biochemical reactions, which usually requires an additional period of incubation. This is the reason that many laboratories take up to 48 hours to return a complete culture report.

■ *Susceptibility of the Organism*

Once identified, the organism's sensitivity to a number of antibiotics must be determined. Many years ago this was less important because bacterial resistance was a rare phenomenon. Now, however, any one species of organism can have widely different patterns of antibiotic susceptibility depending on a number of factors:

1. If the organism was acquired in the community, it tends to be more sensitive to antibiotics. However, even this once hard-and-fast rule is changing. Increasing incidence of resistant organisms such as methicillin-resistant *Staphylococcus aureus* (MRSA) is being reported from the community.
2. Infections acquired in the hospital or nursing home, the so-called nosocomial infections, are generally resistant to a large number of antibiotics. There are nosocomial organisms that are resistant to all known antibiotics. These are especially pervasive in intensive care units (ICUs) of major teaching hospitals.

3. Patients having received previous antibiotic therapy tend to have selected more resistant organisms.

Susceptibility patterns also vary widely from one community to another and even from one hospital to another within the same community. For this reason many hospital laboratories will publish an *antibiogram,* which shows any trends developing in antibiotic resistance to aid in empiric therapy. It includes the following:

1. All of the organisms isolated over a given period of time
2. How many of each species are isolated
3. The percentage of each species susceptible to all of the antibiotics that are normally tested

There are two primary methods by which laboratories determine antibiotic sensitivity of various organisms: the disc-diffusion or Kirby-Bauer method and the determination of the minimal inhibitory concentration (MIC), usually through a microdilution technique. Each has its benefits and drawbacks. As previously mentioned, most laboratories are using some type of automated sensitivity device using commercially available antibiotic panels. Because the antibiotic susceptibility panels run by the machines are preset, it may be necessary to order a disc-diffusion test for the organism against a drug not found on the panel. Therefore it is still important to understand the test.

Disc-Diffusion Method

1. The isolated organism is plated onto an antibiotic-free agar plate.
2. Small discs containing a set amount of various antibiotics are laid onto the plate.
3. The plate is incubated for 18 to 24 hours (although some organisms, such as methicillin-resistant *S. aureus*, require longer incubation).
4. A "zone of inhibition" or circle of agar clear of bacterial growth develops around some of the discs.
5. The diameter of this zone is measured in millimeters.
6. The measured diameter is then compared against a standard set by the National Committee for Clinical Laboratory Standards (NCCLS). This standard describes zone diameters for what is considered sensitive, intermediate, and resistant to the antibiotic.

7. The zones must be measured and compared against the standard. A zone that may appear small may define a sensitive strain for that particular antibiotic. Likewise, a large zone around one antibiotic does not mean that the drug is any more effective.

Pros
1. It is easy to perform.
2. It is inexpensive.
3. It seems to give clinically relevant information.
4. It is easy to interpret. All the information given to the physician is a clear-cut answer: yes, it is sensitive, or no, it is not.

Cons
1. The method is strictly qualitative. It cannot determine exactly how effective a drug will be.
2. The technique is more labor-intensive and takes a longer time period than the automated tests.

Minimal Inhibitory Concentration
The MIC is the concentration of antibiotic needed to inhibit visual growth of an organism.

Broth Tube Dilution Technique
The MIC is determined by the broth tube dilution, microdilution, or agar technique. The test employed by the commonly used automated devices is a microdilution method, and all of the following steps are automated as opposed to being performed by hand. All three yield similar results, so the differences are academic and technical rather than practical.

1. An increasing amount of antibiotic is added to each series of tubes containing media.
2. These antibiotic dilutions (in micrograms per milliliter) are generally doubling (i.e., 0.1, 0.2, 0.4, 0.8, 1.6, and so on).
3. A set amount of isolated organism is inoculated into each tube.
4. The tubes are incubated for 18 to 24 hours in a manual method. If automated, the results can be significantly faster.
5. After incubation, the tubes are examined for visual evidence of bacterial growth.
6. The lowest concentration of antibiotic that does not show visual evidence of bacterial growth is determined to be the MIC.

7. The susceptibility of the organism to that drug is determined by comparing the MIC to a set of NCCLS breakpoints. These breakpoints are based on achievable serum levels of the antibiotic.

Pros

1. The method is very precise.
2. It is quantitative. It tells exactly how much antibiotic is needed to inhibit the growth of the organism. Note the use of *inhibit*. The MIC by definition does not determine the amount of antibiotic necessary to *kill* the organism.
3. It is useful in antibiotic selection in very serious infections caused by multiresistant organisms.
4. It is relatively rapid if done by the automated device as opposed to the slower, less specific disc-diffusion method.

Cons

1. It is difficult to interpret unless one is familiar with the technique.
2. If done by hand, it is more expensive to perform and requires more expertise than the disc-diffusion method.
3. The information provided by this method is not really necessary in the treatment of most infections.

MIC Interpretation and Breakpoint

There is much confusion as to what an MIC really means in a clinical setting. Furthermore, the term *breakpoint* has been used when discussing whether an organism will be susceptible to a particular antibiotic. This is true regardless of which technique is used. It is important to understand both of these issues because they are interrelated.

As a raw number, the MIC is useful for comparing the relative effectiveness of one antibiotic to another in an in vitro setting. The MIC number by itself, however, means little in an in vivo clinical setting. When treating a live person with an infection, who really cares if a tube of broth is clear or not?

Traditionally, clinicians are taught that the lower the MIC, the more effective the drug. This would only seem to make sense. If less of a drug is needed to inhibit growth, then it must be "more powerful." Using this logic:

1. Drug A with an MIC against *S. aureus* of 0.1 µg/ml would be much more effective than drug B with an MIC of 1.0 µg/ml (10 times higher). Unfortunately, it is not that easy. The MIC

determination doesn't include some vital information, such as if the drug gets high enough concentrations in the body to be effective. What is its achievable serum level?

2. Using the same example, what happens if drug A is poorly absorbed from the gastrointestinal tract and only achieves a serum level after dosing of 0.4 µg/ml, while drug B is well absorbed and can achieve 256 µg/ml in the serum? Drug A can only achieve a serum level two dilutions (doublings) above its MIC, while drug B's serum level is eight full dilutions above its MIC.

Which would be the smarter choice? Clearly, there is more of drug B available to work against the organism and a greater safety net between how much it would take to inhibit the bug versus how much is in the body.

Because it would be impossible for anybody to have all the facts about serum levels and MICs immediately available when it came time to clinically select an antibiotic, this information has all been calculated and standardized beforehand. The NCCLS has set guidelines (breakpoints) for each drug against each type of organism. These numbers are then used to make a clinical determination as to whether the organism is sensitive or resistant to a given antibiotic. This is then programmed into the laboratory computer that generates the culture and sensitivity (C & S) report. For instance, if the MIC for drug A against another tested organism is found by the machine to be 1 µg/ml, and the NCCLS has set the susceptibility breakpoint at 32 µg/ml, then the computer prints out an "S" for sensitive. If the MIC is found to be 64 µg/ml, then this is greater than the breakpoint and results in the printing of an "R" for resistant.

The bottom line of this discussion is that, when used in a vacuum, MIC numbers are of limited value in selecting an antibiotic for most lower extremity infections. They are frequently misinterpreted and can lead to more trouble than good. Because the laboratory issuing the report has figured the NCCLS guidelines into its database, using the "S" or "R" is generally sufficient information.

Minimum Bactericidal Concentration

As previously mentioned, the MIC only relates how much antibiotic is needed to *inhibit* the growth of an organism. In the clinical setting, the patient's immune system should be capable of phagocytizing and killing the inhibited organisms. In some cases, however, either the patient's system is not functioning correctly or it may be desirable to kill the organism with an antibiotic. To determine how much antibiotic is needed to actually kill the organism, the minimum bactericidal concentration (MBC) is needed. The MBC is the concentration of antibiotic necessary to kill 99.9% of the organism.

MBC Determination
1. Following the MIC test, any tube without visible growth of organisms is plated onto antibiotic free media.
2. The plates are incubated overnight.
3. The lowest concentration to show no colony formation is determined to be the MBC.

Significance
1. The MBC will determine at what concentration the antibiotic will actually kill the organism, not just "stun" it.
2. If the MBC is within two dilutions of the MIC, the antibiotic is said to be *bactericidal* (i.e., the antibiotic inhibits and kills the bacteria at similar concentrations).
3. If the MBC is significantly greater than the MIC, then the drug is said to be *bacteriostatic*. The patient's immune system is then required to kill the organism.
4. This is not a test run routinely by the local hospital microbiology laboratory and would most likely have to be ordered from a reference laboratory.

Serum Bactericidal Titer
Another test, closely related to the MBC in technique, is the serum bactericidal titer (SBT), also known as the *Schlicter test*. Basically, an SBT is an MBC run on the patient's serum to guarantee that there is sufficient antibiotic in the serum to kill the infecting organism. Furthermore, there are a number of factors in the serum that make it significantly different from laboratory media. It is therefore necessary to make sure that the antibiotic will maintain activity in this environment.

SBT Determination
1. Approximately 20 to 30 minutes following dosage of an antibiotic, the patient's serum is drawn. This is known as the *peak specimen*.

2. Right before a subsequent dose is given, another serum is drawn. This is the trough specimen.
3. Using media, both sets of serum are then serially diluted (i.e., 1:1 [undiluted], 1:2, 1:4, 1:8, and so on).
4. An inoculum of the infecting organism is then placed into each tube.
5. The greatest dilution without growth is determined to be the SBT.
6. This is performed for both peak and trough specimens to ensure activity throughout the entire dosing interval.

Significance
1. The SBT will determine whether the antibiotic maintains activity in the patient's serum.
2. Clinical relevance is still questionable because of a lack of standardization.
3. The SBT seems to be most useful in following the therapy of endocarditis and osteomyelitis.
4. Maintaining a titer of 1:8 probably correlates best with clinical success.

■ *Drug Factors*

Although each class of antibiotics has its own unique properties, a few of these properties are common to all antibiotics. It is the clinician's responsibility to become familiar with all of them so that the proper decision can be made when selecting the most appropriate agent. As a secondary benefit, knowledge of all these factors makes it easier to interpret the literature being published about new drugs and therefore easier to stay abreast of developments.

In Vitro Activity
1. In vitro activity determines how well the antibiotic is performing in the laboratory against common pathogens.
2. Testing is performed against all bacteria for which the drug is potentially targeted.
3. MICs are run against a large number of each type of organism.
4. This is reported as MIC_{50}, MIC_{90}, and the range of MICs.
5. MIC_{50} refers to that MIC at which 50% of the tested isolates were inhibited.
6. MIC_{90} refers to that MIC at which 90% of the tested isolates were inhibited.

7. MIC_{90} is of the most clinical significance. MIC_{50} amounts to the proverbial toss of a coin.
8. The clinical significance of in vitro data is questionable. The data should be only one factor in selecting a possible agent.

In Vivo Activity

1. In vivo activity determines a drug's ability to perform against a given organism in a clinical situation.
2. It is usually reported in the literature in the form of clinical trials.
3. It can also be based on an individual clinician's experience with an agent.
4. A review of a clinical trial in the literature should show that the study was well controlled, randomized, and statistically significant.
5. One should look cautiously at studies supported by pharmaceutical companies. A disclaimer listed along with the author affiliations usually identifies these. Although many of them are legitimate, well-performed trials, some have questionable results. Since the company usually maintains right of first refusal on publication, it is rare to see a study sponsored by a drug company that is not favorable to its product.
6. The study should have been pertinent to the proposed usage. Just because similar organisms are found in intraabdominal infections and diabetic foot infections, does not mean that an antibiotic that is appropriate for one will be appropriate for the other.

Resistance

Two major mechanisms exist for the development of antibiotic resistance.

1. The first and most troublesome is the exchange of genetic information between organisms on plasmids.
   a. A plasmid is extrachromosomal DNA.
   b. It may travel between organisms of the same or different species.
   c. It can code for antibiotic-destroying enzymes (e.g., ß-lactamases).
   d. It causes most hospital outbreaks of resistance.

2. The second mechanism is through alterations in chromosomal DNA via mutation.
   a. It decreases permeability of the bacteria to the antibiotic.
   b. It can cause alteration in binding sites.
   c. It usually is not transferred between species.
3. Probably the most notorious example of this second mechanism is the development of methicillin-resistant *S. aureus*. This resistance is mediated by an increase in the number of low-affinity PBP 2a found on the cell walls of staphylococci, not by an increase in ß-lactamase.
4. Some organisms have the capability to "turn on" the development of ß-lactamases when exposed to ß-lactam agents. These are known as *inducible ß-lactamases*. Although initially reported as sensitive to ß-lactams, these organisms become rapidly resistant.
5. Extended spectrum ß-lactamases (ESBL) are of growing concern in clinical practice. These enzymes, found in gram-negative organisms such as *Escherichia coli, Klebsiella,* and the Enterobacteriaceae, render these fairly common organisms more resistant than may even show up on laboratory-sensitivity panels. These bacteria are generally sensitive to ß-lactamase inhibitor compounds.
6. Prevention of resistance can be accomplished in two ways:
   a. Proper use of antibiotics
   b. Proper "barrier" techniques, such as hand washing

Pharmacokinetics

1. The pharmacokinetics of an antibiotic determines its dosage. It is not within the scope of this chapter to examine all of the parameters. However, some definitions are warranted. Clinical relevance is explained as needed.
2. The *bioavailability* of an antibiotic refers to the amount of drug available to treat an infection. This is calculated by the "area under the curve" on a graph of antibiotic levels versus time.
3. The *half-life* is the amount of time required for one half of the antibiotic to be eliminated from the body. Its clinical significance is its use in calculating the interval between doses.
4. *Tissue penetration* is the level of antibiotic that is achievable in any given body tissue. For some tissues, such as muscle, skin, and plasma, the determination is relatively easy. Bone penetra-

tion studies, on the other hand, have been notoriously unreliable. This is more completely covered in the section on osteomyelitis therapy.

5. The *protein binding* of an antibiotic refers to how much drug is bound to albumin and other plasma proteins versus the amount of freely circulating drug. It is known that only the free drug has antimicrobial activity. The true clinical significance of the percentage of bound versus unbound drug is still being debated. It is possible that highly protein-bound antibiotics may be less active.

Cost

1. Purchase prices of antibiotics range from a few cents to more than $50 for a single dose of some agents.
2. The cost of an antibiotic does not just refer to purchase price. It also takes into account the monitoring of possible toxicities. For example, although gentamicin is inexpensive to buy, the patient's creatinine and antibiotic levels must be monitored frequently. This adds significant cost to the regimen.
3. If a patient taking gentamicin does develop nephrotoxicity, the cost of the extra days in the hospital must also be added to the drug cost.
4. Dosing costs are also added to overall drug costs. It has been estimated that it costs between $10 and $20 per dose to give an antibiotic. This takes into account pharmacy time, nursing time, bags, solutions, and tubing. Therefore even an inexpensive drug given q6h to q8h may cost more per course of therapy than a relatively expensive drug given q12h to q24h.

Antibiotic-Killing Effects

There are two distinct pharmacodynamic ways in which an antibiotic will kill an organism.

1. Concentration-dependent killing occurs when there is a direct correlation between the level of the drug above the MIC and the drug's ability to kill the organism. As the concentration continues to increase, so does the killing. This is usually found in quinolones and aminoglycosides.
2. Time-dependent killing occurs whenever the drug is above the MIC; however, there is minimal increase in the rate of killing as the level rises further above the MIC. This effect is found most commonly with penicillins and cephalosporins.

Postantibiotic Effect

1. The postantibiotic effect (PAE) refers to the antibiotic's ability to stun the organism even after the levels of the antibiotic have decreased below the MIC, preventing the organism from entering a growth phase.
2. Antibiotics with a significant PAE, such as the aminoglycosides and quinolones, can be administered less frequently than their half-lives would normally suggest. This is because the organism is incapable of multiplying for the duration of the PAE.
3. Few if any ß-lactams demonstrate a PAE.
4. Postantibiotic effects are most commonly found in concentration-dependent killing agents.

Inoculum Effect

1. Some antibiotics have decreased activity in the presence of large numbers of organisms yet work well under laboratory conditions. This is known as an *inoculum effect*.
2. The laboratory will usually test antibiotic MICs at a fixed bacterial inoculum of 10^5 or 10^6.
3. In abscesses, for example, the inoculum can exceed 10^8. Therefore when choosing an antibiotic in this situation, one with no inoculum effect should be selected.

Toxicity

The toxicity of an antibiotic agent is an important drug factor to consider (see Adverse Effects, subsequently).

■ *Host Factors*

Everybody is different. For this reason each individual will handle an antibiotic differently. These individual quirks will have a direct effect on antimicrobial activity, toxicity, absorption, and excretion of different drugs.

Age

The Older Adult

1. The likelihood of the presence of other host factors, such as decreased renal or liver function, is greater in the older adult patient. Also, other chronic diseases may be present that affect host defenses.
2. Older patients may be more prone to hypersensitivity.

3. There is good evidence of diminished immune function in older adults.
4. Gastrointestinal absorption may be altered because of changes in gastric pH.
5. Atrophy of muscle and fat make intramuscular injection more difficult.
6. Older patients have usually been exposed to more antibiotics and more organisms, especially if they live in a nursing home. This will lead to more resistant infections.
7. Infections present differently in older patients, so diagnosis may be more difficult. For example, fever and cardinal manifestations may be diminished.

The Young Patient

1. Infants and children are susceptible to totally different organisms that affect different sites from adults (e.g., hematogenous osteomyelitis of the long bones). In fact, the specialty of pediatric infectious diseases is totally separate from adult infectious diseases.
2. Antibiotic dosing requirements are more critical because of size differences.
3. Gastric pH differences in small children may modify oral absorption.
4. Tetracycline will permanently stain bones and teeth.
5. As with the elderly patient, there is a higher probability of other host factors being present.

Genetic Abnormalities

Glucose-6-phosphate dehydrogenase deficiency will lead to hemolysis when the patient is given sulfonamides.

Metabolic Abnormalities

1. Diabetes mellitus frequently causes renal disease, which will change antibiotic excretion and force modification of the dosing.
2. Some antibiotics, such as the sulfonamides, can cause hypoglycemia in diabetics taking sulfonylureas.

Renal Insufficiency

1. Most commonly used antibiotics are cleared through the kidney. Therefore, in the face of renal insufficiency, many antibiotic dosing regimens must be altered.

2. These alterations may take the form of decreasing the dose or increasing the time interval between doses.
3. Information concerning these changes is usually available in the package insert of the antibiotic or in the *Physicians' Desk Reference* and in Appendix 7.

Hepatic Dysfunction
Those antibiotics that are not handled by the kidney are inevitably metabolized or otherwise handled by the liver. These include the following:

1. Clindamycin
2. Erythromycin
3. Chloramphenicol
4. Cefoperazone

Dosing of these agents should probably be reduced in patients with abnormal liver function.

Pregnancy
1. The use of any antibiotic should be avoided, if possible.
2. The teratogenic potential of most antibiotics is not known.
3. Most penicillins, cephalosporins, and erythromycin are probably safe.
4. Ticarcillin and metronidazole should be avoided because of teratogenicity seen in animals.
5. Tetracycline is contraindicated because of staining of fetal bone and the possibility of fatty necrosis of the liver in pregnant women.

Immune Status
1. The patient's immune status will determine how the patient handles an infection.
2. Immune deficit is seen in a number of conditions:
    a. Uncontrolled diabetes mellitus
    b. Acquired immune deficiency syndrome
    c. Long-term corticosteroid use
    d. Advanced age
    e. Acute alcohol abuse
3. If the patient is immunocompromised, the body may not be able to adequately kill invading organisms. Therefore the use of bactericidal antibiotics is recommended.

Site of Infection

1. An adequate level of antibiotic must be able to reach the area of infection.
2. The antibiotic must be able to penetrate into the site, such as an abscess.
3. The environment may be hostile to the antibiotic (e.g., aminoglycosides do not work well in an acid pH).
4. There may be a local immune deficit in the site, such as around an implant.

Miscellaneous Host Factors

1. Anatomic variation may cause spread of infection along unusual fascial planes.
2. Physiologic alterations, such as poor circulation, may alter antibiotic delivery to the site of infection.
3. A history of adverse reaction to an antibiotic may force a change in proposed therapy (see Adverse Effects).

■ *Antibiotic Combinations*

Despite all the broad-spectrum antibiotics on the market, no single drug can always be counted on. In some situations, two or more antibiotics have to be combined to treat the patient appropriately. This can be true with either oral or parenteral therapy. When any antibiotics are combined, three possible interactions can occur:

1. Synergy, which occurs when the combination of the two drugs yields better results than could be predicted by their individual activities (AB > A + B, where A and B are the two drugs and AB is the combination).
2. Indifference (additive effect), which occurs when the combined activity is what could have been predicted based on each individual activity (AB = A + B). This by far is the most common reaction.
3. Antagonism, which occurs when the combined activity is actually less than could have been predicted (AB < A + B).

Indications for Antibiotic Combinations
Synergy

By using antibiotic combinations, it is hoped that synergy will occur. This should allow better clinical efficacy. The classic example of a synergistic combination is the use of a penicillin plus an aminoglycoside in the treatment of the enterococcus. The penicillin is only bacteriostatic against enterococcus. The addition of the aminoglycoside makes the combination bactericidal.

Prevention of Resistance

The combination of two antibiotics causes the organism to have a more difficult time becoming resistant. More mutation steps are needed or more enzyme must be produced to inactivate both drugs. This resistance rarely has a chance to develop. The best example of this indication is the use of rifampin for infections caused by *S. aureus*. As a single agent, the organism develops rapid resistance, rendering the drug rapidly ineffective. When combined with vancomycin, for example, resistance to the combination rarely occurs.

"Shotgun Therapy"

Before the culture reports are received from the laboratory, a polymicrobial infection may be suspected. In order to hit it hard, frequently multiple agents are empirically begun. The therapy is then tapered once laboratory results are returned.

Polymicrobial Infection

Once the culture results are returned, there may be multiple organisms isolated from the infection. It is conceivable that even with a broad-spectrum single agent there may be a "therapeutic hole" in the coverage. A second or third agent may need to be added.

Filling Therapeutic Holes

One way to consider whether to add an additional antibiotic or to change current combinations is to evaluate the need to plug therapeutic holes or gaps in coverage.

1. Example 1. The patient is on clindamycin and ciprofloxacin. The culture returns with organisms well covered by these two agents but also *Enterococcus*. *Enterococcus* represents a therapeutic hole in this combination because it is not covered. Consider changing the clindamycin to a drug such as amoxicillin/clavulanic acid to plug the hole. Another option would be to continue the current regimen and add a third drug, such as vancomycin.
2. Example 2. The patient is on piperacillin/tazobactam for a diabetic foot infection. What are some of the therapeutic holes? If the culture comes back with MRSA, this represents a hole in the coverage. It may be necessary to add vancomycin.

Contraindications to Antibiotic Combinations

Antagonism

Although synergy is the goal when two antibiotics are combined, antagonism may occur. Despite culture reports of the individual agents claiming sensitivity of the organism, treatment may fail. Antagonism can occur on two levels:

1. Molecular, in which the two chemicals are noncompatible.
2. Microbial, in which one agent makes the organism resistant to the other.

The best example of molecular antagonism is the combination of an aminoglycoside with a penicillin. When mixed in the same bag, or when together in the patient's serum for a prolonged period, the penicillin will inactivate the aminoglycoside. For this reason they should be dosed at different time intervals.

An example of microbial antagonism is the combination of two ß-lactam agents. Theoretically, one drug can induce the organism to produce ß-lactamase, rendering one or both agents ineffective.

Cost

In this age of cost containment, the addition of multiple anti-biotics may not be viewed favorably by the hospital. As previously discussed, the purchase price of the antibiotic is only a small fraction of the cost of administration. Multiple agents multiply the cost.

Adverse Effects

Antibiotics are foreign substances. They can have significant toxicities. The use of multiple agents exposes the patient to a greater likelihood of developing one of these adverse effects. Although penicillin may not be bactericidal against enterococci, it is a relatively safe drug. The addition of an aminoglycoside significantly raises the possibility of toxicity.

■ *Home Intravenous Antibiotics*

It seems like the first individual to visit a patient in the hospital is not the attending physician or the resident but rather someone from discharge planning. This phenomenon began over a decade ago with the advent of the dreaded diagnosis-related groups

(DRGs) system of determining reimbursement to a hospital. Before the initiation of DRGs, it was relatively easy to keep a patient in the hospital for as long as necessary, even if it meant 4 to 6 weeks for intravenous (IV) antibiotic therapy. Now the patients are expected out almost before they are admitted.

In response to this new paradigm, home intravenous antibiotic companies sprouted up like weeds. Some offered physicians questionable deals from consultantships to billing for telephone "visits" to partnerships in order to get business. Fortunately most are now long gone.

Home IV antibiotics are still useful for some conditions, such as endocarditis. But the availability of newer antibiotics that have similar bioavailability in both oral and parenteral forms has rendered most of their usage for lower extremity infections moot. If for some reason the patient cannot be placed on one of these oral regimens, then indications include the following:

1. The major indication for home intravenous therapy is osteomyelitis. Following the definitive surgical debridement and/or initial antibiotic course, the patient receives intravenous therapy at home to complete the 4- to 6-week course of antibiotics.
2. Patients with diabetic foot infections, once medically and surgically stable, may benefit from home intravenous therapy. The home-care nurse can usually follow the patient's medical status with the appropriate laboratory tests ordered by the physician.
3. Patients who refuse to be hospitalized yet require a course of intravenous therapy for any type of infection are candidates. To watch for untoward reactions, most home health services require that at least one dose of the drug be given in the presence of a physician.

Requirements
1. The patient or a family member must be able to learn to administer the therapy. The patient will be required to "plug himself in" on a daily basis. Nurses usually are only necessary on an every-other or third-day basis to check the line and restock the patient with supplies.
2. The patient must have venous access. This is usually accomplished by placement of a central line, such as a Hickman or Groshong catheter, a peripherally inserted central catheter (PICC) line, or through a peripheral heparin lock.
3. A history of intravenous drug abuse is a strict contraindication.

4. The patient should have at least one dose in the hospital or the physician's office.
5. The patient's health insurance must cover the home care.

ADVERSE EFFECTS OF ANTIBIOTICS

As a class of drugs, antibiotics are relatively safe when given at the proper dosage with proper patient selection. Unfortunately, even with these precautions, adverse effects will occasionally occur. For semantic purposes, these effects can be divided into three types of reactions:

1. Toxicity reactions caused by excessive amounts of the agent. This can occur by either administering too much or by the body's inability to metabolize or excrete the antibiotic, thereby causing accumulation.
2. Side-effect reactions that may occur at normal therapeutic levels. By definition, these are not immunologically mediated.
3. Allergies, which are immunologic side effects.

■ *Toxicities and Side Effects*

Ototoxicity

Ototoxicity is one of the most severe adverse effects attributed to antibiotics. The two common manifestations of this effect are deafness and vestibular impairment. Deafness may or may not be reversible, depending on the drug.

1. This toxicity is attributed to exposure to prolonged elevated levels of various agents.
2. High-frequency hearing is usually lost first.
3. Hearing deficit in the normal speaking range is a late complication, making early detection possible only by audiometry.
4. Tinnitus and "fullness" are two early symptoms.
5. Renal impairment, previous ear disease, the concomitant use of two or more ototoxic agents, and the use of loop diuretics are all major risk factors.
6. Damage may not be evident until after the drug is discontinued.
7. The damage may progress despite discontinuation of the drug.

8. Vestibular damage begins as mild vertigo and can progress to ataxia.
9. The vestibular damage is usually partially reversible.

Antibiotics Associated with Ototoxicity

1. Aminoglycosides. All agents in this class have the potential to cause both types of ototoxicity. Studies have shown small differences in potential for each drug, but the clinical relevance of these findings is questionable.
2. Erythromycin. Unlike the irreversible condition seen with aminoglycosides, erythromycin can produce a temporary deafness. The onset is usually within 48 hours of initiation of therapy. Risk factors include high doses, renal and hepatic dysfunction, and advanced age. Discontinuation of the drug usually returns hearing.
3. Vancomycin. Early experience with vancomycin led to the widespread belief that this agent could cause deafness. It is now believed that this was due more to the impurities in those early preparations than to the drug itself. There is little to substantiate ototoxicity with vancomycin at this point. However, there may be a synergistic effect in increasing ototoxicity between vancomycin and aminoglycosides when given together.

Other Neurologic Effects

Besides ototoxicity, there are a number of other neurologic sequelae attributable to the administration of antibiotics. Although less common in both prevalence and number of agents that cause them, these neurotoxicities are no less important.

Neuromuscular Blockade

1. It is generally attributed to the aminoglycosides.
2. It affects acetylcholine release and uptake in the synapse.
3. It is brought on by rapid administration of the drug. Aminoglycosides should always be administered over a 30-minute period and never in a bolus.
4. It is potentiated by general anesthetics, sedatives, and narcotics.
5. It is reversible with calcium administration.

Seizures

1. These are most commonly associated with penicillin, ampicillin, and imipenem.

2. High dosage and impaired renal function are two major risk factors.
3. Previous seizure history or any damage to the blood-brain barrier can potentiate the seizures.

Peripheral Neuropathy
1. This is seen in patients who have been on isoniazid and griseofulvin for prolonged periods.
2. It presents as a stocking-glove distribution.
3. Pyridoxine may be helpful in reversal.

Nephrotoxicity

Probably the most worrisome and bothersome toxicity caused by antibiotics is nephrotoxicity. More has been written and discussed about this effect than any other. Furthermore, more time is probably spent calculating dosage adjustments than actually examining the patient.

1. The major risk factor is preexisting renal impairment.
2. Other risk factors include advanced age, recent or concurrent administration of another nephrotoxic agent, and concomitant hepatic disease.
3. The earliest clinically relevant indication is an increase in serum creatinine.
4. When faced with a patient with diminished renal function for whom use of a potentially nephrotoxic agent is being contemplated, the physician has three options:
   a. Decrease the dose of the drug.
   b. Increase the time interval between dosings.
   c. Choose a drug handled by the liver.
5. Nephrotoxic agents can be used safely in patients with impaired kidneys if dosage reduction recommendations are followed.
6. Dialysis is not a contraindication to the use of nephrotoxic agents. Most antibiotics are cleared, to some extent, by dialysis. Check the recommended dosage for patients undergoing this procedure and modify accordingly.
7. Onset of the nephrotoxicity can begin as early as 3 to 4 days following initiation of therapy. However, it may not begin or be recognized until after therapy has been discontinued.
8. The nephrotoxicity caused by most agents is reversible. If there are no alternatives, a patient should not be denied a potentially life- or limb-saving drug based on the fear of renal damage.

Antibiotics Associated with Nephrotoxicity

1. Aminoglycosides. All aminoglycosides are nephrotoxic. Small variations between each member of the group are not clinically significant. The damage appears to be located in the proximal tubules and leads to a decreased glomerular filtration rate. Dosing recommendations and calculations are covered in the section on aminoglycosides.
2. Vancomycin. As with vancomycin-induced ototoxicity, the nephrotoxicity is probably more a function of earlier formulations. In renally compromised patients, however, close monitoring of serum creatinine and drug levels is still recommended.
3. Penicillins and cephalosporins. Both of these classes of drugs have been reported to have a potential to cause interstitial nephritis. This appears to be a hypersensitivity reaction to the agent. The classic cause is the use of methicillin. Because this drug is no longer in wide clinical use, its importance is questionable. However, other members of this class, including penicillin G and ampicillin, can also cause interstitial nephritis.

Hepatotoxicity

Liver toxicity is a relatively rare effect of drugs used in the treatment of lower extremity bacterial infections. Only two commonly used drugs have potential to cause hepatotoxicity:

1. Tetracycline, especially in pregnant women, can cause a fatty degeneration of the liver that may be fatal. There is a possibility that this will also be seen in patients taking excessive doses (both oral and parenteral) or in patients with preexisting hepatic disease.
2. Erythromycin, when formulated as the estolate or ethyl succinate salts, may produce jaundice and hepatocellular damage. This is related to prolonged courses of therapy and is reversible.

Antibiotic-Associated Diarrhea

Antibiotic-associated diarrhea (AAD) can be caused by two major mechanisms:

1. Alterations in the gut microbiologic flora, causing incomplete metabolism and absorption of food.

2. Selection and overgrowth of a toxin-producing strain of *Clostridium difficile*.

Although both can cause marked diarrhea, the latter is the more severe. *C.-difficile*–associated diarrhea (CDAD), also generically known as *pseudomembranous colitis* because of its potential to form pseudomembranes in the colon, potentially can cause severe illness and death. Fortunately, true pseudomembranous colitis is only present in about 30% of cases of AAD.

1. Any antibiotic can cause CDAD. Although there is a common belief that clindamycin is the major cause, a whole list of cephalosporins and penicillins have been indicted.
2. Clinical illness can occur following oral or parenteral therapy. There appears to be no definitive prevalence for one route or the other.
3. Recent studies suggest that the probability of developing true CDAD is extremely rare unless the patient has been hospitalized or in a long-term care facility. Therefore most cases of diarrhea following oral outpatient therapy are probably *not* CDAD.
4. Disease is independent of dosage.
5. Risk factors include old age, cancer chemotherapy, and abdominal surgery.
6. Onset seems to be independent of duration of antibiotic treatment. AAD can occur after a few doses or weeks after the regimen has been discontinued.

Clinical Presentation
1. The clinical picture of CDAD usually includes crampy diarrhea with profuse watery or mucoid stools.
2. Actual diarrhea may be absent. Vague abdominal complaints may be the only indication.
3. Pseudomembranes visualized in the colon or rectum on proctoscopy/sigmoidoscopy or, best of all, endoscopy, are diagnostic. The use of these modalities, however, is not cost-effective and may be unnecessary.
4. Diagnosis is usually made on clinical picture, examination of the stool for white blood cells, and a titer for *C. difficile* toxin.
5. Toxin titers may be misleading, because the large majority of hospitalized patients will be colonized with the organism and therefore will be toxin-positive.

6. Culture for *C. difficile* is sometimes performed but is more technically challenging than the use of ELISA toxin detection. Furthermore, a positive culture will not tell whether the isolated organism is actually producing toxin or just colonizing.

Treatment
1. Discontinuation of the offending antibiotic, if clinically possible, is the easiest treatment. Up to about 25% to 30% of cases will resolve with no further therapy.
2. Fluid and electrolyte support.
3. Do not use antidiarrheal agents. These agents decrease gut motility and can cause an increase in toxin in the bowel. This increase has been reported to lead to a toxic megacolon, which is fatal in more than 80% of cases.
4. In refractory or severe cases or in cases in which the antibiotic cannot be stopped, initiation of empiric antibiotic therapy against the CDAD is the next step.
5. Antibiotic therapy.
   a. Metronidazole, 500 mg PO q8h × 10 days is considered first-line therapy in most cases because of its much lower price.
   b. Vancomycin, 125 mg PO q6h × 10 days. Although potentially slightly more efficacious than metronidazole, its excessive price relegates it to second-line therapy. Furthermore, oral vancomycin is a major factor in the development of vancomycin-resistant enterococcus (VRE).
   c. Recurrence can occur in up to 50% of cases. These usually respond to a second course of therapy.
   d. Parenteral therapy should be avoided except in patients with no oral access. Most antibiotics do not achieve sufficient levels in the colon following parenteral administration. In fact, intravenous vancomycin can cause AAD. The use of parenteral metronidazole has been successful in a few reported cases. Instillation of drug via a nasogastric tube or even an enema has been reported.

Other Gastrointestinal Effects
Although AAD is by far the most severe and therefore clinically important GI adverse effect, there are a few other minor adverse GI effects:

1. Nausea, vomiting, and diarrhea unrelated to pseudomembranous colitis can be caused by almost any drug, whether orally or

parentally administered. The most notorious are erythromycin and tetracycline.

2. Glossitis and stomatitis can be caused by superinfection with a yeast, particularly in the case of tetracycline use.

Neutropenia

Treating an infection with antibiotics will cause an elevated white blood cell count (WBC) to decrease. On occasion, however, the drop in the WBC will continue to a below-normal level. This is not due to the infection resolving but rather to the adverse effect of one of several antibiotics:

1. Sulfonamides can cause an agranulocytosis unrelated to the blood level of the drug.
2. Chloramphenicol, notorious for causing aplastic anemia, can also cause a selective chronic granulocytopenia. This depression is related to high dosing levels.
3. The most common neutropenia seen with the treatment of lower extremity infections is caused by the ß-lactams.
4. Almost any penicillin or cephalosporin can cause this neutropenia.
5. ß-Lactam neutropenia appears to be immunologically mediated, causing a destruction of circulating neutrophils and a depression of their production.
6. For a review of the method of calculating the absolute neutrophil count and determining whether the patient has sufficient neutrophils, see Chapter 1.
7. The ß-lactam neutropenia is reversible with discontinuation of the antibiotic.
8. Vancomycin can also cause a reversible neutropenia.

Bleeding

Bleeding disorders caused by antibiotics have been attributed to a number of possible mechanisms. Two of these have withstood the most scrutiny and are now accepted as the most common etiologies:

1. Platelet dysfunction
2. Suppression of vitamin K-dependent factors, which causes hypoprothrombinemia

Platelet Dysfunction
1. Most common with ß-lactam antibiotics, especially the penicillins

2. Causes increased bleeding time
3. Due to abnormal aggregation of platelets
4. Ticarcillin, ampicillin, and penicillin seem to have the greatest effect
5. Mezlocillin has the least effect

Vitamin K Metabolism
1. It is due to inhibition of carboxylation of vitamin K-dependent coagulation factors.
2. Secondarily, it may be due to inhibition of vitamin K-producing microbes in the gut.
3. It is closely related to antibiotics containing the n-methylthiotetrazole (MTT) sidechain:
   a. Cefoperazone
   b. Cefamandol
   c. Cefotetan
   d. Cefmetazole
4. It is usually reversible with vitamin K administration.
5. Vitamin K should be given prophylactically if these agents are used.
6. It can be detected by elevation in prothrombin time and/or partial thromboplastin time.
7. It may or may not cause clinical evidence of hemorrhage. The clinical importance is not fully known.

Other Hematologic Effects
In addition to neutropenia and bleeding, there are a few less common adverse effects on the hematologic system.

1. Chloramphenicol can produce two distinct hematopoietic depressions:
   a. A reversible depression that is dose dependent.
   b. An idiosyncratic aplastic anemia that is fatal in more than 50% of cases. This may appear weeks or months after discontinuation of the therapy. It is not dose related but may be more prevalent following prolonged therapy.
2. The sulfonamides and chloramphenicol can produce hemolytic anemia in patients with glucose-6-phosphate dehydrogenase deficiency.
3. An elevated Coombs test results with the use of some cephalosporins.

Disulfiram or "Antabuse" Reaction

A number of antibiotics will cause the patient to become very ill when alcohol is ingested during therapy. Symptoms of this disulfiram-like reaction include:

1. Nausea and vomiting
2. Hypotension
3. Peripheral vasodilatation with flushing and sweating
4. Tachycardia

Other important points to remember:

1. It is most closely associated with antibiotics containing the MTT sidechain (see bleeding, covered previously).
2. Metronidazole has also been implicated.
3. Effects may be present for a week or more following discontinuation of the antibiotic.
4. Avoidance of alcohol extends not only to liquor but to any medication in an alcohol base (elixirs).
5. Treatment consists of electrolyte and fluid support.

Red Man (or Red Neck) Syndrome

1. It is unique to vancomycin.
2. It is not a true allergic response; it is called *anaphylactoid*.
3. It is directly related to speed of infusion.
4. Other less significant factors that lead to susceptibility are not clearly understood. The amount of the dose may be one of them.
5. Rapid infusion causes a release of histamine from mast cells.
6. It is characterized by pruritus, flushing with a "hot" sensation, and erythema, especially around the face and neck.
7. Severe cases may result in hypotension.

Treatment

1. Prevention is by far the best treatment. Always administer vancomycin slowly over 1 hour.
2. The condition is usually self-limiting.
3. Antihistamines may make the patient more comfortable until the condition clears up.
4. Prophylactic antihistamines are not recommended.

Dermatologic Side Effects

Any antibiotic can cause a dermatologic reaction. These range from benign rashes and photosensitivities common with tetracyclines to life-threatening exfoliations. Fortunately, these severe reactions are extremely rare. They are listed here for the sake of completeness.

1. Systemic lupus erythematosus
2. Stevens-Johnson syndrome
3. Toxic epidermal necrolysis
4. Exfoliative dermatitis

Antibiotic Monitoring
Antibiotic serum levels are usually monitored for two reasons:

1. To ensure that therapeutic levels of the drug are present
2. To prevent excessive levels that may lead to toxicities

Because most antibiotics are relatively safe, the need for monitoring against the possibility of toxicities is not useful for most drugs used in lower extremity infections (individual monitoring guidelines are included in the discussion of each drug).

1. Aminoglycosides are currently the only class of drug that needs to be routinely monitored. However, some data suggest that monitoring does not necessarily ensure safety or efficacy.
2. Vancomycin is a safe drug that does not need to be monitored from a safety standpoint.

■ *Allergies*

At the initial interview, frequently patients will declare that they are "allergic" to a particular antibiotic. They were inevitably instructed by the physician making the diagnosis to "never let anybody give you this drug." Careful questioning of the patient will reveal some of these responses:

1. They were not able to breathe and almost died.
2. They developed a terrible itch and became covered with blotches.
3. When they took the drug 20 years ago they developed an upset stomach.
4. They had some other nondescript "reaction" such as induration at the site of injection.

The third and fourth scenarios are easy to discount. Frequently patients became ill from impurities found in early formulations.

The first two, however, cause endless concern for physicians when prescribing antibiotics.

Any antibiotic can cause an allergic response. The ß-lactams are by far the most frequent instigators. For this reason, this discussion focuses on this class of agents. There are a number of different classification systems for reactions to antibiotics. Primarily, reactions can be broken down into two types.

Immediate Hypersensitivity

Also known as a type I reaction or anaphylaxis, immediate hypersensitivity is of the greatest clinical concern. This is mediated through immunoglobulin E (IgE).

1. This reaction can occur within 30 minutes of the beginning of a new course of therapy.
2. Although relatively rare, it carries significant mortality.
3. Symptoms include bronchospasm, laryngospasm, laryngeal edema, and cardiac arrhythmias.
4. Treatment consists of intramuscular, intravenous, or subcutaneous administration of epinephrine. Usual dosage is 0.5 mg (5 ml of a 1:10,000 solution or 0.5 ml of a 1:1000 solution) q 10 minutes IV prn or q 30 minutes SQ prn.
5. Desensitization to penicillin can be performed if there are no alternative therapies. This procedure consists of administering extremely small doses initially and gradually increasing the dose hourly. Because this is very rarely used and potentially deadly, the exact technique is not covered.
6. Testing for penicillin allergy can be performed using any of a number of commercially available kits. Skin testing in only good for detecting an immediate hypersensitivity. If there is no response to the challenge, there is only minimal risk of the patient developing a reaction.
7. There are no kits available for testing cephalosporin sensitivity. Immediate reactions to cephalosporins are rather rare.

Delayed Hypersensitivity

Although not medically correct terminology, most other allergic reactions to antibiotics are categorized as a "delayed hypersensitivity." In fact, some of the rashes seen are not really an "allergic" response but rather an idiosyncratic reaction of unknown mechanism.

1. Reactions usually occur within 48 to 72 hours after therapy is begun, although longer delays are possible.

2. Symptoms include urticaria, especially on the trunk and arms, and pruritus.
3. Treatment consists of discontinuation of the offending agent. Antihistamines may be useful in making the patient more comfortable.
4. Ampicillin or amoxicillin are very common causes of rash, particularly in patients with coexistent viral infections such as Epstein-Barr or cytomegalovirus.

Miscellaneous Allergic Reactions

Although the aforementioned two are the most commonly encountered antibiotic allergies, there are other side effects also thought to be immunologically mediated:

1. Interstitial nephritis
2. Granulocytopenia
3. Hemolytic anemia
4. Serum sickness
5. Drug fever

Cross-Reactivity of ß-Lactam Antibiotics

Penicillins and cephalosporins have become the most frequently used classes of antibiotics. If a patient relates an "allergy" to penicillin, cephalosporins are *not* ruled out as alternative therapy. Some data support a much lower figure of "crossover allergy" than the often-cited 10%. Some studies actually point to a cross-reaction rate for immediate hypersensitivity at closer to 1%.

1. If the symptom of penicillin "allergy" is questionable (e.g., an upset stomach) or is temporally distant, cephalosporins can be used with little worry.
2. If there is a history of "rash" with penicillin, cephalosporins can still be used.
3. In the previous two cases, one suggestion is to watch the patient carefully when first giving the cephalosporin. This is best accomplished when parenteral therapy is used. Administration can be stopped immediately if the patient reacts to the drug. Proper supportive therapy should be available. For oral therapy in an outpatient setting, the first dose should be administered before the patient leaves. Have supportive therapy available.
4. Cephalosporins should be avoided entirely in patients with a history of anaphylaxis to penicillin. This recommendation is more based on common practice than medical fact. The risk of

immediate hypersensitivity for cephalosporins in a patient with penicillin allergy is extremely low. Furthermore, as the cephalosporin "generation" increases, the rate of reaction decreases. There are significantly fewer cross-reactions when using second- and third-generation drugs as opposed to first-generation drugs.

5. For imipenem and other penem antibiotics, the same guidelines as those for cephalosporins should be followed.

6. There is little to no evidence of any cross-reactions between the penicillins and the monobactams, such as aztreonam.

SUGGESTED READINGS

Amsden GW, Ballow CH, Bertino JS: Pharmacokinetics and pharmacodynamics of anti-infective agents. In Mandell GL, Bennett JE, Dolin R, editors: *Principles and practice of infectious diseases,* ed 5, p 253, Philadelphia, 2000, Churchill Livingstone.

Brown RB, Levin J, Morris A: Adverse effects of antibiotics, *J Am Podiatr Med Assoc* 79:500, 1989.

Kendler JS, Hartman BJ: Beta-lactam antibiotics. In Armstrong D, Cohen J, editors: *Infectious diseases,* p. 7.5.1, St Louis, 1999, Mosby.

MacGregor RR, Graziani AL: Oral administration of antibiotics: a rational alternative to the parenteral route, *Clin Infect Dis* 24:457, 1997.

Thielman NM: Antibiotic associated colitis. In Mandell GL, Bennett JE, Dolin R, editors: *Principles and practice of infectious diseases,* ed 5, p. 1111, Philadelphia, 2000, Churchill Livingstone.

Johnson S, Gerding DN: *Clostridium difficile* associated diarrhea, *Clin Infect Dis* 26:1027, 1998.

Fekety R: Guidelines for the diagnosis and management of *Clostridium difficile* associated diarrhea and colitis. American College of Gastroenterology, Practice Parameters Committee, *Am J Gastroenterol* 92:739, 1997.

Yoshikawa TT, Norman DC, editors: *Antimicrobial therapy in the elderly patient,* New York, 1994, Marcel Dekker, Inc.

Yoshikawa TT: Epidemiology and unique aspects of aging and infectious diseases, *Clin Infect Dis* 30:931, 2000.

CHAPTER 9

Antibiotic Agents

This chapter presents outlines of various antibiotics commonly used in the treatment of lower extremity infections. Each class of antibiotic is described in terms of its mode of action, spectrum, and toxicities. Then each individual agent is discussed in terms of its indications, dosing, and adverse reactions. Drugs within each class are listed either in order of availability or in order of importance in the treatment of lower extremity infections as opposed to alphabetically. All dosages are for adult patients unless otherwise stated. When one or more agents in a given class are very similar, they are covered together. Trade names are listed when a drug is primarily a proprietary product.

PENICILLINS

First isolated in 1929 by Sir Alexander Fleming, penicillin did not become commercially available until Florey and associates developed a practical way of producing the agent in the early 1940s. The "acid test" of the original agent, penicillin G, came during World War II when the drug was used by the U.S. Army. Originally penicillin G was useful in treating staphylococcal, streptococcal, and gonococcal infections.

Staphylococcal resistance, mediated by the production of ß-lactamase, forced the production of antibiotics resistant to this enzyme. The first semisynthetic penicillin, methicillin, was introduced in the late 1950s. This event was followed by the develop-

213

ment of the expanded-spectrum agents capable of activity against the gram-negative organisms.

■ *Mechanism of Action*

It is clear that penicillins are cell-wall-active agents. Exactly how they affect the cell wall has not been completely elucidated. In gram-positive bacteria, the drug has to fight its way past extracellular ß-lactamase to bind to a site on the cell wall known as a *penicillin-binding protein* (PBP). These PBPs mediate various cell wall functions. The number and affinity of the PBPs varies with each organism.

Gram-negative bacteria pose a more difficult challenge. The drug must first pass through the outer portions of the cell membrane into the periplasmic space. This periplasmic space has a concentration of ß-lactamase that is much higher than that found in the gram-positive organisms. If the agent survives the enzyme, it then must bind with the appropriate PBP.

Resistance to penicillins is mediated by a number of factors:

1. Most commonly the production of ß-lactamase, which can hydrolyse the antibiotic.
2. Alteration in the PBP site.
3. Changes in the cell membrane (of gram-negative organisms) that keep the antibiotic from passing through to reach a target site.

■ *Classification*

The penicillins are classified into a number of subgroups on the basis of their structure and their antimicrobial activity (Box 9-1).

■ *Spectrum of Activity*

General trends of susceptibility can be noted for each class of penicillin. Specific variations for individual agents are noted when each agent is discussed. The penicillins are bactericidal against all bacteria except Enterococci.

1. Natural penicillins.
   a. Streptococci.
   b. Most enterococci.
   c. Non–penicillinase-producing staphylococci (rarely found, constituting less than 10% of all staphylococci).

BOX **9-1**

Classification of Penicillins

Natural Penicillins	**Expanded-Spectrum and**
Penicillin G	**Antipseudomonal Penicillins**
Penicillin V	**(Ureido- and**
	Carboxypenicillins)
Aminopenicillins	Carbenicillin
Ampicillin	Ticarcillin
Amoxicillin	Mezlocillin
	Piperacillin
Semisynthetic (Penicillinase-	
Resistant) Penicillins	**Penicillin/ß-Lactamase**
Methicillin	**Inhibitor Combinations**
Nafcillin	Ticarcillin/clavulanic acid
Oxacillin	Amoxicillin/clavulanic acid
Cloxacillin	Ampicillin/sulbactam
Dicloxacillin	Piperacillin/tazobactam

    d. Non–penicillinase-producing gonococci (also becoming a rare find).

    e. Anaerobes other than *Bacteroides*, especially gram-positive.

2. Aminopenicillins.

    a. Streptococci (no more active than natural penicillin).

    b. Slightly more active against the enterococci.

    c. Gram-negative organisms, including many *Escherichia coli, Proteus mirablis, Shigella,* and *Salmonella.* Significant resistance has now developed in many of these organisms.

    d. Not active against penicillinase-producing (most) staphylococci.

3. Semisynthetic or penicillinase-resistant penicillins.

    a. Staphylococci (all but methicillin-resistant strains).

    b. Streptococci (no more active than natural penicillin).

4. Expanded-spectrum penicillins.

    a. Increased gram-negative spectrum, including most Enterobacteriaceae and some *Pseudomonas aeruginosa.* More and more resistance has developed by these gram-negatives.

    b. Not active against penicillinase-producing staphylococci.

    c. Streptococci (no more active than earlier penicillins).

5. Penicillin/ß-lactamase inhibitor combinations.

    a. Staphylococci (all but methicillin-resistant strains) including "hyperproducers" of ß-lactamase.

b. Anaerobes, including *Bacteroides*.

c. Gram-negative organisms (similar to those covered by the expanded-spectrum penicillins).

■ *Adverse Reactions*

The penicillins are one of the safest classes of antibiotics. They have been used for more than 40 years and have not caused any major toxicity problems. However, they are not entirely free from adverse reactions. (Most of these reactions are described in detail in Chapter 7.)

1. Hypersensitivity—by far the most common adverse reaction. However, even the prevalence of this effect seems to have declined in recent years.
2. Neutropenia.
3. Bleeding and thrombocytopenia.
4. Interstitial nephritis because of a hypersensitivity reaction.
5. Myoclonic seizures.
6. Diarrhea with or without enterocolitis.
7. Elevations in liver function tests (usually transient).
8. Electrolyte imbalances because of the high sodium concentration of some preparations.

■ *Natural Penicillins*

Penicillin G
Penicillin G comes in a number of forms:

1. Aqueous penicillin G for intravenous (IV) use. It can also be used intramuscularly (IM) but offers no advantage over repository forms.
2. Procaine penicillin, one repository form, is available for intramuscular use. It achieves levels detectable for about 12 hours.
3. Another repository form, benzathine penicillin, achieves levels detectable for up to 1 month.
4. Oral penicillin G is available but is infrequently used because of the improved bioavailability of penicillin V.

Spectrum of Activity
1. The drug of choice for most streptococcal infections.
2. Some group B streptococci may be resistant (rare).

3. Although effective against enterococci, ampicillin is slightly preferred.
4. When used against non–penicillinase-producing staphylococci (which constitute less than 10%), therapy must be monitored for the development of resistance because of inducible ß-lactamase production.
5. Non–penicillinase-producing gonococci.
6. Most anaerobes except bacteroides. This includes clostridia.

Dosage and Administration (Note: 1 million U = 625 mg)

1. Aqueous penicillin: up to 20 to 24 million U/day (5 to 6 million q4h) intravenously. Lower doses and IM administration can be used for less severe infections.
2. Aqueous penicillin can also be given intramuscularly in doses of up to 1.2 million U/day.
3. Procaine penicillin: up to 1.2 million U q12h to q24h IM.
4. Benzathine penicillin: a single dose of 1.2 to 2.4 million U IM. Can be repeated weekly to biweekly as required. Commercially prepared mixtures combining procaine and benzathine penicillin are available.
5. Concomitant administration of probenecid, 1 to 2 g/day, will markedly increase the duration of serum levels of all penicillins.
6. Moderate dosage reduction is needed in the presence of renal insufficiency (i.e., creatinine clearance of less than 30 ml/min).

Clinical Usage

Natural penicillins are not used frequently in the treatment of lower extremity infections. Most of these infections are caused by bacteria resistant to this class of drug. Furthermore, although inexpensive, their short half-life and frequent dosage requirements make these agents expensive and bothersome to administer. In most cases alternatives are available that are easier to give and just as effective or even more so. Some potential uses include:

1. Superficial cellulitis of the foot with a Gram stain showing gram-positive cocci in chains.
2. Osteomyelitis or another infection in which the streptococci are the sole pathogens.
3. Septic arthritis in a young individual in which gonococcus is suspected by history and by Gram stain. Even in this case, given

the potential for resistance, other drugs may be easier to administer and may be more effective.

4. Clostridial cellulitis, also called *gas gangrene.* High-dose penicillin, 2 million U q2h to q4h IV, is the traditional therapy.

Penicillin V

Penicillin V, also known as *phenoxymethyl penicillin*, is only available as an oral preparation. It comes as both a potassium and a sodium salt, with the potassium salt being the most commonly used because it produces higher serum levels. The spectrum of activity, adverse effects, and clinical indications are almost identical to those of penicillin G. Penicillin V can be used whenever treatment with an oral form of penicillin is appropriate.

Dosage and Administration

1. 250 to 500 mg qid. The dosage can be elevated to 4 g/day in more severe infections.
2. As with penicillin G, only minor dosing adjustments must be made in patients with impaired renal function.
3. Serum levels are slightly higher if taken on an empty stomach.

■ Aminopenicillins

Ampicillin

Ampicillin is available in the following forms:

1. Intramuscular and intravenous preparations, with intravenous administration being the most common.
2. Oral capsules. Oral preparations of ampicillin are not particularly well absorbed from the gastrointestinal tract and therefore are not commonly used.

Spectrum of Activity

Aminopenicillins were developed to increase the gram-negative coverage of the penicillins, although increases in ß-lactamase production are rendering these drugs less useful.

1. Similar activity to penicillin against most streptococci.
2. Slightly improved coverage of the Enterococci. Ampicillin is only bacteriostatic against these organisms. Bacterial killing is achieved by the combination with an aminoglycoside, although this may not be clinically relevant in lower extremity infections.

3. Some community-acquired *E. coli* are still sensitive. Many hospital-acquired *E. coli* have become resistant.
4. Some *Haemophilus influenzae, P. mirablis, Salmonella*, and *Shigella* are sensitive, although even these are now becoming fairly resistant.
5. Because ampicillin is not penicillinase-resistant, almost all staphylococci are resistant.

Adverse Reactions
Along with the reactions listed for the penicillins as a class, ampicillin has increased incidence of two others worth noting:

1. Drug rash, which is of undetermined origin but is probably not allergic. This is a particular problem when there is a coexisting viral infection such as Epstein-Barr or cytomegalovirus (CMV).
2. Diarrhea, which may or may not be due to pseudomembranous colitis.

Dosage and Administration
1. 250 to 500 mg qid PO.
2. Should be taken on an empty stomach because food decreases absorption.
3. 2 g q4h to q6h IV.
4. Probenecid will increase and prolong serum levels.
5. Only minor dosing changes are required when creatinine clearance drops below 30 to 50 ml/min.

Clinical Usage
As with the natural penicillins, ampicillin is of limited use in lower extremity infections. Even in cases infected with sensitive organisms, such as *P. mirablis*, there are alternatives that are given less frequently and are therefore less expensive to administer. Furthermore, most of the organisms susceptible to ampicillin are found in mixed infections with those organisms (i.e., *Staphylococcus*) that are resistant. Therefore other single agents that can cover all of the organisms are widely available. Some potential uses include the following:

1. Infection with a community-acquired gram-negative that is susceptible.
2. Superficial infection or contamination with an *Enterococcus*.

Amoxicillin

Amoxicillin is a semisynthetic ampicillin that differs only in the presence of a hydroxy group, thereby increasing its ability to be absorbed orally. In fact, levels achieved following oral administration of amoxicillin are almost twice that of the same dose of ampicillin. Spectrum of activity, adverse reactions, and clinical usage are the same as those for ampicillin. It is available in 250- and 500-mg capsules.

Dosage and Administration
1. 250 to 500 mg tid PO.
2. Food has minimal effect on serum levels.
3. Probenecid will increase and prolong serum levels.
4. Dosage adjustment in renal failure is similar to that of ampicillin.

■ Semisynthetic (Penicillinase-Resistant) Penicillins

Nafcillin

Being inherently more effective against staphylococci than methicillin, and also less toxic, nafcillin has become the parenteral penicillinase-resistant penicillin of choice. Although also available in an oral form, nafcillin is administered exclusively parenterally because of its poor absorption and low tissue levels.

Spectrum of Activity
1. *Staphylococcus aureus*, both penicillinase and non–penicillinase-producing.
2. Not effective against methicillin-resistant staphylococci.
3. Not as effective as natural penicillin or aminopenicillins against streptococci. Not effective against enterococci.
4. Ineffective against gram-negative rods.

Adverse Reactions
The incidence of neutropenia is slightly higher than with other penicillins; otherwise their incidences of adverse reactions are similar.

Dosage and Administration
1. 1 to 2 g q4h to q6h IV or IM for most infections.
2. Serum levels are increased by probenecid.

3. Because nafcillin is metabolized by the liver, little or no adjustment is needed in renal failure.
4. Some dosage adjustment is probably required in hepatic failure.

Clinical Usage
1. Parenteral penicillin of choice for moderate to severe staphylococcal infections.
2. Because of the necessity of frequent dosing and its subsequent high cost, there are alternatives that may be more cost-effective and equally efficacious.

Cloxacillin and Dicloxacillin
These agents, known as the *isoxazolyl penicillins*, are covered together because they are both administered orally, and, although there are differences in protein binding and absorption, their achievable levels are similar. Oxacillin is not included here because it has no advantage as a parenteral agent over nafcillin and no advantage as an oral agent over these two drugs.

Spectrum of Activity
The spectrum of activity is the same as that of nafcillin.

Adverse Reactions
See the discussion of adverse reactions for penicillins in the introduction.

Dosage and Administration
1. 250 to 500 mg qid PO for most infections.
2. 500 mg to 1 g qid PO for more severe infections.
3. Most effective when taken on an empty stomach 1 to 2 hours before eating. Serum level of dicloxacillin is more affected by food than is cloxacillin.
4. Probenecid will increase serum levels.
5. Little or no dosage reduction is required with renal insufficiency.

Clinical Usage
Cloxacillin and dicloxacillin are the oral penicillins of choice for mild to moderate staphylococcal infection. They are inexpensive, safe, and effective.

■ *Expanded-Spectrum Penicillins*

Carbenicillin

Although carbenicillin was the first penicillin developed with activity against *P. aeruginosa,* it has no use in the treatment of lower extremity infections. The drugs that have been developed subsequently are safer, require a lower dosage, and are more effective against the same organisms. Before the development of the quinolones, indanyl carbenicillin had been used, inappropriately, as an oral therapy for pseudomonal soft tissue infections. Oral carbenicillin is not absorbed and does not achieve therapeutic levels in the tissues. Its sole indication is urinary tract infection.

Ticarcillin

Ticarcillin is a parenteral antibiotic that is twofold to fourfold more active against *Pseudomonas* than carbenicillin. It therefore requires a lower dosage for comparable efficacy.

Spectrum of Activity

1. *P. aeruginosa*, indole-positive *Proteus, Morganella*, and the Enterobacteriaceae. Resistance can develop in all of these via ß-lactamase induction if the drug is used as a single agent.
2. Less active against the streptococci than penicillin.
3. Less active against the enterococci than mezlocillin.
4. Active against some anaerobes.
5. Not active against most staphylococci.

Adverse Reactions

1. Very high sodium load: 120 mg/g (although less than carbenicillin). This leads to the possible development of hypokalemia, hypernatremia, and fluid retention problems.
2. Possibility of bleeding secondary to platelet dysfunction.
3. Otherwise adverse reactions are the same as those of other penicillins.

Dosage and Administration

1. 3 g q4h to q6h IV for most infections.
2. Requires moderate to major dosage reductions with creatinine clearance below 60 ml/min. The interval should be increased to q8h to q12h.
3. Probenecid increases serum levels.

Clinical Usage
1. Because of the increased activity and decreased sodium load of the ureidopenicillins, ticarcillin has been relegated to a "back shelf" position in the treatment of most lower extremity infections. It has no place as a single-agent drug.
2. Traditionally combined with an aminoglycoside (such as tobramycin, the so-called "T&T" combination) for serious gram-negative infections. There are now safer single agents that have relegated this usage to primarily historic interest.
3. Combined with clindamycin and an aminoglycoside for severe mixed infections. Again, single agents should be considered in place of this usage when possible.

Mezlocillin (Mezlin)
The first of the ureidopenicillins, mezlocillin is described separately because of some important differences in spectrum and side effects. All ureidopenicillins are available as parenteral agents only. All have significantly less sodium than ticarcillin.

Spectrum of Activity
1. Similar to ticarcillin against most gram-negative organisms.
2. Less active against *P. aeruginosa* than piperacillin.
3. More active against the enterococci than any other expanded-spectrum penicillin.
4. More active against *Bacteroides* than other penicillins.
5. Not active against most staphylococci.

Adverse Reactions
1. Less bleeding is seen with mezlocillin than with any other expanded-spectrum penicillin.
2. Otherwise, adverse reactions are the same as those of penicillin.

Dosage and Administration
1. 3 g q4h to q6h IV.
2. Probenecid increases serum levels.
3. Only minor dosage reductions are required when creatinine clearance drops below 30 ml/min.

Clinical Usage
1. Seldom used as a single agent.

2. Single-agent use may be possible in mild-to-moderate entero-coccal infections.
3. Combined with an aminoglycoside or quinolone and an anti-staphylococcal agent for severe mixed infections. However, this can usually be accomplished much easier with fewer drugs.

Piperacillin (Pipracil)

This drug, along with the previously marketed azlocillin, constitutes the other members of the ureidopenicillins. They are considered together because, except for some differences in spectrum, they are very similar.

Spectrum of Activity

1. Both have very good activity against *P. aeruginosa*. They are both more effective against this organism than any other penicillin.
2. Both have activity similar to ampicillin against the streptococci.
3. Neither works against staphylococci.

Adverse Reactions

Adverse reactions are similar to those of other penicillins.

Dosage and Administration

Dosage and administration are similar to those of mezlocillin, 3 to 4 g q4h to q6h.

Clinical Usage

1. Combined with an aminoglycoside for severe pseudomonal infections. Again, single agents have basically supplanted combinations for these infections in the lower extremity.
2. Neither of these drugs should be used unless there is a documented or highly suspected pseudomonal infection.
3. Seldom used as a single agent.

■ ß-Lactamase Inhibitor Combinations

The three currently available ß-lactamase inhibitors, clavulanic acid, sulbactam, and tazobactam, have similar mechanisms of action. These agents are all ß-lactam antibiotics with weak intrinsic antibacterial activity. All, however, have a high affinity for ß-lactamase. When combined with a more active antibiotic, the inhibitor will bind up any ß-lactamase released from the organism. This effectively destroys the inhibitor (thus the nickname "suicide agent") while allowing the other drug to work against the organism unimpeded by the enzyme. This action enhances the spectrum of activity of the antibiotics with which the inhibitor is combined. These agents can now work against many ß-lacta-mase–producing bacteria formerly resistant to them.

None of the currently available agents can inhibit the inducible (Richmond-Sykes I) chromosomal ß-lactamase produced by such organisms as *Pseudomonas, Citrobacter, Serratia, Enterobacter*, or *Morganella*. For this reason, these combination drugs are no more effective against these organisms than the original antibiotic.

This last point is clinically important because many clinicians have been detailed by pharmaceutical representatives on the antipseudomonal activity of these agents. They incorrectly assume that these drugs can be used as single agents against this organism. As a rule, only use these combinations as single agents if the "parent" compound could be used as a single agent. For example, ticarcillin would not be an adequate therapy for most infections caused by *P. aeruginosa*. Therefore ticarcillin/clavulanic acid should not be used in the same situation.

Ticarcillin/Clavulanic Acid (Timentin)

Ticarcillin/clavulanic acid was the first parenteral drug to come on the market that used the inhibitor combination approach to therapy. It is generally available as a fixed combination of 3 g ticarcillin plus 100 mg clavulanic acid. This is commonly ordered as a 3.1-g dose.

Spectrum of Activity

1. Most staphylococci (although not methicillin-resistant staphylococci).
2. Activity against streptococci is similar to that of ticarcillin.
3. Activity against gram-negative organisms is similar to that of ticarcillin, with additional activity against ß-lactamase-producing strains of *E. coli, Klebsiella, Haemophilus*, gonococci, and *Salmonella*. Also effective against any other gram-negative organism with plasmid-mediated production of enzymes.
4. No more effective than straight ticarcillin against organisms with chromosomal ß-lactamase. See the introduction above for a list of these organisms.
5. Excellent activity against anaerobes, including *Bacteroides fragilis*.

Adverse Reactions
1. Similar to those of ticarcillin. Sodium loading is the major concern. Therefore electrolyte imbalance and the development of hypokalemia should be monitored. There is a potential for fluid retention sequelae (i.e., congestive heart failure).
2. See other penicillins for additional adverse reactions.

Dosage and Administration
1. 3.1 g q6h to q8h IV for most infections.
2. Dosage reduction in renal failure follows the same guidelines as with ticarcillin.

Clinical Usage
1. One potential drug of choice for empiric therapy of moderate to severe diabetic foot infections.
2. One potential drug of choice for parenteral therapy of human and animal bite wounds.
3. Useful when the Gram stain shows mixed gram-positive and gram-negative flora. Also of use when anaerobic organisms are highly suspected.
4. Not as widely used anymore since the introduction of piperacillin/tazobactam (see p. 228).

Amoxicillin/Clavulanic Acid (Augmentin)

Amoxicillin/clavulanic acid was the first oral agent developed using the ß-lactamase inhibitor concept. It is available in 250-, 500-, and 875-mg tablets. All contain the same amount of clavulanic acid, 125 mg. Therefore two 250-mg tablets *do not* equal one 500-mg tablet.

Spectrum of Activity
1. Staphylococci (although not methicillin-resistant staphylococci).
2. Antistreptococcal activity is similar to that of amoxicillin.
3. Enterococci.
4. Gram-negative organisms that produce plasmid-mediated ß-lactamase (see ticarcillin/clavulanic acid) including the extended spectrum ß-lactamases (ESBLs).
5. Excellent anaerobic coverage, including *B. fragilis*.

Adverse Reactions
1. Possibly higher incidence of diarrhea than with amoxicillin. Somewhat decreased since the common dosing interval was decreased from three times a day to twice a day.

2. Otherwise, adverse reactions are the same as those of amoxicillin.

Dosage and Administration
1. 500 to 875 mg bid PO. Should be given with food and a full glass of water to minimize the potential for diarrhea.
2. Serum levels are not affected by food.
3. Dosage in renal failure is the same as that for amoxicillin.

Clinical Usage
1. Outpatient therapy of mild-to-moderate diabetic foot infections (i.e., infected ulcerations).
2. Skin and soft tissue infections caused by mixed flora, including staphylococci, sensitive gram-negative organisms, anaerobes, and enterococci.
3. The oral drug of choice for empiric therapy of animal and human bite wound infections.
4. Should not be used as oral therapy of monomicrobial infections (e.g., those caused by staphylococci alone). There are less expensive, equally efficacious oral drugs for these infections.

Ampicillin/Sulbactam (Unasyn)
Ampicillin/sulbactam was the first agent developed using the inhibitor sulbactam. It is available only in a parenteral form in a fixed ampicillin:sulbactam ratio of 2:1. It comes in 3 g (2 g ampicillin, 1 g sulbactam) and 1.5 g (1 g ampicillin, 0.5 g sulbactam) doses.

Spectrum of Activity
1. Similar to that of amoxicillin/clavulanic acid.
2. Slightly more active than ticarcillin/clavulanic acid against the gram-positive organisms, including the enterococci.
3. Less active than ticarcillin/clavulanic acid and piperacillin/tazobactam against the gram-negative organisms.

Adverse Reactions
Adverse reactions are similar to those of ticarcillin/clavulanic acid, although with a slightly lower sodium load.

Dosage and Administration
1. 1.5 to 3 g q6h IV or IM for most infections.
2. The 1.5-g size is used for less severe infections.
3. Dosage in renal failure is the same as that of ampicillin.

Clinical Usage
1. Empiric therapy of moderately severe diabetic foot infections when the Gram stain reveals predominately gram-positive organisms.
2. Mixed infections, including enterococcal, staphylococcal, and anaerobic organisms.
3. Empiric therapy of bite wound infections.

Piperacillin/tazobactam (Zosyn)

Piperacillin/tazobactam is the most recent of the inhibitor compounds to reach the market. It has generally supplanted ticarcillin/clavulanic acid in many hospitals, although the spectrum of activity is very similar.

Spectrum of Activity
1. Similar to ticarcillin/clavulanic acid. May be slightly broader spectrum.
2. Enhanced activity against *Enterococcus*. This may be due to inherent activity of piperacillin as opposed to the addition of the tazobactam.

Adverse Reactions
Similar to other drugs in this class.

Dosage and Administration
1. 3.375 g q6h IV.
2. 4.5 g q8h dosing may save money and is just as effective.

Clinical Usage
1. One of the empiric drugs of choice for moderate to severe diabetic foot infections.
2. Empiric therapy of presumed mixed aerobic, anaerobic infection where a broader-spectrum agent is desired.
3. Severe bite wound infections.

CEPHALOSPORINS

Giuseppe Brotzu is responsible for discovering the precursor to almost all subsequent cephalosporins. This agent, cephalosporin C, was isolated from raw sewage in Sardinia. From these modest beginnings, the most commercially successful class of antibiotics was launched. Physicians who have attempted to stay current with all of the advances in these agents most likely curse that fateful day in 1945. That being said, the proliferation of new drugs that was seen throughout the 1980s and early 1990s has slowed considerably. Whereas new drugs seemingly appeared daily, the flow is currently at a trickle only to be superseded by other classes such as the quinolones.

All cephalosporins share a similar basic structure: a four-member ß-lactam ring attached to a six-member dihydrothiazine ring. Modifications, by the addition of various sidechains to different locations on the parent molecule, are responsible for the individual characteristics of each agent.

■ *Mechanism of Action*

The mechanism of action of the cephalosporins appears to be similar to that of the penicillins. Originally thought to directly interfere with cell wall synthesis, they are now known to interact with the PBPs found on the cell wall or membrane. Which particular type of PBP the agent binds with determines what the spectrum of activity will be. For example, first-generation drugs have a higher affinity for the PBP of *S. aureus* than do some later-generation drugs.

Resistance to the cephalosporins is also mediated in much the same way as that of the penicillins. Decreased binding to the PBP is one common mechanism of resistance. Either the drug cannot reach the PBP or the PBP site is altered. The other common cause of resistance is the production of ß-lactamase enzymes capable of hydrolyzing the agent. Cephalosporins have variable susceptibility to these enzymes. First-generation cephalosporins are more resistant to hydrolysis by staphylococcal enzymes, whereas later-generation drugs are more resistant to gram-negative enzymes. Some gram-negative organisms, including *Enterobacter, Citrobacter, Serratia, Morganella, Pseudomonas, Providencia,* and *Acinetobacter,* produce a chromosomal ß-lactamase, the Richmond-Sykes type 1, that is capable of inactivating all cephalosporins. The production of these enzymes can be "induced" or "derepressed" when an organism is subject to treatment with a ß-lactam antibiotic. Therefore an organism that appears initially sensitive may develop rapid resistance.

■ *Classification*

The cephalosporin antibiotics are classified into four groups or "generations," based loosely on their antibacterial spectrum (Box 9-2). Some general statements can be made about each

---

BOX 9-2

Commonly Used Cephalosporin Antibiotics

First-Generation—Parenteral
Cefazolin   (Ancef, Kefzol)
Cephaparin   (Cefadyl)

First-Generation—Oral
Cephalexin   (Keflex, Keftab)
Cephradine   (Velosef)
Cefadroxil   (Duricef)

Second-Generation—Parenteral
Cefoxitin   (Mefoxin)
Cefuroxime   (Zinacef)
Cefotetan   (Cefotan)
Cefamandole   (Mandol)

Second-Generation—Oral
Cefaclor   (Ceclor)
Cefuroxime axetil   (Ceftin)
Cefprozil   (Cefzil)

Third-Generation—Parenteral
Cefotaxime   (Claforan)
Ceftizoxime   (Cefizox)
Ceftriaxone   (Rocephin)
Ceftazidime   (Fortaz, Tazicef, Tazidime)
Cefoperazone   (Cefobid)

Third-Generation—Oral
Cefdinir   (Omnicef)
Cefpodoxime proxetil   (Vantin)
Cefixime   (Suprax)

Fourth-Generation—Parenteral
Cefepime   (Maxipime)

group. It should be remembered that there is some overlap in this system. Individual drugs of any given group may not fit the general statement.

1. It has been traditionally taught that first-generation cephalosporins have better overall activity against the gram-positive cocci than later generations. Although this was initially true, some of the newer second-, third-, and even fourth-generation drugs have activity that is equal to if not better than the first-generation agents.
2. Second-generation cephalosporins were developed specifically for increased activity against *H. influenzae.*
3. As a side benefit, second-generation drugs also have increased activity against a few other gram-negative organisms, including some indole-positive *Proteus* and resistant *E. coli.*
4. Some third-generation cephalosporins have less gram-positive activity than earlier generations, although, as previously mentioned, this distinction has blurred. However, it is still a truism that these drugs have increased gram-negative coverage. They were specifically designed to be effective against the "nosocomial" pathogens. Unfortunately, many of the gram-negative nosocomial pathogens have developed resistance to even these later-generation drugs.
5. The newest group, the fourth-generation cephalosporins, have the benefit of the gram-negative coverage of the third generation, including excellent activity against *P. aeruginosa*, a trait not even shared by all third-generation drugs, *plus* the gram-positive activity of the first generation.

■ *Spectrum of Activity*

General trends in microbial susceptibility can be stated for each generation of cephalosporin. Any variation from these trends is noted under each individual agent.

1. First generation.
   a. Staphylococci (penicillinase and non–penicillinase-producing, except for methicillin-resistant organisms).
   b. Streptococci.
   c. Gram-negative organisms, including many *E. coli, P. mirablis, Shigella,* and *Salmonella* that do not produce ESBL.
   d. Anaerobes other than *Bacteroides.*

2. Second generation.
   a. Staphylococci.
   b. Streptococci (similar to first-generation drugs).
   c. Expanded gram-negative coverage, including *H. influenzae*, some indole-positive *Proteus*, *Klebsiella*, and some resistant *E. coli*.
   d. Anaerobic coverage similar to that of first-generation drugs, with cefoxitin and cefotetan both active against some *Bacteroides*.
3. Third generation.
   a. Staphylococci (but most are less active than earlier agents).
   b. Streptococci (similar to both first- and second-generation drugs).
   c. Generally more active against gram-negative rods. Sensitivity varies with each individual agent and each organism because of the development of the aforementioned ß-lactamases.
   d. Excellent coverage against most gonococci.
   e. The anaerobic spectrum is similar to that of other cephalosporins. *Bacteroides* coverage varies with each agent.
   f. There is variable coverage of *P. aeruginosa* depending on the drug, with ceftazidime having the best coverage.
4. Fourth generation.
   a. Staphylococci comparable to first generation.
   b. Streptococci.
   c. Gram negatives including *P. aeruginosa*.

Some organisms are generally resistant to all cephalosporins:

1. Methicillin-resistant organisms, including *S. aureus* and *Staphylococcus epidermidis*.
2. Enterococci.
3. *Clostridium difficile*.
4. *Acinetobacter*.

■ *Adverse Reactions*

Because cephalosporins are structurally related to the penicillins, their observed adverse reactions are similar. As is the case with penicillins, cephalosporins are relatively safe agents. This is not to say that these drugs are free from adverse effects. Any of the following can be seen. Any adverse reaction peculiar to a particular agent is included in the discussion of that agent.

1. Hypersensitivity reactions are by far the most common effect seen with cephalosporin use. These "allergies" can take any form, from rare life-threatening anaphylactic reactions, which are less common with cephalosporins than penicillins, to the more common "rash." The true etiology of this skin reaction is not known. A more complete discussion on hypersensitivity, and in particular, cross-reactions between ß-lactams, can be found in Chapter 8.
2. Diarrhea with or without enterocolitis.
3. Bleeding, especially with those agents that contain the n-methylthiotetrazole (MTT) sidechain structure.
4. Neutropenia.
5. Phlebitis with intravenous administration.

■ *First-Generation Cephalosporins—Parenteral*

Cefazolin (Ancef, Kefzol)

Although other agents, such as cephalothin, were developed first, cefazolin has become the clear parenteral first-generation cephalosporin of choice. The main reason for this preference is its longer half-life, which allows less frequent dosing compared to its competitors.

Spectrum of Activity

1. *S. aureus* (non–methicillin-resistant staphylococci). The one disadvantage of this drug is that it may be slightly less active, at least in vitro, against staphylococci than other first-, and even some later-generation drugs. The clinical relevance of this difference is not clear, and this has clearly become the drug of first choice for most staphylococcal infections.
2. Streptococci. May be slightly less effective than penicillin, but, because of the less frequent dosing, it is frequently useful.
3. Gram-negative organisms, including *E. coli, P. mirablis*, some *Klebsiella* (not generally *Klebsiella pneumoniae*).
4. Anaerobes, including *Peptococcus* and *Peptostreptococcus*. Not *B. fragilis* or other *Bacteroides*.

Adverse Reactions

Adverse reactions are the same as those of other cephalosporins.

Dosage and Administration

1. 1 g q8h IM or IV for most infections. For more severe infections should be increased to 2 g q8h. Should not be shortened to q6h.

2. Moderate to major dosage reduction is required with renal failure.

3. Probenecid will increase serum levels of almost all cephalosporins. Because of cefazolin's prolonged half-life, the addition of probenecid is not as important as with the penicillins and is practically never used.

Clinical Usage

1. The drug of choice for initial empiric treatment of many community-acquired infections of the lower extremity. As with all antibiotics, treatment should be modified with receipt of the culture report and clinical findings.

2. Can be used effectively to treat most infections caused by sensitive staphylococci. Because of its lower dosage and less frequent dosing interval, it is more cost-effective than even significantly less-expensive penicillins.

3. May be used for infections caused by streptococci. However, for the same reasons as stated previously, cefazolin may be less expensive than penicillin, penicillin seems to be more active clinically and should still be considered the drug of choice.

4. Most commonly used drug for prophylaxis of lower extremity surgery.

■ *First-Generation Cephalosporins—Oral*

Cephalexin (Keflex, Keftab)/Cephradine (Velosef)

Cephalexin and cephradine are two orally available cephalosporins having a spectrum of activity and adverse effects similar to those seen with cefazolin. Keftab is a hydrochloride salt of cephalexin that is approved for less-frequent dosing but has recently been withdrawn from the market.

Dosage and Administration

1. 250 to 500 mg bid–qid PO. The lower dosage should be used for less severe infections. The dosage may be increased to as high as 3 to 4 g/day for more severe cases. Cephalexin hydrochloride is dosed 500 mg twice a day.

2 Moderate dosage reduction is required with renal failure.

3. Probenecid will increase serum levels but is rarely used.

Clinical Usage

1. Outpatient therapy of many community-acquired infections.

Especially useful if there is a mix of gram-positive and some susceptible gram-negative organisms.
2. For infections caused solely by staphylococci, one of the semi-synthetic penicillins may be less expensive, but its more frequent dosing makes it less convenient.
3. Usefulness for prophylaxis in outpatient surgery has not been proven, but these drugs are frequently used for this purpose.

Cefadroxil (Duricef)
The addition of a hydroxyl group to cephalexin yields cefadroxil. The sole difference between these agents is that cefadroxil has prolonged serum levels when compared to cephalexin, thereby altering dosing schedules. All other parameters are the same. It offers no real advantage over cephalexin.

Dosage and Administration
1. 500 mg q12h PO or 1 g q24h PO for most infections.
2. 1 g q12h PO for more severe infections.

■ Second-Generation Cephalosporins—Parenteral

Cefoxitin (Mefoxin)
First released in 1978, cefoxitin was one of the first second-generation cephalosporins. Actually a cephamycin rather than a cephalosporin, cefoxitin has some interesting characteristics that differentiate it from other members of this class. Most of these differences are in the area of spectrum. Cefoxitin is available only in a parenteral form.

Spectrum of Activity
1. More active against the gram-negative organisms than cefazolin.
2. Less active against the gram-positive organisms than either cefazolin or the other second-generation cephalosporins.
3. Cefoxitin has been shown consistently to be the most active cephalosporin against the anaerobic organisms. This spectrum includes most members of the *Bacteroides* family.

Adverse Reactions
Adverse reactions of cefoxitin are similar to those of other cephalosporins.

Dosage and Administration
1. 2 g q6h to q8h for most infections. Usually given intravenously.
2. When to be injected intramuscularly, the drug should be diluted in lidocaine to decrease pain.
3. Moderate dosage reduction is required in renal insufficiency.

Clinical Usage
1. Empiric therapy of infections that frequently include anaerobic pathogens (i.e., diabetic foot infections). Much of its use in these cases has been superseded by the ß-lactamase inhibitor compounds.
2. In areas where *Enterococcus* is endemic, cefoxitin should be used cautiously to prevent selection of those resistant organisms.

Cefotetan (Cefotan)
Cefotetan is another second-generation cephalosporin (also technically a cephamycin) developed to compete with cefoxitin. They both have a relatively similar spectrum of activity, with the exceptions listed subsequently. Cefotetan also has a longer half-life, allowing less-frequent dosing. Unfortunately, cefotetan also contains an MTT sidechain, so there may be an increased potential for adverse events related to this moiety. It is available only in a parenteral form.

Spectrum of Activity
1. Anaerobic spectrum similar to that of cefoxitin but less active against non-*fragilis* species of *Bacteroides*.
2. More active against the gram-positive and gram-negative organisms than cefoxitin, with activity approaching that of the third-generation drugs.

Adverse Reactions
Cefotan contains an MTT sidechain with all of the corresponding side effects. These include possible bleeding and alcohol intolerance, although the true clinical importance of the MTT sidechain may be minimal.

Dosage and Administration
1. 1 to 2 g q12h IV for most infections.
2. Moderate dosage adjustment is required in renal insufficiency. The interval should be increased from 12 to 24 hours.

Clinical Usage
1. Settings similar to those of cefoxitin.

Cefuroxime (Zinacef)

Cefuroxime is a second-generation cephalosporin that has all of the "traditional" benefits of this class of agents. It also has improved activity against the gram-positive organisms. It is available in both a parenteral form and an oral form, which will be covered separately.

Spectrum of Activity
1. Excellent coverage against *H. influenzae*. Also, other gram-negative organisms are usually sensitive to this class of agents.
2. Staphylococcal coverage is the best of any parenteral second-generation drug. Some evidence points to staphylococcal coverage at least comparable to the first-generation agents.

Adverse Reactions
Adverse reactions are similar to those of other cephalosporins.

Dosage and Administration
1. 750 mg q12h IV or IM for most infections.
2. 1.5 g q12h for more severe infections.
3. Moderate dosage reduction in renal insufficiency.

Clinical Usage
1. Because of the rarity of infections caused by organisms such as *H. influenzae*, cefuroxime has limited use in the lower extremity.
2. Because of its good staphylococcal coverage and relatively long half-life, there is a possible place for this drug in surgical prophylaxis, although the advantage over less expensive, first-generation agents has not been proven.

Cefamandole (Mandol)

Along with cefoxitin, cefamandole was one of the earliest second-generation cephalosporins. Because of the potential for side effects caused by its MTT sidechain, and no clear-cut therapeutic advantage over other agents, this drug has gradually fallen into disfavor in the treatment of lower extremity infections. Its use has been limited to mostly surgical prophylaxis. The reason for this use is its in vitro advantage against some resistant staphylococci compared with other drugs. The clinical relevance of this finding is unclear.

■ *Second-Generation Cephalosporins—Oral*

Cefaclor (Ceclor)
Although considered a first-generation agent by some, cefaclor's expanded coverage against *Haemophilus* has led to general consideration that it is a second-generation drug. It is available in 250- and 500-mg capsules.

Spectrum of Activity
Its spectrum of activity is similar to that of most first-generation agents, except for slightly more activity against *H. influenzae*.

Adverse Reactions
Adverse reactions are similar to those of other cephalosporins.

Dosage and Administration
250 to 500 mg three times a day.

Clinical Usage
Cefaclor offers no advantage over other oral cephalosporins in the treatment of lower extremity infections.

Cefuroxime Axetil (Ceftin)
Cefuroxime axetil is the oral form of the parenteral drug cefuroxime. It is available in 125-, 250-, and 500-mg tablets. Its long half-life allows for twice-daily dosing.

Spectrum of Activity
1. Like the parent compound, the oral form is more active in vitro against gram-positive organisms than some of the first-generation drugs.
2. Gram-negative and anaerobic spectrum is similar to that of the parenteral form.

Adverse Reactions
Adverse reactions are similar to those of other cephalosporins.

Dosage and Administration
1. 125 to 250 mg twice a day for most infections.
2. The 500-mg tablet is seldom needed.

Clinical Usage
1. Can be used in place of older oral cephalosporins for empiric therapy of many mild-to-moderate community-acquired lower extremity infections.
2. Although relatively expensive, it can be cost-effective compared to other nongeneric oral cephalosporins because of its twice-daily dosing and excellent staphylococcal coverage.
3. Once cultures are received, the patient should be switched to a narrower-spectrum, less-expensive agent.

Cefprozil (Cefzil)

Very similar in many respects to cefuroxime axetil, this second-generation oral cephalosporin actually has better activity against staphylococcus and streptococcus than do some of the first-generation drugs. It also can be dosed as a true, twice-a-day, drug.

Spectrum of Activity
Similar to cefuroxime axetil.

Adverse Reactions
Adverse reactions are similar to those of other cephalosporins.

Dosage and Administration
250 to 500 mg twice a day.

Clinical Usage
Same as cefuroxime axetil.

Loracarbef (Lorabid)

Considered by many to be nothing more than a twice-a-day version of cefaclor, this drug, a carbacephem antibiotic, has minimal use in the treatment of lower extremity infections. See discussion concerning cefaclor for more information.

Dosage and Administration
400 mg twice a day.

■ *Third-Generation Cephalosporins—Parenteral*

Cefotaxime (Claforan)

Released in the early 1980s, cefotaxime was the first third-generation cephalosporin available for use. It has all of the prototypical activities of this group of agents. One unusual aspect of this drug is that it is metabolized to desacetyl cefotaxime, which is also an active antibiotic. There is evidence that this metabolite may interact synergistically with the parent compound to increase its half-life and antimicrobial spectrum.

Spectrum of Activity
1. May be slightly more active against the gram-positive organisms than other third-generation agents.
2. Gram-negative spectrum includes all the typical organisms against which these drugs were originally targeted. Caution should be used in treating gram-negative organisms with inducible type I ß-lactamase.
3. Not effective against *P. aeruginosa*.
4. Activity against the anaerobes, especially *Bacteroides*, has been shown in vitro when cefotaxime is combined with its metabolite.

Adverse Reactions
Adverse reactions are similar to those of other cephalosporins.

Dosage and Administration
1. 1 to 2 g q8h to q12h IV or IM for most infections.
2. 2 g q6h IV or IM for severe infections.
3. Unlike most cephalosporins, dosage has to be decreased only in severe renal failure (creatinine clearance less than 20 ml/min).

Clinical Usage
1. Because of the potential for an enhanced anaerobic spectrum, cefotaxime may be useful in treating diabetic foot infections either as a single agent or combined with clindamycin. However, there are better drugs for this indication.
2. Useful as a "workhorse" third-generation agent with infections that are caused by susceptible organisms. Overall usefulness of most agents in this class of drugs is relatively limited. This is especially true with the increase in resistant organisms and the advent of the quinolones.

Ceftizoxime (Cefizox)
Ceftizoxime is similar to cefotaxime in most parameters. Although not metabolized in the same fashion as the other drug, studies have shown that ceftizoxime may have some inherent activity against the *Bacteroides*. Unfortunately, these studies have been largely in vitro, and a significant effect has been noted with

changes in the media in which the studies have been run. The clinical relevance of this activity is not clear.

Dosage and Administration
1. 1 to 2 g q8h to q12h for most infections.
2. Moderate dosage reduction is required in renal insufficiency.

Clinical Usage
The clinical usage is similar to that of cefotaxime.

Ceftriaxone (Rocephin)
Ceftriaxone has the longest half-life of any cephalosporin, about 7 to 8 hours. This allows a much longer interval between doses compared to other drugs. In fact, once-daily dosing has been the most accepted dosing for this drug. The drug is extensively protein bound, which may limit the amount of freely circulating drug available to kill the organism, especially at lower dosages. Another distinction of this drug is its significant biliary elimination.

Spectrum of Activity
Similar to cefotaxime. Possibly less active against the gram-positive organisms.

Adverse Reactions
Because of biliary elimination, there may be a higher incidence of diarrhea with this drug.

Dosage and Administration
1. 1 to 2 g q12h to q24h IV or IM. For most infections 1 to 2 g/day is the maximum required dosage. There is little or no indication for dosages as high as 4 g/day.
2. Minimal to no dosage adjustment is required in renal insufficiency because of biliary elimination.

Clinical Usage
1. The drug of choice for infections caused by gonococci. Should be used empirically in a young adult presenting with the clinical symptoms of septic arthritis.
2. Has become the drug of choice for more advanced cases of Lyme borreliosis.
3. Outpatient therapy of susceptible infections. Can be given as a daily intramuscular injection/intravenous infusion in the office setting. Although frequently used as outpatient, long-term

therapy for *S. aureus* osteomyelitis, there may be better selections with more activity against that pathogen.
4. Should not be used for surgical prophylaxis because of its high cost and relatively weak antistaphylococcal activity when compared to first-generation agents.

Ceftazidime (Fortaz, Tazicef, Tazidime)

Ceftazidime has the distinction of being the most active cephalosporin against *P. aeruginosa*. The tradeoff for this expanded spectrum is significantly less activity against the gram-positive organisms. Otherwise the gram-negative spectrum is similar to that of cefotaxime. Adverse reactions are also similar to those of other cephalosporins.

Dosage and Administration
1. 1 g q8h IV or IM for skin and skin structure infections.
2. 2 g q12h IV or IM for bone and joint infections.
3. Moderate dosage adjustment is needed in renal insufficiency.

Clinical Usage
Reserved as single-agent therapy in many infections caused by *P. aeruginosa*. This includes most skin infections and osteomyelitis. (Note: This may not be a popular view with those physicians who claim that all pseudomonal infections must be treated with at least two antibiotics.)

Cefoperazone (Cefobid)

The first cephalosporin with activity against *P. aeruginosa*, cefoperazone has a sufficiently long half-life to allow less frequent dosing. Unfortunately, cefoperazone contains an MTT sidechain and is highly protein bound. It also has some interesting quirks in its spectrum that limit its use.

Spectrum of Activity
1. Activity against *P. aeruginosa* is twofold to fourfold less than ceftazidime.
2. Cefoperazone is significantly less active than cefotaxime against other gram-negative and gram-positive organisms.

Adverse Reactions
1. Because of its MTT sidechain, there is a potential for bleeding and a disulfiram-like (Antabuse) reaction.

2. Because of biliary elimination, there is a potential for increased incidence of diarrhea.

Dosage and Administration
1. 2 g q12h IV for most infections.
2. The interval should be decreased to q8h for pseudomonal infections.
3. No dosage adjustment needed in renal insufficiency, but liver function must be monitored.

Clinical Usage
The clinical usage of this drug is limited by its side effect profile and the fact that its spectrum offers no advantage over any other cephalosporin. If *P. aeruginosa* is the organism of concern, then ceftazidime or a quinolone would be better choices.

■ *Third-Generation Cephalosporins—Oral*

Cefdinir (Omnicef)
Cefdinir is a third-generation oral cephalosporin that was originally marketed primarily as once-daily therapy for upper respiratory tract infections. It is now also being marketed as twice-daily therapy for lower extremity skin and skin structure infections. It has some interesting properties that make it a promising drug in this situation.

Spectrum of Activity
1. Better activity against staphylococci and streptococci than the first-generation drugs such as cephalexin. This has been shown both in vitro and in at least one clinical trial.
2. Good activity against the common community acquired gram-negatives while not being as broad spectrum as other third-generation cephalosporins against the Enterobacteriacaeae. Not effective against *P. aeruginosa*.

Adverse Reactions
Similar to earlier generation cephalosporins.

Dosage and Administration
1. 300 mg twice a day for skin and skin structure infections.
2. 600 mg once a day has been found effective in respiratory tract infections. This also may eventually be shown to be effective as once-daily therapy in skin and skin structure infections.

Clinical Usage

A potentially useful first-line empiric therapy for skin and skin structure infections of the lower extremity given the increased gram-positive activity versus first-generation drugs and the true twice-a-day (possibly, eventually qd) dosing.

Cefpodoxime Proxetil (Vantin)
Spectrum of activity
1. Somewhat less effective in vitro than cefdinir against staphylococcus and streptococcus.
2. Slightly broader spectrum against some of the Enterobacteriaceae than cefdinir.

Adverse Reactions
Similar to other cephalosporins.

Dosage and Administration
400 mg twice a day for skin and skin structure infections.

Clinical Usage
It has few advantages that would make it useful for lower extremity infections. There are alternatives for better gram-positive and gram-negative activity.

Cefixime (Suprax) and Ceftibuten (Cedax)
These drugs are considered together because of similar spectrum and usage. Cefixime was the first of the oral third-generation agents. The spectrum of these drugs is interesting in that they have no activity against staphylococci or *P. aeruginosa*. Otherwise, their spectrum is similar to other third-generation drugs. They are being marketed mainly for use in respiratory infections. There is almost no indication for these drugs in the treatment of lower extremity infections.

■ *Fourth-Generation Cephalosporins—Parenteral*

Cefepime (Maxipime)
Combines the advantages of antipseudomonal third generations with the anti-gram positive activity of earlier-generation drugs. All with twice-daily convenience.

Spectrum of activity
1. Good activity against staphylococci and streptococci approaching that of the first-generation drugs.

2. Activity against *P. aeruginosa* and other gram-negatives that is comparable if not better than ceftazidime.

Adverse reactions
Similar to other cephalosporins.

Dosage and Administration
1 to 2 g q12h IV for most infections.

Clinical Usage
1. A very broad-spectrum antibiotic that should be reserved for mixed infections in which *S. aureus* along with *P. aeruginosa* and other Enterobacteriaceae are playing a major role.
2. For pure infections caused by Pseudomonas, there are other agents, such as ciprofloxacin, that may be preferable.

CARBAPENEM ANTIBIOTICS

The carbapenem antibiotics are ß-lactam drugs containing a five-member ring attached to the ß-lactam ring structure, not unlike the cephalosporins. These are potent, broad-spectrum agents, derivatives of the compound thienamycin. They are resistant to most ß-lactamases, including the chromosomal-induced enzymes that are so effective in inactivating the later-generation cephalosporins. There are currently three compounds commercially available, with a third that may be released by the time of publication.

■ *Imipenem/Cilastatin (Primaxin)*

Imipenem was the first commercially available member of the carbapenem group of antibiotics. Initially it was found that imipenem was destroyed in the kidney. Cilastatin, a renal dehydropeptidase inhibitor, was added to the active drug to prevent this hydrolysis at the brush border of the renal tubule. Unlike clavulanic acid and sulbactam, cilastatin is not an antibiotic and does not affect the activity of imipenem.

Imipenem is an extremely potent antibiotic with the broadest spectrum of any available drug. Its spectrum is so broad that it is jokingly referred to as "gorillamycin." This broad spectrum comes at a significant cost because this drug is not inexpensive. However, when used in place of expensive and potentially toxic combination therapy, this drug can actually become cost-effective.

Spectrum of Activity

1. Most gram-positive aerobes and anaerobes. Some Enterococci are resistant. Although in vitro imipenem will inhibit many strains of methicillin-resistant staphylococcus, its activity is not dependable enough for infections caused by these organisms.
2. The only significantly resistant gram-negative organisms are *B. cepacia* and *S. maltophilia*. Resistance has also increased to *P. aeruginosa,* although it may still have clinically useful activity for mixed infections.
3. *Acinetobacter baumanii,* resistant to most antibiotics, is mostly susceptible to imipenem.
4. Imipenem has been shown to be the most effective ß-lactam antibiotic against clinically important strains of anaerobic bacteria. This includes all bacteroides and clostridia, with the exception of *C. difficile*.

Adverse Reactions

1. Imipenem has been shown to cause seizures in patients with a history of seizure disorders and in patients with markedly reduced renal function. This has been a problem especially in intensive care unit patients with multiple medical problems. The problem also becomes more prevalent with increased dosing.
2. Nausea and vomiting associated with infusing the drug too rapidly have been reported.
3. Cross-reactivity is possible in patients with a history of penicillin allergy.

Dosage and Administration

1. 500 mg q6h to q8h for most infections. If the patient's seizure history or renal function is unknown, therapy should be begun empirically with the less-frequent dosage.
2. Lesser dosages of 250 mg q6h have been used in less severe infections.
3. Dosages as high as 4 g/day have been used but may result in a significant increase in seizure potential and are not indicated in the treatment of lower extremity infections.
4. Moderate to major dosage adjustment is required in patients with renal insufficiency.

Clinical Usage

1. A very effective drug for the empiric therapy of life- or limb-threatening infections in the diabetic patient. This includes gas-forming infections such as necrotizing fasciitis.

2. Treatment of infections caused by traditionally multiresistant organisms such as *Acinetobacter*.
3. Because of the cost and potential for resistance development, imipenem is often reserved for severe life-threatening infections and is frequently under the restriction for use by the infectious disease section at most hospitals.

■ *Meropenem (Merrem)*

Unlike imipenem, meropenem does not require the addition of a renal dehydropeptidase inhibitor such as cilastatin. It also can be given less frequently. Otherwise, they are fairly similar drugs.

Spectrum of Activity
Slightly more effective than imipenem against some of the gram-negative organisms, including resistant *P. aeruginosa*. Less active against gram-positives. The clinical significance of these differences is not known.

Adverse Reactions
Similar to imipenem but may cause fewer seizures.

Dosage and Administration
1 to 2 g q8h IV.

Clinical Usage
See imipenem.

■ *Ertapenem (Invanz)*

The newest of the carbapenem antibiotics, this drug had been specifically studied in diabetic foot infections before its approval. It also has the advantage of once-daily dosing.

Spectrum of Activity
1. Slightly less active against gram-positive organisms than imipenem, but probably not of clinical significance.
2. More effective against the Enterobacteriaceae and at least equal against the anaerobes.
3. Not effective against *P. aeruginosa*.

Adverse Reactions
See meropenem.

Dosage and Administration
1 g q24h IV or IM.

Clinical Usage
1. In a large clinical trial against piperacillin/tazobactam for diabetic foot infections, ertapenem was found to be at least as effective. Therefore with its once-daily dosing and the ability to give IV or IM, this drug may prove very useful for this clinical situation.
2. Other mixed infections where broad gram-positive, gram-negative, and anaerobic coverage is needed.

OTHER ß-LACTAM ANTIBIOTICS

■ *Aztreonam (Azactam)*

Aztreonam is the first of a unique group of antibiotics known as the *monobactams*. They derive this name from their structure, which is a single ß-lactam ring without the corresponding five- or six-member ring seen with other ß-lactam drugs. Not only is the structure of aztreonam interesting, so is its antimicrobial spectrum and side effect profile.

Spectrum of Activity
1. Aztreonam is only active against gram-negative aerobes. This includes most *P. aeruginosa.*
2. The only resistant gram-negative organisms include *B. cepacia, S. maltophilia*, and *Acinetobacter*.
3. There is no activity against gram-positive organisms or anaerobes.

Adverse Reactions
1. A relatively safe drug with no major side effects.
2. Despite its being a ß-lactam, there have been no reports of cross-reactivity between aztreonam and any penicillin or cephalosporin.

Dosage and Administration
1. 1 to 2 g q8h IV. The 2-g dose should be reserved for the most severe cases.
2. Moderate dosage reductions are required in renal insufficiency.

Clinical Usage

1. In place of aminoglycosides for severe gram-negative infections.
2. In combination with clindamycin when a mixed infection including gram-negative organisms, gram-positive organisms, or anaerobes is suspected.
3. In penicillin- or cephalosporin-allergic patients to treat a susceptible infection.

AMINOGLYCOSIDES

Since its discovery in the 1940s, the aminoglycoside family of antibiotics has remained a mainstay in the treatment of severe gram-negative infections. Until the mid-1980s, these drugs were the only available therapy for infections caused by such organisms as *P. aeruginosa* and *A. baumanii*. With the availability of safer broad-spectrum agents, the role of aminoglycosides is now less defined. Despite significant toxicity and tricky dosing schedules, some physicians still only feel comfortable while using these agents when a gram-negative is present. There is still a school of thought that *P. aeruginosa* must always be treated with a combination including aminoglycosides. Although the need for these drugs is still fairly clear in life-threatening, systemic gram-negative infections, their use in the vast majority of lower extremity infections is mostly unnecessary and severely limited by the potentials for toxicity.

Only three aminoglycosides, *gentamicin (Garamycin), tobramycin (Nebcin),* and *amikacin (Amikin)*, have any indications for lower extremity use. Because all these drugs have similar spectrums of activity, adverse reactions, dosing principles, and clinical usages, they are considered jointly. When significant differences exist, they are listed.

Spectrum of Activity

1. Excellent coverage of the aerobic gram-negative bacteria. Although slight in vitro differences do exist, the clinical significance of these is difficult to prove. Some generalizations about each agent's gram-negative spectrum include the following:
   a. Gentamicin has the best activity against *Serratia*.
   b. Tobramycin is the most effective against *P. aeruginosa*.
   c. Amikacin is reserved for infection caused by gram-negative organisms resistant to gentamicin and tobramycin.

2. These drugs are effective against staphylococci. The reason they are not used against these organisms is that safer, equally effective agents are available.
3. Although some or most streptococci are susceptible, these agents are seldom used against these organisms. The exception to this is the common use of aminoglycosides in combination with a ß-lactam for synergy against the enterococci and some tolerant strains of streptococci.
4. These drugs have no activity against the anaerobes. Aminoglycosides require oxygen to cross the cell membrane.

Adverse Reactions

Serious adverse effects are the major reason for the decline of aminoglycosides' popularity. A number of risk factors predispose a patient to these toxicities:

1. Advanced age.
2. Previous therapy with aminoglycosides.
3. Concurrent use of certain drugs, including loop diuretics.
4. Chronic illness.
5. Genetic predisposition to develop toxicity.

There are three adverse effects most commonly mentioned.

Nephrotoxicity

Aminoglycoside nephrotoxicity is one of the most feared side effects. All three drugs are capable of producing this condition with only slight, probably insignificant, differences in potential. The onset of nephrotoxicity usually begins several days after initiation of therapy but may also be seen more rapidly or not until after the antibiotic has been discontinued. The first indication is usually a significant increase in serum creatinine. Unfortunately, by the time this occurs, significant damage may already have been done. Some clinicians have attempted to use early indicators such as urine casts and enzymes with mixed results. These tests are usually too nonspecific. Fortunately the damage is usually reversible. Concurrent use of vancomycin may potentiate this nephrotoxicity.

Ototoxicity

Probably the most devastating side effect of aminoglycoside use is ototoxicity. Unlike the nephrotoxicity, this condition is generally irreversible. Ototoxicity can manifest as either auditory or vestibular damage.

Symptoms of auditory toxicity include the following:

1. A feeling of fullness in the ears.
2. Tinnitus.
3. Loss of auditory acuity, especially in high frequencies.

Because the high-frequency hearing is the first affected, the patient normally has no difficulty hearing voices and may not perceive a problem. Audiometric testing is the most sensitive way to detect the loss.

Symptoms of vestibular toxicity include the following:

1. Dizziness.
2. Nausea.
3. Inability to maintain balance in a dark room.
4. Nystagmus.

As with nephrotoxicity, ototoxicity can occur at any time following initiation of therapy, but it generally is not seen until after the patient has been taking the drug for a number of days. Ototoxicity appears to be less connected to excessive serum levels of antibiotic than the nephrotoxicity.

Neuromuscular Blockade

When excessive levels of the antibiotic accumulate at the neuromuscular junction, acetylcholine release from the nerve is inhibited and paralysis results. The only mechanism for achieving such high levels is through rapid administration of the drug via an intravenous bolus injection. For this reason, aminoglycosides should always be infused over 30 minutes.

Dosage and Administration

Aminoglycosides are all available in a parenteral form. Gentamicin is also available in a topical cream. Aminoglycosides are not absorbed from the stomach and therefore are not available in an oral form.

There has been significant literature and debate in past years about the possible increased safety and efficacy of once-daily dosing for aminoglycosides as opposed to the more traditional multiple doses. It is becoming increasingly clear that the single daily dose is best. In order to be complete, however, a discussion on the traditional multidose regimen will be presented first.

■ *Multiple Daily Doses*

Entire books and chapters in books have been devoted to the dosing of these agents. There is a fairly clear correlation between excessive dosing and increased incidence of side effects. Furthermore, the patients who most frequently need these drugs are usually the ones with the most underlying medical problems, further complicating the dosing. It is hoped that these guidelines simplify the use of these drugs.

1. A course of aminoglycoside therapy should always be started with a "loading dose." This stays the same regardless of the patient's renal function. The loading dose can be compared to filling a new car tank with gasoline before driving it home. Loading doses are generally as follows:
   a. Gentamicin or tobramycin, 2 mg/kg
   b. Amikacin, 7.5 mg/kg
2. Following the loading dose, "maintenance doses" are calculated. The maintenance dose can be compared to the fill-up for the car after driving. Maintenance doses are dependent on renal function as described subsequently. In patients with normal function, the usual doses are as follows:
   a. Gentamicin or tobramycin, 5 to 7 mg/kg/day q8h to q12h.
   b. Amikacin, 15 mg/kg/day, usually q12h.
3. Before a decision is made on the maintenance dose, the patient's creatinine clearance must be calculated using the following equation:

$$\text{Creatinine clearance} = \frac{(140 - \text{age}) \times \text{weight (in kg)}}{\text{Serum creatinine} \times 72}$$

$$(\text{for women} = \times 0.85)$$

Technically, the weight should be "lean body weight." So, for an obese patient, the ideal weight should be estimated.
4. Another method for calculating creatinine clearance is by the use of the "dosing nomogram" found in many drug inserts and textbooks.
5. Assuming "normal renal function" is defined as a creatinine clearance of around 100 ml/min (it can be much higher), there is a linear relationship between clearance and percentage of renal

function. For example, if the clearance is 50 ml/min, 50% renal function may be assumed and therefore 50% of the full dose calculated. If the full dose is 5 mg/kg/day, then 2.5 mg/kg/day twice to three times a day should be administered.

6. All of the aforementioned guidelines are only applicable pending the determination of antibiotic blood levels. Antibiotic blood levels are determined as follows:

   a. Peak levels are drawn immediately following administration of a dose.

   b. Trough levels are drawn 20 to 30 minutes before the administration of the next dose. These levels should be ordered initially after the third dose of aminoglycoside. If within normal range, the levels need not be ordered again unless there is a rise in the serum creatinine level. (Serum creatinine should be monitored about three times a week when the patient is receiving these drugs.) The following are normal ranges for peak and trough levels:

   c. Gentamicin and tobramycin: peak = 6 to 10 µg/ml; trough = less than 2 µg/ml.

   d. Amikacin: peak = 20 to 30 µg/ml; trough = less than 10 µg/ml.

7. Two techniques can be used to change the dose of an aminoglycoside when inappropriate levels are found:

   a. Raise or lower the amount of the dose.

   b. Increase or decrease the time interval between doses. The following are recommendations with various combinations of peak and trough results:

      1. If the peak is high and the trough is normal, decrease the amount.

      2. If the peak is low and the trough is normal, increase the amount.

      3. If the peak is OK and the trough is high, increase interval.

      4. If the peak is high and the trough is high, decrease the dose and increase the interval.

Although data are inconclusive, there does appear to be a correlation between excessive levels and nephrotoxicity. The correlation with ototoxicity is less clear. Generalizations such as "a high peak is more predictive of nephrotoxicity and a high trough is more predictive of ototoxicity" have not been clearly proven.

8. If aminoglycosides are given concurrently with a penicillin, there will be a decrease in aminoglycoside levels because of competition between the two drugs.

■ *Single Daily Dose*

The rationale behind using a single daily dose is based on three premises.

1. Observations that a single daily dose may decrease toxicity.
2. Aminoglycosides posses a significant postantibiotic effect (PAE) so that the organisms are still "stunned" even after the drug is no longer above the MIC.
3. Aminoglycosides posses "concentration-dependent killing." Therefore the higher the level, the better the microbial kill.

Multiple studies have established the fact that giving a single daily dose of an aminoglycoside can decrease toxicity and increase efficacy. It is rapidly becoming the standard dosing regimen in most hospitals. Essentially there is minimal dosage calculation required. The patient receives the entire daily dose at one time.

1. Gentamicin and tobramycin, 5 to 7 mg/kg.
2. Amikacin, 15 mg/kg.

There are no hard-and-fast rules for monitoring the levels. It is assumed that the patient will develop a significant peak given the large amount of drug administered. Probably more important is the trough monitoring to assure that the patient is able to excrete the drug. Recommendations run from 18 to 24 hours after the dose. Expected trough levels should be less than 1 µg/ml.

In varying degrees of renal failure, recommendations again run from a decrease in the total overall dose proportionate to the degree of renal insufficiency to simply increasing the interval to q48h.

Clinical Usage

Acceptable settings for the use of aminoglycoside antibiotics in lower extremity infections are hard to find. In light of the development of newer, safer agents, arguments for the use of these drugs are evaporating. One argument, the low cost of aminoglycosides versus these newer drugs, has been shown not to stand scrutiny. It is true that the per-gram cost of these drugs is low, but the cost of monitoring for toxicities and the cost of extra days in the hospital should more than compensate for the price of the drug if toxicity occurs.

The following are some potential uses:

1. Treatment of severe gram-negative infection or sepsis. Especially indicated when organisms multiresistant to the newer agents are present.
2. In combination with a ß-lactam, such as ampicillin or mezlocillin, for severe infections caused by the enterococci or tolerant species of Streptococcus. When used for synergy, as in these cases, full dosing levels of the aminoglycoside are not used.
3. Some clinicians still use triple-agent combinations with a ß-lactam and an antianaerobic agent for shotgun therapy of the diabetic foot infection. The use of an aminoglycoside in these patients is questionable. Diabetic feet have been shown to contain a large number of anaerobes, and aminoglycosides are ineffective against these organisms. Diabetic feet frequently form large abscesses that aminoglycosides cannot penetrate because of the low pH in pus. Finally, the diabetic patient is renally compromised and more prone to aminoglycoside toxicities.

ANTIANAEROBIC AGENTS

Two drugs, metronidazole and clindamycin, are grouped under this heading because traditionally their use has been predominately against anaerobic organisms. This does not mean that their spectrum or clinical use is limited to these organisms. Clindamycin in particular is also an extremely good choice against gram-positive organisms.

■ *Metronidazole (Flagyl)*

First developed for the treatment of infections caused by *Trichomonas vaginalis* and amoebae, metronidazole has been found to be one of the most active antibiotics against the anaerobic bacteria. The drug is available in oral and parenteral forms. Oral absorption is excellent and gives serum levels that parallel those seen with parenteral dosing.

Spectrum of Activity

Metronidazole is bactericidal against almost all gram-negative anaerobes, including *B. fragilis*. It is somewhat less effective against some gram-positive anaerobes.

Adverse Reactions

1. Generally a well-tolerated antibiotic.
2. Dry mouth with a metallic taste is the most common side effect.
3. Disulfiram-like or Antabuse reaction occurs with alcohol ingestion.
4. May cause seizures in patients with a history of seizure disorder.
5. Some questionable evidence points to the drug as a possible carcinogen. This has mostly been shown in animals with prolonged exposure.

Dosage and Administration

1. 500 mg three to four times a day PO for most infections. Because the serum levels following oral dosing are so good, this is the recommended route for all but the most severe infections.
2. Parenteral dose is generally stated as being a 15-mg/kg loading dose followed by 7.5 mg/kg q6h to q8h.
3. Dosage reduction is not usually needed in impaired renal function. Impaired hepatic function may require some dosage adjustment.

Clinical Usage

1. Because of its narrow spectrum, lower extremity use of metronidazole is limited. There are a number of other agents with excellent anaerobic activity that also work against other common lower extremity pathogens (i.e., the ß-lactamase inhibitor compounds).
2. As one component of combination therapy in the treatment of anaerobic lower extremity infections, particularly diabetic foot infections. Even though the drug is very inexpensive, this need to combine it with another drug defeats the benefit.
3. As the treatment of choice (orally) for pseudomembranous colitis caused by *C. difficile*.

■ *Clindamycin (Cleocin)*

Frequently grouped in with the macrolides due to a similar molecular structure and mechanism of activity, clindamycin is well known as an effective drug against the anaerobes, so it is placed here. A very effective antibiotic for lower extremity infections, clindamycin has received some negative attention because of its side effect profile. This has caused many physicians to not use this drug. The parent compound of this drug, lincomycin, although once widely used, has mostly been replaced by clindamycin. Clindamycin, like the macrolides, works by binding to the 50S ribosome. It is available in both an oral form and a parenteral form.

Spectrum of Activity

1. Most gram-positive organisms, including *S. aureus* and the streptococci. Not effective against enterococci and most strains of methicillin-resistant *S. aureus* (MRSA). Although generally considered bacteriostatic, at least against many strains of staphylococci minimal inhibitory concentrations are quite close to minimum bactericidal concentrations.
2. Most anaerobes, including the *Bacteroides*. Not quite as effective as metronidazole against these organisms. More than 20% of *Bacteroides* may be resistant. Only moderate activity against most *Clostridia* and no activity against *C. difficile*.

Adverse Reactions

The main side effect of this drug is diarrhea. It is well known to be the most common predisposing factor to *C. difficile* colitis, although any drug can cause this condition. It is estimated that as many as 20% of patients may experience diarrhea while receiving therapy. Of these, most cases are insignificant and transient, resolving promptly upon discontinuation of the drug. Severe colitis is much more uncommon.

Dosage and Administration

1. 600 to 900 mg q8h IV or IM. Until recently this drug was dosed q6h. It is now known that this is unnecessary. The latest data show that even q12h to q24h dosing may be effective.
2. 150 to 300 mg two to three times a day PO for outpatient therapy.
3. Because the drug is metabolized in the liver, no dosage change is needed in renal failure unless there is concomitant hepatic failure.

Clinical Usage

1. Outpatient oral therapy of staphylococcal infections in patients allergic to penicillins and cephalosporins.
2. Oral therapy of mildly infected diabetic ulcerations.
3. Combined with an agent effective against the gram-negative organisms, such as a quinolone, for treatment of severe diabetic infections.

4. There are some interesting data that point to clindamycin as the possible drug of choice for staphylococcal osteomyelitis. It is postulated that this is because of its excellent penetration into bone and leukocytes and its unique ability to dissolve the glycocalyx, or slime layer.

ANTI–GRAM-POSITIVE ANTIBIOTICS

Early antibiotic development was directed against *Staphylococcus* and *Streptococcus*. Penicillin was considered the miracle drug that it was because it could prevent deaths caused by these organisms. As they became somewhat resistant, new gram-positive antibiotics, such as the penicillinase-resistant penicillins, were developed. Vancomycin became available for the tougher organisms. Then, throughout the 1980s and into the 1990s, most of the development of new antibiotics was directed against gram-negative organisms. The later-generation cephalosporins, the quinolones, carbapenems, monobactams, all came to market during this period. Much concern was generated over the resistance development in *Pseudomonas* and the Enterobacteriaceae. Gram-positives were covered by most of these new antibiotics to varying degrees, but no real emphasis was placed on these bacteria because pretty much all isolates were susceptible to readily available antibiotics. Things have now come full circle. MRSA has proliferated to the point that it is now a common community organism, not strictly a nosocomial pathogen. Frank vancomycin resistance has developed in some species of *Staphylococcus* and in *Enterococcus*. Others demonstrate vancomycin tolerance. The organisms have once again "outsmarted" the best efforts to destroy them. Over the past few years, new developments in antibiotic therapy have concentrated on new drugs to counter the resistant gram-positive organisms. Linezolid and quinupristin/dalfopristin were the first of this new breed. A few that were once forgotten, such as daptomycin and teicoplanin, seem to have risen like a phoenix and are again being studied.

■ *Vancomycin (Vancocin)*

Vancomycin was the prototype of the truly effective anti–gram-positive antibiotics. It is currently the only available member of the glycopeptide antibiotics. Although introduced in the mid-1950s, the drug did not see much use because of its perceived side effects, high cost, and the general susceptibility of organisms to other cheaper, safer antibiotics. Because of the problem with MRSA and ampicillin-resistant enterococci, this drug has seen tremendous use over the past 10 to 15 years. Along with the increased use came the inevitable problem of resistance to the point that the Centers for Disease Control and Prevention had to issue guidelines on its use. Vancomycin is available for intravenous use and in an oral form. Absorption from the stomach is virtually nonexistent. The oral form is indicated strictly for the treatment of colitis.

Spectrum of Activity
1. Bactericidal against all gram-positive organisms, including MRSA and MRSE; enterococci (against which it may only be bacteriostatic); other streptococci; gram-positive anaerobes, including clostridia; and corynebacteria.
2. No gram-negative aerobic or anaerobic spectrum.
3. Resistance in Enterococcus (VRE) and some tolerance in staphylococcus (VISA) is becoming a major clinical problem.

Adverse Reactions
1. Most of the side effects recognized early on with vancomycin were more the result of impurities in the preparation of the drug than inherent failings with the drug itself.
2. Nephrotoxicity, although no longer common, can still occur with elevated serum levels. Renal function should be followed while the patient is taking vancomycin.
3. Likewise, ototoxicity is very rare and has probably been more related to impure early formulations. In fact, most studies that look at vancomycin ototoxicity have not been able to conclusively point to a direct correlation. When it does occur, it tends to be reversible.
4. The most significant side effect of vancomycin is known as "red man" or "red neck" syndrome. This syndrome is caused by a release of histamine from mast cells, although the full mechanism has not been discovered. It is directly related to speed of intravenous infusion. It is also more common once a single infusion go above 1 g. For this reason, vancomycin should always be infused over at least 45 to 60 minutes.

Clinical presentation of red man syndrome includes flushing, a hot feeling, and pruritus. Although self-limiting, oral antihistamines may make the patient feel more comfortable. Prophylactic use of antihistamines may decrease the incidence, but the data are inconclusive.

Dosage and Administration

1. Various dosing schemes will work with vancomycin. The maximum dose should be kept at 2 g/day. The currently most common dosing is 1 g q12h for severe infections.
2. Oral dosage for *C. difficile* colitis is 125 mg four times a day. This is significantly more expensive and marginally more effective than metronidazole.
3. Intravenous vancomycin should always be administered slowly over 45 to 60 minutes. Vancomycin should never be administered in a bolus.
4. There has been great debate in the literature about the need for peak and trough serum levels when dosing vancomycin. The overall consensus seems to be that monitoring is not necessary when using this drug. There is no benefit because it is safer than originally thought, and, when giving a full 1-g dose, peak levels are reliable. The only possible benefit of monitoring is following a trough level to ensure that the body is clearing the drug. Normal serum levels of vancomycin are peak, 20 to 50 µg/ml; and trough, less than 10 µg/ml, depending on the laboratory.

Clinical Usage

1. The drug of choice for MRSA and MRSE infections.
2. For the treatment of normally susceptible gram-positive infections in patients with an allergy to penicillin or cephalosporins.
3. Surgical prophylaxis for prosthetic joint implants when MRSE is a problem pathogen.
4. Surgical prophylaxis for any lower extremity surgery in centers with significant MRSA problems or in patients with ß-lactam allergy.
5. Can be used either as a single agent or combined with an aminoglycoside for severe enterococcal infections. Aminoglycoside/vancomycin combinations may potentiate nephrotoxicity.
6. Oral therapy for *C. difficile* colitis when metronidazole fails.

■ *Quinupristin/dalfopristin (Synercid)*

The synergistic combination of quinupristin and dalfopristin, two streptogramin antibiotics, was the first FDA-approved therapy for

VRE. The drug had significant clinical usage in "compassionate care" cases and clinical trials before its somewhat delayed release. It provided the first truly life-saving compound for serious gram-positive infections that could not be treated by more conventional therapies.

Spectrum of Activity
1. Approved for use against *Enterococcus faecium*, including vancomycin-resistant strains. *E. faecalis* is generally resistant.
2. Also effective against *S. aureus* including MRSA. Interestingly, its labeling is only for non-MRSA infections.

Adverse Reactions
1. Local inflammation and phlebitis at the IV site. This drug needs to be given through a central line or PICC line only.
2. Myalgias and arthralgias are fairly common.

Dosage and Administration
7.5 mg/kg q8h to q12h given through a central IV line.

Clinical Usage
1. The clinical usage of this drug is severely limited by its toxicity profile and its high cost. A 10-day course of therapy will cost more than $3000 at current pricing.
2. There is some debate as to whether skin and skin structure infections with VRE even need to be treated. If it is decided to treat them, there is now a better, safer, less expensive, oral alternative.

■ *Linezolid (Zyvox)*

The first commercially available oxazolidinone antibiotic, linezolid offers a truly exciting advance in the treatment of gram-positive infections. It was released not long after the release of quinupristin/dalfopristin, and because of its superior activity, safety profile, and availability in oral form, it has quickly become the drug of choice for these infections.

Spectrum of Activity
Extremely effective against all gram-positive organisms including routine Enterococcus and staphylococcus and MRSA and VRE strains. The FDA labeling includes all of these in the indication.

Adverse Reactions

This is a fairly safe-looking drug with initial usage. There have been some reports of thrombocytopenia, especially with usage longer than 10 to 14 days. As with any new drug, other safety issues may arise with experience.

Dosage

600 mg twice a day IV or PO. As with some other drugs like the quinolones, serum levels are nearly identical given either IV or PO.

Clinical Usage

1. A promising drug for very resistant gram-positive infections of the lower extremity. The caveat about the real need to treat VRE from the skin and skin structures still stands. Only treat if the organism is isolated from a reliable deep culture.
2. Because of its high cost even for PO usage (approximately $120/day) it should not be used for routine gram-positive infections, including MRSA, when less-expensive alternatives such as minocycline or TMP/SMX can be used. This is a drug that needs to be used only when absolutely necessary.
3. Clinical trials against diabetic foot infections are underway, and preliminary results look promising.

■ *Rifampin*

Traditionally used in combination therapy for tuberculosis, rifampin has had a renaissance of late because of its excellent activity against staphylococci. The one problem with the drug is the propensity for rapid development of resistance to it. For this reason it is never used alone. Rifampin is only available in an oral form.

Spectrum of Activity

1. Very active against staphylococci and streptococci.
2. Active against all mycobacteria.
3. Some gram-negative activity, especially against *Neisseria* and *Haemophilus*.

Adverse Reactions

1. Red discoloration of all body fluids. Will permanently stain soft contact lenses.
2. Skin rash.
3. Flu-like symptoms with high, prolonged dosages.

Dosage and Administration

1. 300 mg twice a day PO for most infections.
2. Minimal or no adjustments need be made in patients with renal insufficiency.

Clinical Usage

1. In combination with vancomycin, minocycline, or trimethoprim/sulfamethaxazole for treatment of MRSA or MRSE. This appears to be a very popular use, but the data are still coming in on the true efficacy of these combinations.
2. Treatment of lower extremity mycobacterial infection in combination with other agents.

■ *New Developments in Anti–Gram-Positive Antibiotics*

It is interesting to note that when the first edition of this book was written the same two antibiotics were listed as "new developments." As discussed previously, these drugs were actually halted in their development at that time because they offered no real advantage over vancomycin. Now, with the increasing concern about gram-positive infection, there is renewed interest. It remains to be seen if either or both ever becomes available in the United States.

1. Teicoplanin, a glycopeptide antibiotic similar to vancomycin, has some potential advantages over vancomycin.
   a. Better activity against the streptococci.
   b. Better activity against the enterococci.
   c. Potential for once-daily dosing.
   d. Activity against the staphylococci appears similar to that seen with vancomycin. All of these advantages are in vitro. Clinical studies performed thus far have yielded mixed results. Early studies showed significant failures, especially in endocarditis patients. It is now known that these studies used too low a dose. High-dose studies are more promising.
2. Daptomycin is a related lipopetide antibiotic. Its in vitro activity against the gram-positive organisms appears similar or slightly better than that of either of the other drugs. In vitro its activity is very dependent on the media in which it is tested, making clinical statements difficult.

QUINOLONES

If the 1980s were the decade of the cephalosporins, then the 1990s were the quinolone decade. New drugs were being studied at a feverish pace. It was not uncommon to see papers in the antibiotic literature that would compare the activity of 20 or so different experimental quinolone compounds at a time. Almost as quickly as they were being studied, they were being released to the market. A flood of new "-oxacins" followed the earlier introductions of norfloxacin and ciprofloxacin. Initially these drugs were promising the world—so-called "one-stop shopping for all of your antibiotic needs." Unfortunately, as with all antibiotic expectations, the luster soon started to dull. A number of drugs were pulled from the market or severely limited in their use for various toxicities, including hepatic and renal failures and QT interval changes. Resistance, especially against *S. aureus* and *P. aeruginosa,* began to be reported, primarily because of incredible overusage.

When used properly, the quinolones are still one of the most important and effective classes of drug available. Some of the newer agents truly do represent vast improvements over earlier compounds. This section will only cover those drugs with utility in the management of lower extremity infections. Drugs that are specific for urinary or respiratory pathogens will not be reviewed.

■ *Ciprofloxacin (Cipro)*

The first of the quinolones approved for skin and skin structure infections, ciprofloxacin still enjoys the distinction of being one of, if not the most, prescribed quinolone antibiotic. Unfortunately, much of its use is unwarranted and unnecessary and has contributed to significant resistance development. Because many of the adverse events with quinolone usage are shared throughout the class, they will only be listed here instead of being repeated for each drug.

Spectrum of Activity
1. The main benefit of ciprofloxacin is its excellent coverage against virtually all common gram-negative bacteria. This coverage extends to usually resistant organisms such as *P. aeruginosa* and those producing an inducible ß-lactamase (*Enterobacter, Citrobacter, Serratia, Morganella, Pseudomonas,* and *Providencia*).

Acinetobacter shows only variable susceptibility, whereas *B. cepacia* and *S. maltophilia* are frankly resistant.

2. Ciprofloxacin has been the most disappointing in its coverage of the staphylococci. Originally touted as being an excellent alternative for staphylococcal infections, including MRSA, a large number of studies have shown significant staphylococcal resistance (up to 90% for MRSA). There may be a benefit to combining ciprofloxacin with rifampin in the treatment of these infections.

3. Ciprofloxacin shows no clinically useful activity against the *Enterococci* or the anaerobes, and its activity against the *Streptococci* is not reliable.

Adverse Reactions

1. A relatively well-tolerated drug. Only a small percentage of patients will have mild complaints, including nausea and headaches. As with all quinolones, some neurotoxicity and photosensitivity are possible.

2. Theophylline and its derivatives, including caffeine, will be potentiated by the use of ciprofloxacin. Patients taking theophylline should have their serum levels checked regularly. Patients should be advised to avoid coffee, tea, or any soft drink containing caffeine.

3. Antacids and iron supplements have been shown to significantly reduce the absorption of ciprofloxacin from the stomach. If needed, the patient should take the drug at least 1 hour before or 2 hours after the antacid.

4. The quinolones have been shown to cause degeneration of cartilage in young animals. For this reason they are contraindicated in children with open growth plates. However, increased experience with this drug in children with pseudomonal infections and cystic fibrosis has not shown any significant cartilage problems.

5. One interesting potential adverse effect of ciprofloxacin and possibly other quinolones is that there has been an association between quinolone usage, tendonopathies, and frank tendon ruptures, particularly of the Achilles tendon. It is believed that this may be related to the same connective tissue toxicity that has been shown in cartilage as discussed previously. This is still a rare occurrence. Given the hundreds of millions of patients treated with these drugs, only very few cases of rupture have been reported in the literature. However, it may be prudent to heed a patient's complaint about tendon pain while taking one

of these drugs. The drug should be discontinued, if possible, and the area placed at rest.

Dosage and Administration

1. 500 mg twice a day PO for mild to moderate infections. It has been shown that the 500 mg PO dose is pharmacokinetically equivalent to the 400 mg IV. For this reason IV dosing is almost always unnecessary unless the patient is NPO or unable to take PO medications.
2. 750 mg twice a day PO for severe infections and osteomyelitis.
3. Decrease to once daily in patients with severe renal insufficiency.

Clinical Usage

Because of overuse of this antibiotic with the resultant resistance development and potential for treatment failures, it is necessary to not only list when this drug *is* indicated but also when it *is not*. When used properly in place of parenteral therapy, this agent can save the hospital and the health care system huge amounts of money along with benefiting the patient.

Indications include the following:

1. Severe gram-negative and nosocomial infections caused by susceptible organisms. Therapy can be inpatient or outpatient.
2. Oral therapy for osteomyelitis caused by gram-negative organisms, including *P. aeruginosa*. The convenience of the oral form will alleviate the need for continuing parenteral antibiotics for 4 to 6 weeks. Note: This drug should not be routinely used for gram-positive osteomyelitis because it has no benefit over other drugs and may promote resistance development.
3. Treatment of diabetic foot infections when combined with either clindamycin (for staphylococci, streptococci, and anaerobes) or metronidazole (for anaerobes). Some studies have actually shown that this drug can be used as a single agent in these infections despite its lack of anaerobic and gram-positive activity. There are clearly two schools of thought on this matter.

Contraindications include the following:

1. Ciprofloxacin should not be thought of as a routine oral antibiotic. It should be thought of as a parenteral antibiotic that just happens to be able to be given orally. Keeping this in mind should help to avoid overuse.

2. The drug is not indicated in a simple community-acquired infection in which a normal oral agent such as a cephalosporin or penicillinase-resistant penicillin would be used. These infections tend to be caused by staphylococci and streptococci, two organisms not covered particularly well by ciprofloxacin.
3. Ciprofloxacin is not indicated for prophylaxis of lower extremity surgery.

■ *Levofloxacin (Levaquin)*

This drug is the L-isomer of the parent compound ofloxacin, still available on the market as Floxin. Given the improvement and advantages of levofloxacin, there is no reason to cover ofloxacin as a separate compound. This drug is steadily surpassing ciprofloxacin as the quinolone of choice for lower extremity infections.

Spectrum of Activity
1. Better activity against both staphylococcus and streptococcus than ciprofloxacin. Less potential for resistance to these organisms because of the more numerous and complicated steps the bacteria have to go through to develop the resistance.
2. Less active against *P. aeruginosa* while still maintaining significant activity against other gram-negatives. The clinical significance of this diminished pseudomonal activity is not clear.

Adverse Reactions
See ciprofloxacin. Significantly less of an interaction (if at all) with the theophylline derivatives.

Dosage and Administration
500 mg once a day PO or IV for mild to moderate infections.

750 mg once a day PO or IV for complicated skin and skin structure infections.

As with any quinolone, IV and PO dosings are fairly equivalent.

Clinical Usage
The once-daily dosing, better gram-positive activity, and FDA approval for complicated skin and skin structure (which by definition includes diabetic foot infections) makes this the quinolone of choice for most lower extremity infections. Only

in the case of a documented infection by *P. aeruginosa* does ciprofloxacin provide a theoretical advantage.

Three of the so-called "fourth-generation" quinolone drugs will be listed here in a slightly abbreviated form. They lack clinical experience in lower extremity infections, have severe restriction on their usage, or do not have the indication at all. For this reason they do not warrant a full description at this time.

■ *Moxifloxacin (Avelox)*

Moxifloxacin may be the most useful of the newer drugs for lower extremity infections. It is currently FDA approved for skin and skin structure infections. It shares many of the advantages of levofloxacin, being better against gram-positive organisms than ciprofloxacin along with enhanced activity against the anaerobes. This bodes well for its possible usage in diabetic foot infections for which it is currently being studied.

Dosage and Administration
400 mg qd PO/IV.

■ *Gatifloxacin (Tequin)*

Similar to moxifloxacin in many ways minus the FDA indication for skin and skin structure infections as of this writing. Also may be slightly less effective against the anaerobes. However, with good gram-positive and gram-negative coverage and once-daily dosing, this drug may still find a place in treating lower extremity infections. The potential for QT interval lengthening has been mentioned with both of these two drugs; however this finding is of questionable clinical importance.

Dosage and Administration
400 mg qd PO or IV.

■ *Trovafloxacin (Trovan)*

This drug provided an exciting "flash in the pan" for the treatment of lower extremity infections during the approximately 1 year it was widely available. Many clinicians used this quinolone for severe diabetic foot infections (a usage for which it had FDA approval) with excellent success. Unfortunately, because of a few deaths from hepatic failure, the drug was severely restricted. It is included here because, contrary to popular opinion, it was not withdrawn completely and is still available on a limited basis. Usage must follow strict criteria that includes "limb-threatening infection," use for less than 14 days in an inpatient facility, and the inability to use alternative therapies given an understanding of the risk-benefit analysis. If the patient fits these criteria, this drug is still a very effective antibiotic.

Dosage and Administration
200 mg qd PO or IV.

SULFONAMIDES

The sulfa drugs were the first antimicrobial agents used. They date back more than a decade before the discovery of penicillin. The intervening years have seen a large number of these agents come and go. Only one, the combination of trimethoprim and sulfamethoxazole (also known as cotrimoxazole), now has clinical significance in the treatment of lower extremity infections.

■ *Trimethoprim/Sulfamethoxazole (Bactrim, Septra)*

Used originally for urinary tract infection, this combination drug is quite well absorbed after oral administration and reaches sufficient levels in tissue to have a wide variety of lower extremity uses. It is available in both oral and parenteral forms in a fixed trimethoprim:sulfamethoxazole ratio of 1:5.

Spectrum of Activity
1. Bacteriostatic against all organisms.
2. Good activity against staphylococci, including MRSA.
3. Limited activity against some groups of streptococci but not the enterococci.
4. Excellent coverage against most gram-negative organisms except *P. aeruginosa*. Variable activity against *Serratia*.
5. One of the drugs of choice against *B. cepacia* and *S. maltophilia*.

Adverse Reactions
1. Hypersensitivity in patients allergic to sulfa products. This can range from a mild rash to a potentially fatal reaction. Stevens-Johnson syndrome is also seen.

2. Hemolytic anemia in patients with glucose-6-phosphate dehydrogenase deficiency. Other hematologic disorders, such as megaloblastic anemia, are rare.
3. Crystalluria, seen with other sulfa products, is less common with this agent.
4. Most side effects are seen in the high doses used in the treatment of acquired immune deficiency syndrome patients with *Pneumocystis* pneumonia.
5. Hyperglycemia is seen in patients on sulfonylureas.

Dosage and Administration
1. One double-strength tablet, containing 160 mg trimethoprim and 800 mg sulfamethaxazole, twice daily PO is sufficient for most infections.
2. Should be increased to three times a day for more severe infections.
3. Because of its excellent oral absorption, the parenteral form is rarely needed. When it is ordered, the dosing is based on the trimethoprim component.

Clinical Usage
1. Oral therapy of susceptible gram-negative and staphylococcal infections in penicillin-allergic patients.
2. Oral therapy for MRSA based on sensitivity report. Combination with rifampin may be beneficial although not really necessary.
3. Treatment of *B. cepacia* and *S. maltophilia* infections of the lower extremity.

MACROLIDES

The macrolide class of antibiotics has shown a tremendous surge in popularity over the past decade with the introduction of a number of newer agents to improve on the venerable erythromycin. All of these newer drugs are improvements over erythromycin because of a better spectrum of activity or fewer adverse events.

■ *Erythromycin*

The first of the macrolide class of antibiotics, erythromycin has been available for almost 50 years. It has a broad spectrum and is available in a large number of preparations. There are numerous oral salts, an intravenous form, and topical forms.

Spectrum of Activity

1. Good activity against staphylococci (except for MRSA) and streptococci (except for enterococci).
2. Activity against a few gram-negative species but not most lower extremity pathogens.
3. Some activity against gram-positive and gram-negative anaerobes but not against *B. fragilis*.

Adverse Reactions

1. Thrombophlebitis and pain on intravenous injection limit its usefulness in the setting.
2. Significant gastrointestinal symptoms including nausea and vomiting.
3. Hepatotoxicity has been seen with the estolate and ethylsuccinate forms. In most cases it is mild and reversible.
4. Allergic reactions are possible.

Dosage and Administration

1. There appears to be no major difference in efficacy of the different preparations.
2. 250 to 500 mg four times a day PO for most infections.
3. 1 g q6h IV diluted in at least 100 ml of solution and infused slowly. Because of pain on administration, the intravenous form should be limited to only when it is absolutely necessary.
4. Intramuscular injection is not given because of pain.
5. No dosage adjustment needed in patients with renal insufficiency.

Clinical Usage

Alternative oral therapy for community-acquired infections involving staphylococci and streptococci in patients allergic to penicillin and cephalosporins.

■ *Azithromycin (Zithromax)*

Azithromycin, one of two clinically important newer macrolides, has significant advantages over erythromycin in terms of safety and convenience. It has a unique dosing form that differentiates it from most other antibiotics currently available.

Spectrum of Activity

1. Sufficient activity against common gram-positive pathogens including staphylococcus and streptococcus.
2. Limited gram-negative activity. Most of the studies have all been done on respiratory pathogens, but some community acquired skin pathogens, such as *Proteus* and *E. coli,* should also be covered.

Adverse Reactions

GI upset is the most common, although this is significantly less of a problem than with other drugs in this class.

Dosage and Administration

500 mg (two pills) day 1, followed by 250 mg once a day for 4 days ("Z-pak"). Taken 1 hour before or 2 hours after meal.

Clinical Usage

1. The very short-term convenient dosing of this drug (once daily for 5 days) makes it a good selection for noncompliant patients in whom taking a drug multiple times per day for 10 or more days would not be feasible.
2. Penicillin-allergic patients with mild-to-moderate skin and skin structure infections.
3. When evaluating efficacy of this agent, the clinician should not make a snap decision after the initial 5 days of dosing. The drug is still in the system and working for up to 10 days. Likewise, if a second course is needed, it should probably be given at day 10, not day 5.

■ *Clarithromycin (Biaxin)*

A wildly popular drug for respiratory infections, clarithromycin has few advantages that would make it particularly useful for lower extremity infections. It does not have the dosing advantage of azithromycin and is sometimes difficult for patients to tolerate.

Spectrum of Activity

1. Similar to other macrolides with better gram-positive activity than azithromycin. The clinical relevance of this finding is not clear.
2. Probably not as effective as azithromycin against some gram-negatives. Again, the clinical relevance is questionable.

Adverse Reactions

1. Similar to other macrolides but may have more problems with tolerance from a gastrointestinal standpoint. Many patients also complain of a bad taste from this drug.
2. More potential for drug interactions than azithromycin. Similar to erythromycin in this respect. Will interact with other drugs metabolized by cytochrome P-450 isoenzyme 3A4. Similar in this regard to azole antifungals such as itraconazole.

Dosage and Administration

250 to 500 mg twice a day PO.

Clinical Usage

Limited in lower extremity infections because it has no clear advantage over azithromycin other than possibly better activity against gram-positives without the dosing advantage.

■ *Dirithromycin (Dynabac)*

Dirtithromycin is another newer macrolide with no discernable advantage over any other drug in its class. It may also have a more frequent incidence of adverse reactions than even erythromycin. It is included for completeness' sake and because there was a limited attempt for a short time to market this drug for use in lower extremity infections. Its one potential advantage would be its dosing of 500 mg once a day PO for 10 days. But even this is longer than azithromycin.

TETRACYCLINES

■ *Tetracycline/Doxycycline/Minocycline*

Tetracycline and its congeners are broad-spectrum, bacteriostatic antibiotics. They share some properties with early macrolides like erythromycin. They have been around a long time, they have problems with patient tolerability, and they have limited, defined roles in lower extremity infections. For most lower extremity pathogens, there are alternative, cidal, safer antibiotics.

Tetracycline comes in many forms. Two longer half-life congeners, doxycycline and minocycline, are the most currently used agents. These two drugs also show a significant increase in their activity compared to the parent compound.

Spectrum of Activity

1. Good activity against most staphylococcal and streptococcal organisms, with the exception of the enterococci. Minocycline has the best activity and is also effective against MRSA.
2. Some activity against clinically relevant gram-negative organisms and anaerobes.
3. Where the tetracyclines have their greatest advantage is in the treatment of "unusual" pathogens. The following are some of these that have lower extremity implications:
   a. *Borrelia burgdorferi*, the causative agent of Lyme disease.
   b. *Actinomyces*, the cause of Madura foot.
   c. *Mycobacterium marinum*.

Adverse Reactions

1. Gastrointestinal irritation with oral therapy.
2. Thrombophlebitis and pain on intravenous administration.
3. Skin reactions, including rash and photosensitivity.
4. Staining of bones and teeth.
5. Superinfection, especially with yeast.
6. Contraindicated in pregnant patients.

Dosage and Administration

1. Minocycline and doxycycline: 100 mg q12h PO.
2. Tetracycline: 250 to 500 mg four times a day PO.
3. All of the above can be given intravenously at similar dosages. They should be diluted in at least 100 ml of solution and infused slowly.

Clinical Usage

1. Minocycline has become one of the oral drugs of choice for MRSA infection when TMP/SMX is resistant or linezolid is too expensive. Rifampin may be added according to some authorities but may not always be necessary.
2. Doxycycline is the drug of choice for early Lyme borreliosis at the erythema migrans stage and even with some localized neurological findings.
3. For treatment of infections caused by any of the "unusual" organisms mentioned above.

4. For treatment of staphylococcal or streptococcal infection in a penicillin-allergic patient when no other alternatives are available.

CONCLUSION

This chapter was not meant to be an exhaustive review of every available antibiotic. Only antibiotics with a potential for direct utilization in the treatment of lower extremity infections were covered. A number of antibiotics were not discussed. Drugs such as chloramphenicol, colistin, and others, while they may have some limited use in lower extremity infections, are so rarely used that it was thought unnecessary to cover them. Further information on the pharmacokinetics of these drugs, including serum peaks, half-lives, and dosing in renal insufficiency, are available in the appendix table.

SUGGESTED READINGS

Burkhardt JE, Walterspiel JN, Schaad UB: Quinolone arthropathy in animals versus children, *Clin Infect Dis* 25:1196, 1997.

Gilbert DN: Aminoglycosides. In Mandell GL, Bennett JE, Dolin R, editors: *Principles and practice of infectious diseases,* ed 5, p 307, Philadelphia, 2000, Churchill Livingstone.

Mingeot-Leclercq M, Tulkens PM: Aminoglycosides: nephrotoxicity, *Antimicrob Agents Chemother* 43(5):1003, 1999.

Part 1, Section E. Anti-infective therapy. In Mandell GL, Bennett JE, Dolin R, editors: *Principles and practice of infectious diseases,* ed 5, Philadelphia, 2000, Churchill Livingstone.

Ryback MJ, Abate BJ, Kang SL et al: Prospective evaluation of the effect of an aminoglycoside dosing regimen on rates of observed nephrotoxicity and ototoxicity, *Antimicrob Agents Chemother* 43(7):1549, 1999.

Shankibaei M, Pfister K, Schwabe R et al: Ultrastructure of Achilles tendons of rats treated with ofloxacin and fed a normal or magnesium-deficient diet, *Antimicrob Agents Chemother* 44(2):261, 2000.

The Johns Hopkins Division of Infectious Diseases On-line Antibiotic Guide. http://hopkins-abxguide.org

PART IV

Microorganisms

CHAPTER 10

Microorganisms

The purpose of this chapter is not to present an exhaustive review of microbiology. It contains no discussions about growth determinants or classification systems. Instead, it is geared to the clinician who has just received a culture report from the laboratory and wants a quick reference to help determine what the presence of the isolated organism means. Most of the clinically important bacteria are listed. Under each organism is a brief discussion of its clinical significance, interesting resistance patterns that are found in nature or may develop on therapy, and a list of antibiotic selections useful in the treatment of that organism. The drugs are listed in relative order of effectiveness. In many cases more than one drug is effective. The equally effective drugs are listed on the same line. When applicable, an oral alternative is listed. If an oral form of one of the parenteral agents exists, it should also be considered effective unless noted otherwise.

GRAM-POSITIVE COCCI

■ *Staphylococcus aureus*

Clinical Significance
Staphylococcus aureus is by far the most common organism isolated from lower extremity infections. It is also known as coagulase-positive staphylococcus for its ability to coagulate rabbit plasma in the laboratory and to differentiate it from the coagulase-nega-

tive species. This organism is a major cause of infection following surgery in osteomyelitis, in diabetic foot infections, and in almost any community-acquired cellulitis.

Resistance Patterns

S. aureus has an interesting history in terms of resistance development and can be held up as an example of how antibiotic selection pressure can cause various changes in a microorganism. Currently *S. aureus* may present with one of four patterns of antibiotic sensitivity. This is a change from the first edition of this handbook, when only three patterns were known.

1. Penicillin-sensitive, also known as *non–penicillinase-producing*. This is the original form of *S. aureus* as seen at the time of the invention and development of penicillin in the 1930s and 1940s. This isolate is now very rare, probably accounting for less than 5% of isolates.
2. Methicillin-sensitive. Also known as *penicillinase-producing*. This is the most common isolate. It is resistant to penicillin because of the production of ß-lactamases, but it is susceptible to penicillinase-resistant penicillins such as nafcillin and oxacillin. It is also susceptible to the majority of cephalosporins and ß-lactamase inhibitor compounds.
3. Methicillin-resistant *S. aureus* (MRSA) can account for a large percentage of isolates depending on the hospital or community. Originally thought to be a nosocomial problem, in recent years disturbing reports have shown this organism to now be the cause of strictly community-acquired infections. True resistance to methicillin is caused by a chromosome-mediated change in penicillin-binding proteins (PBPs) on the cell wall leading to an excess expression of the low penicillin affinity PBP-2a. By definition, this organism is resistant to all penicillins and cephalosporins. ß-lactamases do not play a role, and therefore ß-lactamase inhibitor compounds will not be useful. In addition, some isolates that are not truly methicillin-resistant are reported as such because of a hyperproduction of ß-lactamase. In these cases the inhibitor containing compounds may work. However, since the standard laboratory is not going to differentiate, their use may be risky.
4. Vancomycin-intermediate *S. aureus* (VISA). Little if any true resistance has developed to vancomycin by *S. aureus*. However, the first report of isolates of only intermediate susceptibility

(MIC = 8 µg/ml) from Japan in 1996 caused widespread concern. Since then VISA has been reported a number of times in both the United States and in Europe. The first reported case in the United States was in Michigan in 1997. These isolates appear to arise from MRSA and develop their lowered susceptibility while on prolonged courses of vancomycin. Also, most cases have been isolated from patients on dialysis. VISA is not easy to detect in the laboratory and may not be reported out on a standard culture report. Fortunately, it is still relatively uncommon and as yet not reported as a problem in the lower extremity.

When determining the sensitivity of any *S. aureus* isolate, the methicillin/nafcillin/oxacillin line of the report should be looked at first. Despite MRSA being a clinical problem for decades, some laboratories still do not report it correctly. Although the organism is shown on the report as resistant to the penicillinase-resistant penicillins (PRPs), it is reported as sensitive to cephalosporins. If the organism is resistant to PRPs, it is not necessary to check any further. The organism is methicillin-resistant and, by definition, cephalosporin-resistant.

Antibiotic Therapy
Antibiotic selection depends on which of the aforementioned resistance patterns is found.

Penicillin-Sensitive
1. Penicillin G. Although traditionally the "silver bullet" for this type of organism because of the need for frequent, inconvenient dosing and the possibility of resistance development, any of the drugs under item 2 may actually be better choices.
2. First-generation cephalosporins, penicillinase-resistant penicillin, clindamycin, vancomycin, macrolides, tetracyclines, or trimethoprim/sulfamethoxazole (TMP/SMX).
3. The oral form of any of the above except vancomycin.

Methicillin-Sensitive
1. Penicillinase-resistant penicillin, first-generation cephalosporins, advanced-generation cephalosporins with expanded antistaphylococcal activity (i.e., cefdinir, cefuroxime, cefepime).
2. Vancomycin, clindamycin, minocycline, macrolides, or TMP/SMX.
3. The oral form of any of the above except vancomycin.

Methicillin-Resistant

1. Vancomycin (parenteral only), linezolid (oral/parenteral).
2. Minocycline, TMP/SMX, both oral and both with or without rifampin added.

Vancomycin-Intermediate

1. No firm treatment recommendations are available. Combinations of vancomycin with rifampin and an aminoglycoside, or the use of vancomycin in combination with a ß-lactam drug have been reported. Also, daptomycin, an experimental glycopeptide antibiotic, may have usable activity, as may TMP/SMX. The best treatment may well be prevention through the use of good infection-control procedures.

■ *"Coagulase-Negative" Staphylococci*

Staphylococcus epidermidis, Staphylococcus hominis, Staphylococcus saprophyticus, Staphylococcus warneri, Staphylococcus haemolyticus, Staphylococcus saccharolyticus, Staphylococcus xylosus, Staphylococcus simulans, Staphylococcus auricularis, Staphylococcus lugdunensis, among others.

Clinical Significance

The "coagulase-negative" staphylococci (CNS), once considered mere contaminants, are now known as a major cause of infection. This is especially true with *S. epidermidis*, which is probably the major cause of infections following any implant surgery. Other species of CNS are less commonly found in lower extremity infections but still have been reported and could be considered potential pathogens if clinical and laboratory evidence points their way. CNS are also the major cause of intravenous line sepsis.

A culture result that shows CNS should be evaluated carefully. The source of the culture must be determined. Was it superficial or deep? Is there heavy growth or only sparse growth? If the specimen was reliable and there are moderate or more organisms, along with the presence of white blood cells on gram stain, a CNS may be assumed to be a pathogen. If the only CNS isolated was from broth subculture of a superficial swab, it may be assumed that the CNS is a contaminant. This call becomes particularly tricky in the situation where a bone culture is harvested to diagnose osteomyelitis. Frequently, sparse growth of CNS is isolated from the bone. Is this a pathogen or a contaminant from when the bone was taken out through potentially contaminated skin and superficial tissue? Unfortunately, there is no easy answer. Each case is different.

Resistance Patterns

CNS can demonstrate all of the same resistance patterns as *S. aureus*. *S. epidermidis* is the most consistently resistant, with some centers reporting greater than 80% methicillin resistance. In fact, if sensitivity results are pending, *S. epidermidis* should be treated empirically as being methicillin-resistant. Other species of CNS tend to be more susceptible to the penicillins. Unlike *S. aureus*, full-fledged vancomycin resistance has been reported with some CNS.

Antibiotic Therapy

The same guidelines as for *S. aureus* should be followed. The caveat needs to be added that empiric therapy for prosthetic joint implant infections or other infections suspected of being caused by CNS should follow the aforementioned guidelines set for MRSA.

■ *ß-hemolytic Streptococci: Groups A and B*

1. *Streptococcus pyogenes* (group A)
2. *Streptoccoccus agalactiae* (group B)

Clinical Significance

These two groups of ß-hemolytic streptococci are the two most commonly found in the lower extremity. Group B streptococci are extremely common in diabetic foot infections to the point of almost being ubiquitous. It is also commonly found in neonatal infections and infections in immunocompromised patients. Group A streptococci are most common in superficial skin infections such as erysipelas. However, group A streptococcus is also the organism synonymous in the mainstream press with "flesh-eating bacteria." It has been implicated as the causative organism for necrotizing fasciitis and toxic shock syndrome. It can cause a rapidly progressive, necrotizing condition in an otherwise normal, healthy host. This has been seen as a postoperative complication in lower extremity surgery. Traditionally, the patient presents with significant pain out of proportion with immediate clinical findings. This can occur as rapidly as a few hours after surgery, making differentiation from normal postoperative pain difficult.

Resistance Patterns

Fortunately, neither of these two groups of streptococcus has developed a significant resistance problem.

Antibiotic Therapy

1. Penicillin. As with the aforementioned listing for staphylococcus, the oral cephalosporins may work as well or better and be easier to administer.
2. First-generation cephalosporins, advanced-generation cephalosporins with expanded antistreptococcal activity (i.e., cefdinir, cefuroxime, cefepime), clindamycin, macrolides, and vancomycin.
3. The oral forms of any of the above except vancomycin.

■ *Other Streptococci*

1. Viridans Streptococci—*Strepcococcus intermedius, Streptococcus mitis, Streptococcus mutans, Streptococcus sanguis,* among others.
2. Group C—*Streptococcus equisimilis,* among others.
3. Group G.

Clinical Significance

All of the aforementioned groups of streptococci can cause lower extremity infections to varying degrees. In particular, groups C and G, both ß-hemolytic organisms, are fairly common causes of skin infections, septic arthritis, and osteomyelitis. Group G is also found frequently in patients with underlying malignancy. Viridans streptococci are alpha-hemolytic organisms that cannot be serogrouped. These are of rather lower virulence and are more commonly found in diseases, such as endocarditis and respiratory infections.

Resistance Patterns and Antibiotic Therapy

Unlike other streptococci, these groups share some interesting resistance patterns, including lower levels of sensitivity to penicillin. In particular, many strains of viridans strep and group G strep show significant penicillin resistance. Of these organisms, only group C shows reliable penicillin sensitivity. The addition of an aminoglycoside along with penicillin may be synergistic in treating all infections caused by these groups because they are sometimes tolerant (not killed) by penicillin alone. Tolerance to varying degrees or frank resistance has also been described with vancomycin, some cephalosporins, and other commonly used antibiotics. Because sensitivities are variable, therapies cannot be simply listed as with other organisms and need to be directed by the culture and sensitivity (C&S) report.

■ *Enterococci*

1. *Enterococcus faecalis*
2. *Enterococcus faecium*

Clinical Significance

Previously known as "group D streptococci" (and still erroneously labeled as such by some laboratories), the enterococci are considered by some to be the emerging pathogen of the future. These organisms make up the predominant flora in the human gut. *E. faecalis* is the most frequently isolated, but *E. faecium* is becoming more common and may be more difficult to treat. When isolated from a wound, these organisms are often considered contaminants, even by authorities in the field, and are not treated. In fact, they are often found as one of many organisms isolated from an infected diabetic foot wound. However, if isolated as a predominant organism from a reliable culture, they cannot be ignored and should be addressed. These organisms are capable of producing infection in soft tissue and bone by themselves or in synergy with other bacteria.

Resistance Patterns

One of the major problems in the treatment of enterococcal infection is that antibiotics bactericidal against most organisms are only bacteriostatic against these. Furthermore, many antibiotics, including all cephalosporins, have no activity at all. Of course, the greatest resistance problem with these organisms is the discovery of vancomycin-resistant enterococcus (VRE). This organism is the darling of the mainstream press and has been dubbed a "superbug."

Antibiotic Therapy

1. Penicillin or ampicillin. Gentamicin can be added for synergy in more severe cases but is usually not required in lower extremity infections.
2. Vancomycin in patients allergic to penicillins.
3. ß-Lactamase inhibitor compounds such as oral amoxicillin/clavulanic acid or parenteral piperacillin/tazobactam or ampicillin/sulbactam can be used in cases of mixed infections, including staphylococcus and/or gram-negatives and anaerobes.

4. VRE: linezolid, either oral or parenteral, is the drug of choice. Quinupristin/dalfopristin is FDA approved and can also be used, but its use is limited by the need for parenteral therapy through a central line and the high cost. Note: Some infectious disease specialists do not believe in treating VRE unless it is isolated from the bloodstream. Use the same criteria for determining the need for treatment of VRE as for any suspected enterococcal infection.

▨ *Anaerobic Gram-Positive Cocci*

1. *Peptostreptococcus*
2. *Peptococcus*

Clinical Significance
The anaerobic cocci play an important role in lower extremity infections. Most of the clinically important organisms previously classified as *Peptococcus* have now been moved to the *Peptostreptococcus* genera. These organisms are some of the most frequently isolated organisms in diabetic foot infections. They have also been implicated in various necrotizing wound infections.

Resistance Patterns
Fortunately, these are very susceptible organisms. Some resistance can be seen to macrolides and tetracyclines.

Antibiotic Therapy
1. Penicillin
2. Clindamycin, metronidazole, ß-lactamase inhibitor compounds

GRAM-POSITIVE BACILLI

▨ *Clostridium tetani*
Clinical Significance
C. tetani is a ubiquitous organism found in the environment. Although it is very susceptible to a number of disinfectants and antibiotics, it forms spores that are extremely resistant. When introduced into a wound, the spores will develop into the vegetative form and produce a powerful neurotoxin. Tetanus is not actually an infection in the strict definition of the word. Rather, it is an intoxication from the neurotoxin. Antibiotic therapy has a doubtful

effect on the course of the disease. Immunization is the primary means of prevention. An immunization protocol is given in Chapter 4.

Resistance Patterns
C. tetani has no resistance pattern.

Antibiotic Therapy
1. Penicillin
2. Tetracycline

■ *Clostridium perfringens*

Clinical Significance
C. perfringens is the most significant of a long list of clostridia capable of producing infections. This organism is extremely fast growing and is able to produce numerous toxins, in particular alpha-toxin, capable of destroying tissue. It is most well-known as the cause of clostridial myonecrosis, or gas gangrene. It may also cause other infections, including localized abscesses and fasciitis. Occasionally isolated from mixed infections, in these cases its pathogenic role is unclear.

Resistance Patterns
Some resistance to antibiotics has been noted but is relatively rare. Some strains of clostridia are resistant to clindamycin.

Antibiotic Therapy
1. Penicillin.
2. Imipenem, ß-lactamase inhibitor compounds, clindamycin, expanded spectrum cephalosporins.
3. Miscellaneous modalities, including surgical debridement and hyperbaric oxygen, are the mainstays of therapy.

■ *Corynebacterium jeikeium* (Group JK or Diphtheroids)

Clinical Significance
A number of organisms that resemble *Corynebacterium diphtheriae* are grouped under the genus *Corynebacterium* and are collectively known as the *diphtheroids*. Of these, the one of most clinical importance in lower extremity infections is *C. jeikeium*. One of the most common culture reports returned from a laboratory reads either "skin flora" or "diphtheroids," followed by "sensitivity not indi-

cated." In most patients diphtheroids represent nothing more than skin flora that contaminate a specimen. Diphtheroids can become pathogenic in severely immunocompromised patients, patients who have been hospitalized and are receiving broad-spectrum antibiotics, or patients who have a prosthetic joint.

Resistance Patterns
Diphtheroids, unlike other gram-positive bacilli, are mostly resistant to penicillins and cephalosporins.

Antibiotic Therapy
1. Vancomycin.
2. Possibly levofloxacin or rifampin. Because of variable sensitivity patterns, laboratory C&S reports should be followed if vancomycin cannot be used.

■ *Corynebacterium minutissimum*
Clinical Significance
Another one of the diphtheroid group of bacteria, this organism is best known as the cause of erythrasma. This disease, covered in Chapter 2, presents as interdigital maceration and scaling. The diagnosis is usually made by the "coral red" florescence on Wood's lamp examination. Deeper abscesses and infections have been reported, particularly in patients with underlying malignancy.

Antibiotic Therapy
1. Oral erythromycin, possibly other macrolides
2. Topical clindamycin

GRAM-NEGATIVE COCCI

■ *Neisseria gonorrhoeae*
Clinical Significance
Depending on the definition of "lower extremity," the gonococcus may or may not be a frequent cause of infection. In a relatively low percentage of patients infected with gonorrhea, a condition known as *disseminated gonococcal infection* (DGI) can occur. The major clinical significance of DGI in the lower extremity is its relation to septic arthritis. Gonococcal infection should be considered in any young adult patient presenting with

septic arthritis. A complete discussion of the clinical features of gonococcal arthritis is found in Chapter 3.

Resistance Patterns
Significant incidence of penicillin-resistant gonococcus has been reported, especially in poor urban areas. Interestingly, the rate of infection by these more resistant organisms has actually decreased over the past few years. Quinolone resistance, although not yet a major problem in the United States, has been reported elsewhere in the world.

Antibiotic Therapy
1. Ceftriaxone given intravenously (IV) or intramuscularly (IM) is now considered the drug of choice for DGI. Other equivalent third-generation cephalosporins may also be as adequate, but ceftriaxone has the advantage of once-daily dosing.
2. Ciprofloxacin or other quinolones should be used if local resistance is not reported.
3. Penicillin (if resistance is not a local problem). Azithromycin has also been reported as effective.

■ *Neisseria meningitidis*
Clinical Significance
Meningococcal disease is not actually a condition of the lower extremity. As its name suggests, it is most commonly a cause of meningitis. This organism most directly affects the lower extremity when it becomes systemic through bloodstream dissemination, or *meningococcemia*. In these cases a very distinct finding is subcutaneous ecchymosis that can occur frequently on the extremities. Frank gangrene of the toes is also a common sequelae of severe disease.

Antibiotic Therapy
1. Penicillin—high dose
2. Ceftriaxone or comparable third-generation cephalosporin

■ *Kingella kingae*
Clinical Significance
Not a particularly common organism, but one of growing importance, *K. kingae* can cause osteomyelitis and septic arthritis, particularly in children.

Antibiotic Therapy
1. Ceftriaxone or comparable third-generation cephalosporins.
2. Penicillin, tetracyclines, macrolides, quinolones, meropenem, and aminoglycosides all have shown activity.

ANAEROBIC GRAM-NEGATIVE RODS

Relatively recently the clinically important gram-negative anaerobic rods were re-categorized. Formerly all in the genus *Bacteroides*, they were split into four distinct genera: *Bacteroides, Prevotella, Porphyromonas, and Fusobacterium*. All play some role in lower extremity infections.

■ *Bacteroides*

1. *Bacteroides fragilis*
2. *Bacteroides thetaiotaomicron*
3. *Bacteroides vulgatus*

Clinical Significance
Bacteroides are the most important causes of anaerobic infections in the lower extremity. They are also some of the most numerous bacteria in the body, being normal flora in the gut, the oral cavity, and female genitourinary system. Many studies point to one or another of this group as being the single most commonly isolated organism in the diabetic foot infection. They have a few virulence factors and other characteristics that make them important pathogens:

1. They act synergistically with other organisms to cause or potentiate infection.
2. They are capable of forming a glycocalyx (slime layer) to protect their colonies.
3. They tend to be resistant to many normally effective anaerobic antibiotics such as penicillin.
4. They produce numerous enzymes and toxins.

Resistance Patterns
The *Bacteroides* tend to be multiresistant. Antibiotics that work against other anaerobes, such as penicillin and first-generation cephalosporins, tend to be ineffective.

Antibiotic Therapy

1. Metronidazole, penems, and ß-lactamase inhibitor compounds
2. Clindamycin, chloramphenicol
3. Antianaerobic cephams–cefoxitin, cefotetan

■ *Prevotella/Porphyromonas/Fusobacterium*

1. *Prevotella melaninogenica* (formerly *Bacteroides melaninogenicus*)
2. *Porphyromonas asaccharolytica* (formerly *Bacteroides asaccharolyticus*)
3. *Fusobacterium necrophorum*

Clinical Significance

Although not as numerous as the *Bacteroides* in lower extremity infections, these organisms may also be found, especially in mixed cultures. They are particularly prevalent in diabetic foot infections, decubitus ulcerations, and following bite wounds.

Resistance Patterns

These tend to be less resistant to penicillin than the *Bacteroides*. *Fusobacterium*, in particular, still remains mostly susceptible to penicillin. More resistance has been noted with the other two genera.

Antibiotic Therapy

Same as previously discussed with *Bacteroides,* although penicillin may still be drug of choice for *Fusobacterium.*

AEROBIC GRAM-NEGATIVE RODS—ENTEROBACTERIACEAE

Discussion of the aerobic gram-negative rods is broken down into two groups. The first, those members of the family Enterobacteriaceae, are by far the most common gram-negative isolates recovered in the clinical bacteriology laboratory. For this reason they are presented first. The second group consists of a diverse group of other clinically important gram-negative rods that may not be isolated nearly as often. All are presented in alphabetical order, not in any order of importance or pathogenicity.

A note about antibiotic selection: particularly with the gram-negative organisms, susceptibility will vary among communities, hospitals, and even among isolates. The production of extended spectrum ß-lactamases (ESBL) will render useless previously very useful drugs, such as third-generation cephalosporins. Make sure to check the laboratory sensitivity results for definitive therapy.

■ *Citrobacter*

1. *Citrobacter freundii*
2. *Citrobacter diversus*

Clinical Significance
The *Citrobacter* species are sometimes found in lower extremity infections. They are most common in patients who have been hospitalized, but can also be found in community-acquired infections. Both species are seen, but *C. freundii* seems to be the more common of the two.

Resistance Patterns
C. freundii is the more resistant of the two organisms. Whereas *C. diversus* may be sensitive to ampicillin and first-generation cephalosporins, *C. freundii* is resistant to all but third-generation agents and is frequently even resistant to those. Antibiotic selection is based on individual sensitivity reports.

Antibiotic Therapy
1. Quinolones, ß-lactamase inhibitor combinations
2. Penems, third-generation cephalosporins, aminoglycosides, extended-spectrum penicillins, aztreonam, TMP/SMX

■ *Enterobacter*

1. *Enterobacter aerogenes*
2. *Enterobacter cloacae*
3. *Enterobacter agglomerans*
4. *Enterobacter sakazakii*

Clinical Significance
All of the aforementioned *Enterobacter* species are capable of causing lower extremity infection, especially in patients who have been on antibiotics. As with the other enteric pathogens, they are most common in debilitated patients who have been in the hospital or nursing home, and in diabetics. In some cases they are also seen in community-acquired infections.

Resistance Patterns

Enterobacter are capable of producing an inducible, chromosomal ß-lactamase when challenged with a ß-lactam antibiotic. For this reason care must be taken when treating these organisms. Isolates that were originally susceptible to a ß-lactam such as a third-generation cephalosporin may become resistant on therapy. Sensitivity reports must be followed carefully. *E. cloacae* is the most notoriously resistant of the *Enterobacter*.

Antibiotic Therapy

See the therapies listed for *Citrobacter*. ß-lactamase inhibitor combinations may not be as effective against *E. cloacae*.

■ *Escherichia coli*

Clinical Significance

Having gained great notoriety in the last few years as a cause of sometimes fatal disease related to hamburger consumption, *E. coli* has always been one of the best-known gram-negative rods. Although not as well known for its capacity to cause lower extremity infections, it still is a regular isolate from these sites. The organism may be considered as the "representative gram-negative" in community-acquired infections. This frequency may be attributed to the infamous "fecal fallout."

Resistance Patterns

For the most part *E. coli* has remained a fairly susceptible organism that is easy to treat. However, because of ESBLs, some strains have become significantly resistant, and these are becoming more commonplace. Long gone are the days of assuming that a first-generation cephalosporin or even ampicillin would be effective.

Antibiotic Therapy

1. ß-lactamase inhibitor combinations, quinolones.
2. Cephalosporins (first- through third-generation, depending on local susceptibility patterns), penems, TMP/SMX, extended-spectrum penicillins, aztreonam, aminoglycosides.

■ *Klebsiella*

1. *Klebsiella oxytoca*
2. *Klebsiella pneumoniae*

Clinical Significance
Of the *Klebsiella, K. oxytoca* is the most frequently seen in lower extremity infections. *K. pneumoniae* is also occasionally isolated from the foot, but it is difficult to determine if it is a pathogen in these infections. Mostly this organism is known for causing lobar pneumonia in special-population patients such as alcoholics.

Resistance Patterns
K. oxytoca is the more susceptible of the two organisms. However, again, both species can develop ESBLs rendering them resistant to a number of drugs.

Antibiotic Therapy
See selections for *E. coli.*

▦ *Morganella morganii*
Clinical Significance
Formerly known as *Proteus morganii, Morganella* is predominantly seen in nosocomial lower extremity infections.

Resistance Patterns
Morganella is capable of producing the same inducible ß-lactamase seen with *Enterobacter* and other organisms.

Antibiotic Therapy
See the therapies listed for *Citrobacter.*

▦ *Proteus*

1. *Proteus mirabilis*
2. *Proteus vulgaris*

Clinical Significance
P. mirabilis is probably the most common gram-negative organism isolated from the lower extremity. Even more so than *E. coli, P. mirabilis* is normal flora of the foot. Frequently found in moist interdigital areas, *Proteus* has a distinctive odor that makes it easy to recognize. Most infections that begin in the digital interspaces have this organism as at least one of the pathogens. The organism is also commonly seen in paronychias, although probably more as a contaminant than a true pathogen. *Proteus* is known as a

"swarming" organism for its ability to totally take over any culture plate or surface on which it grows. This may account for some of the frequency of isolation.

P. vulgaris (also known as indole-positive *Proteus*) is fortunately much less common than *P. mirabilis*. It is considered mostly a nosocomial pathogen and is rarely community acquired. It also has a high degree of antibiotic resistance.

Resistance Patterns
Fortunately, *P. mirabilis* remains a fairly susceptible organism. Some strains are beginning to show resistance to ampicillin. *P. vulgaris* is much more resistant to antibiotics than *P. mirabilis*.

Antibiotic Therapy
For *P. mirabilis*:
1. First-generation cephalosporin, ß-lactamase inhibitor combinations
2. Second-, third-generation cephalosporins, quinolones, TMP/SMX

For *P. vulgaris*:

1. Quinolones, ß-lactamase inhibitor combinations
2. Penems, third-generation cephalosporins, aminoglycosides, aztreonam

■ *Providencia*

1. *Providencia stuartii*
2. *Providencia rettgeri*

Clinical Significance
Providencia are nosocomial organisms that are occasionally seen in lower extremity infections. Of the two common species, *P. stuartii* is by far the more frequently found.

Resistance Patterns
These organisms tend to have resistance patterns similar to those of *P. vulgaris*, to which it is closely related.

Antibiotic Therapy
See the therapies listed for *P. vulgaris*.

■ *Salmonella*

Clinical Significance

Mostly known as a cause of acute gastroenteritis, *Salmonella* is the most common cause of osteomyelitis of the lower extremity in patients with sickle cell disease. The etiology is thought to be as a result of sickle-cell–induced thromboses of the gut, allowing the *Salmonella* to become blood borne.

Resistance Patterns

Resistance has begun to develop in some countries to quinolones, penems, and third-generation cephalosporins, probably due to ESBLs. The use of antibiotics in animal feed is believed to be a major mechanism of this resistance development.

Antibiotic Therapy

1. Quinolones
2. Later-generation cephalosporins

■ *Serratia*

1. *Serratia marcescens*
2. *Serratia liquefaciens*

Clinical Significance

For many years *Serratia* was thought to be a harmless contaminant and was used as a marker dye because of its red pigment. It is now known to cause infections in the lower extremity and other areas of the body. It is most commonly considered a nosocomial pathogen but can occasionally be seen in community-acquired infections. *S. marcescens* is by far the most frequent pathogen of this group. (As an interesting sidelight, since this organism was named after a man named Serrati, the proper pronunciation is probably with a hard "t" sound as opposed to the more commonly heard "sh" sound.)

Resistance Patterns

As is the case with some of the other gram-negative organisms, *Serratia* is capable of producing an inducible ß-lactamase. See *Enterobacter* for the clinical significance of this enzyme.

Antibiotic Therapy

See the therapies listed for *Citrobacter*.

OTHER AEROBIC GRAM-NEGATIVE RODS

■ *Acinetobacter*

1. *Acinetobacter baumanii* (formerly *A. calcoaceticus* var. *anitratus*)
2. *Acinetobacter lwoffi*, among others

Clinical Significance

Acinetobacter is an opportunistic pathogen that has become a major problem in some institutions. This is probably because of antibiotic selection pressures, as this organism is generally found in the intensive care units of tertiary care hospitals. For this reason, the organism has become very resistant. Some strains are reported to be resistant to all known antibiotics. It is also occasionally seen in community-acquired infections including soft tissue infections of the lower extremity, especially following trauma.

Resistance Patterns

A. baumanii is a very resistant organism. Most strains are only sensitive to one or two antibiotics. *A. lwoffi* tends to be more susceptible to a broader range of drugs. Therapy needs to be based on the laboratory sensitivities for each particular isolate.

Antibiotic Therapy

1. Imipenem, meropenem, ampicillin/sulbactam (other ß-lactamase inhibitor combinations are less effective because it is the sulbactam with the inherent activity)
2. Quinolone (with or without the addition of an aminoglycoside)

■ *Aeromonas hydrophilia*

Clinical Significance

As its name implies, *A. hydrophilia* is a "water-loving" organism. It is most associated with lower extremity infections following trauma occurring in fresh water such as a pond or a lake. The infection can be rapidly progressive and is very similar to *Vibrio* infection in similar circumstances.

Resistance Patterns

Aeromonas tends to be resistant to most penicillins and many early generation cephalosporins.

Antibiotic Therapy

1. Quinolones
2. TMP/SMX, penem, aminoglycosides, third- or fourth-generation cephalosporins

■ *Alcaligenes*

1. *Alcaligenes xylosoxidans*
2. *Alcaligenes faecalis*

Clinical Significance

Although rarely found and of questionable significance as a pathogen, *Alcaligenes* species have been seen in lower extremity infections. They are primarily nosocomial organisms and are found colonizing hospital equipment and fluids. They are also normal flora of the gastrointestinal (GI) tract.

Resistance Patterns

A. xylosoxidans is the more resistant of the two, being more resistant to the early spectrum cephalosporins than *A. faecalis*. Since sensitivities vary widely, the culture report becomes important in determining therapy.

Antibiotic Therapy

1. Penems
2. Some quinolones; some cephalosporins, particularly third generation; some aminoglycosides; ß-lactamase inhibitor compounds

■ *Bartonella henselae*

Clinical Significance

Formerly known as the "cat scratch organism," this bacterium is found fairly commonly in domestic cats. It is most common in kittens and wild cats. Since typical cat scratch disease is caused by a scratch or bite, it can occur in the lower extremity. A localized lesion followed a few weeks later with lymph node involvement is the usual course of events.

Antibiotic Therapy

1. Azithromycin, clarithromycin
2. TMP/SMX, doxycycline, quinolones

■ *Capnocytophaga canimorsus (Formerly DF-2)*

Clinical Significance

Literally from the latin for the "dog bite" organism, this was previously known by the CDC alphanumeric Dysgonic Fermenter-2. It is normal flora of a dog's mouth and is mostly associated with dog-associated bites or contact. It can cause systemic disease without bites, especially in immunocompromised or asplenic patients.

Antibiotic Therapy

1. ß-lactamase inhibitor combinations, penicillin
2. Quinolones, third-generation cephalosporins, clindamycin, erythromycin

■ *Eikenella corrodens*

Clinical Significance

Like *C. canimorsus*, *E. corrodens* is primarily a bite wound pathogen. The difference is that *Eikenella* is found mostly in human bites. It is usually one of many organisms found in a human bite infection.

Resistance Patterns

E. corrodens is usually resistant to first-generation cephalosporins and penicillinase-resistant penicillins. The organism is also resistant to clindamycin, metronidazole, and erythromycin.

Antibiotic Therapy

1. Penicillin, amoxicillin/clavulanic acid
2. TMP/SMX, quinolones, doxycycline, impanel, later-generation cephalosporins

■ *Homophiles influenza*

Clinical Significance

Most common in the upper respiratory tract, *H. influenza* has been occasionally isolated from the lower extremity. It may be found in community-acquired or nosocomial settings. It can cause cellulitis, osteomyelitis, or septic arthritis, particularly in children.

Resistance Patterns

H. influenza is generally resistant to first-generation cephalosporins and ampicillin. In fact, the second-generation cephalosporins were developed specifically with this organism in mind.

Antibiotic Therapy
1. Third-generation cephalosporins, ß-lactamase inhibitor combinations
2. Quinolones, TMP/SMX, azithromycin, clarithromycin

▪ *Pasteurella multocida*

Clinical Significance
This is a common pathogen recovered from cat bites and other animal bite wound infections. Even patients exposed to animals but not bitten may develop infection with this organism. It can cause the entire gamut of lower extremity infections, including cellulitis, septic arthritis, and osteomyelitis.

Resistance Patterns
It is generally resistant to first-generation cephalosporins and penicillinase-resistant penicillins.

Antibiotic Therapy
1. Third-generation cephalosporins, ß-lactamase inhibitor combinations, penicillin, ampicillin
2. Quinolones, doxycycline, TMP/SMX

▪ *Pseudomonas aeruginosa*

Clinical Significance
Volumes have been written about this organism. It is the scourge of many a clinician. It can present with a wide range of lower extremity manifestations, from the most common presentation as a harmless superficial contamination of a wound, as green-nail syndrome, as osteomyelitis, or even as life-threatening sepsis. It is predominantly a water-dwelling organism that is common in sinks, faucets, and even tap water. Fresh fruits and vegetables are heavily contaminated with the organism and should be kept out of the patient's room when an open wound is present.

Resistance Patterns
One of the reasons for the widespread fear of this organism is its resistance patterns. For this reason some clinicians believe that any infection caused by *P. aeruginosa* requires combination therapy with an aminoglycoside. Although that may have been the case 15 years

ago, or in systemic or pulmonary infections, newer antibiotics have been shown to be extremely effective as single-agent therapy. This is particularly true when dealing with lower extremity skin, skin structure, and bone and joint infections. Despite these advances, however, *Pseudomonas* continues to develop resistance. In some hospitals, strains resistant to all known antibiotics have been isolated. Conversely, there are some community-acquired strains that remain exquisitely susceptible. Antibiotic therapy should be guided by a knowledge of what resistance patterns are like in a particular community and the laboratory sensitivity results.

Antibiotic Therapy
See Appendix 4.

■ *Stenotrophomonas (formerly Pseudomonas and then Xanthomonas) maltophilia and Burkholderia (formerly various Pseudomonas species) cepacia*

Clinical Significance
These two organisms are usually considered together. They are infrequent causes of lower extremity infections. Nonetheless, they are occasionally found and are notable for their resistance to antibiotics. These tend to be opportunistic pathogens found in patients on multiple previous courses of antibiotics. They are also occasionally found in compromised patients.

Resistance Patterns
Both are resistant to most cephalosporins (some ceftazidime sensitivity), penicillins, and ciprofloxacin. Since sensitivity varies widely from strain to strain, reports for the specific organism are very helpful.

Antibiotic Therapy
1. TMP/SMX (*Stenotrophomonas* or *Burkholderia*), ceftazidime (*Burkholderia*)
2. Minocycline, doxycycline, penems, ticarcillin/clavulanic acid

■ *Vibrio vulnificus*

Clinical Significance
This is one of the few *Vibrio* species that is not known as a major cause of diarrhea. Rather, it causes a severe, necrotizing skin and

skin structure infection along with sepsis. It can be acquired through the consumption of raw oysters, in which it is a very frequent contaminant, especially in warm-water months. The organism finds its way out of the gastrointestinal tract and into the bloodstream, where it can be fatal in about one half of the cases. It can also directly contaminate open wounds exposed to warm saltwater. There have also been cases reported of necrotizing fasciitis caused by *V. vulnificus* following puncture wounds of the extremities by fish spines and fins. As with any severe, necrotizing infection, surgical incision and drainage plays a major role in the treatment.

Antibiotic Therapy
1. Doxycycline
2. Ceftazidime, cefotaxime, ciprofloxacin

NONTUBERCULOUS MYCOBACTERIA

The nontuberculous mycobacterium, sometimes referred to as *atypical mycobacterium*, can occasionally cause lower extremity infections. These organisms are ubiquitous in the environment and consist of more than 65 different species. They are mostly considered nosocomial pathogens and are very prevalent in water systems in hospitals and homes. They frequently infect immunocompromised patients. There are a few species that are of particular interest in the lower extremity.

■ *Mycobacterium marinum*

Clinical Significance
This organism is most commonly associated with fish tanks or trauma that occurs in saltwater. It usually presents as a localized granuloma as opposed to a spreading infection. The infection usually occurs 2 to 3 weeks after contact with contaminated water such as that found when cleaning a fish tank. Treatment is primarily through surgical excision of the lesion.

Antibiotic Therapy
1. Clarithromycin, minocycline, doxycycline, TMP/SMX
2. Combination of rifampin plus ethambutol
3. All treatment for a minimum of 3 months

■ *"Rapid growing" mycobacteria*

1. *Mycobacterium fortuitum*
2. *Mycobacterium chelonae*
3. *Mycobacterium abscessus*

Clinical Significance

These are the nontuberculous mycobacteria most likely to cause infections in the lower extremity. They are known as rapid growing because they can usually be isolated and identified within 7 days of being cultured. They have been reported to cause surgical wound infections, but their propensity for causing septic arthritis following intraarticular injection is their most interesting trait. These organisms have been reported to cause series of infections through contaminated solutions, in particular injectable steroids, and contaminated injecting devices. Surgical debridement or drainage is an important aspect of treatment.

Antibiotic Therapy

1. Clarithromycin seems to be the best single agent, especially for *M. chelonae* and *M. abscessus.*
2. There is various single agent use of or combinations of amikacin, cefoxitin, TMP/SMX, doxycycline, imipenem, depending on individual sensitivities.

SUGGESTED READINGS

Bacterial Diseases. In Mandell GL, Bennett JE, Dolin R, editors: *Principles and practice of infectious diseases,* ed 5, Philadelphia, 2000, Churchill Livingstone.

Fridkin SK: Vancomycin-intermediate and -resistant *Staphylococcus aureus:* what the infectious disease specialist needs to know, *Clin Infect Dis* 32(1):108, 2001.

Phillips MS, Fordham von Reyn C: Nosocomial infections due to nontuberculous mycobacteria, *Clin Infect Dis* 33:1363, 2001.

Update: *Staphylococcus aureus* with reduced susceptibility to vancomycin—United States, 1997, *MMWR Morb Mortal Wkly Rep* 46(35):813-815, 1997.

Appendix

Commonly Used Oral Antibiotics and Their Usual Dosages*

ANTIBIOTIC	DOSAGE
Penicillins	
Amoxicillin	250-500 mg tid
Amoxicillin/clavulanic acid (Augmentin)	500-875 mg bid (two 250-mg tablets *do not equal* 500 mg)
Cloxacillin	250-500 mg qid
Dicloxacillin	250-500 mg qid
Penicillin VK	250-500 mg qid
Cephalosporins	
Cephalexin	250-500 mg bid-qid
Cephradine	250-500 mg tid-qid
Cefadroxil	500-1000 mg qd-bid
Cefaclor (Ceclor)	250-500 mg tid
Cefuroxime axetil (Ceftin)	250 mg bid
Cefprozil (Cefzil)	250-500 mg bid
Cefdinir (Omnicef)	300 mg bid

*Brand names are given when the drug is proprietary. For spectrum of activity and specific clinical usage recommendations, see Chapter 8.

Continued

APPENDIX 1

Commonly Used Oral Antibiotics and Their Usual Dosages—cont'd

ANTIBIOTIC	DOSAGE
Quinolones	
Ciprofloxacin (Cipro)	500-750 mg bid
Levofloxacin (Levaquin)	500-750 mg qd
Moxifloxacin (Avelox)	400 mg qd
Gatifloxacin (Tequin)	400 mg qd
Trovafloxacin (Trovan)	200 mg qd
Other Oral Agents	
Clindamycin (Cleocin)	300 mg bid-tid
Doxycycline (Vibramycin)	100 mg bid
Erythromycin	500 mg qid
Metronidazole (Flagyl)	500 mg tid
Minocycline (Minocin)	100 mg bid
Tetracycline	250-500 mg bid
Trimethoprim/sulfamethoxazole(Bactrim/Septra)	1 DS bid

*Brand names are given when the drug is proprietary. For spectrum of activity and specific clinical usage recommendations, see Chapter 8.

APPENDIX 2

Generic and Trade Names of Antibiotics Commonly Used in Foot Infections

GENERIC	TRADE
Amikacin	Amikin
Amoxicillin	Amoxil, Polymox, Trimox, Wymox
Amoxicillin/clavulanic acid	Augmentin
Ampicillin	Omnipen, Polycillin
Ampicillin/sulbactam	Unasyn
Azithromycin	Zithromax
Aztreonam	Azactam
Carbenicillin	Geopen
Carbenicillin (oral)	Geocillin
Cefaclor	Ceclor
Cefadroxil	Duricef, Ultracef
Cefazolin	Ancef, Kefzol
Cefdinir	Omnicef
Cefepime	Maxipime
Cefixime	Suprax
Cefoperazone	Cefobid
Cefotaxime	Claforan
Cefotetan	Cefotan
Cefoxitin	Mefoxin
Cefprozil	Cefzil
Ceftazidime	Fortaz, Tazicef, Tazidime
Ceftibuten	Cedax
Ceftizoxime	Cefizox
Ceftriaxone	Rocephin
Cefuroxime	Zinacef
Cefuroxime axetil	Ceftin
Cephalexin	Keflex, Keflet, Keftab
Cephradine	Anspor, Velocef
Chloramphenicol	Chloromycetin
Ciprofloxacin	Cipro
Clarithromycin	Biaxin
Clindamycin	Cleocin
Cloxacillin	Tegopen
Dicloxacillin	Dynapen, Pathocil
Dirithromycin	Dynabac
Doxycycline	Vibramycin, Doryx, Vibratab

Continued

Generic and Trade Names of Antibiotics Commonly Used in Foot Infections—cont'd

GENERIC	TRADE
Ertapenem	Invanz
Erythromycin(s)	Eryc, Erythrocin, Ilosone, E-Mycin, EES
Gatifloxacin	Tequin
Gentamicin	Garamycin
Imipenem/cilastatin	Primaxin
Kanamycin	Kantrex
Levofloxacin	Levaquin
Lincomycin	Lincocin
Linezolid	Zyvox
Meropenem	Merrem
Methicillin	Staphcillin
Metronidazole	Flagyl, Protostat
Mezlocilin	Mezlin
Minocycline	Minocin
Moxalactam	Moxam
Moxifloxacin	Avelox
Mupirocin	Bactroban
Nafcillin	Nafcil, Unipen
Oxacillin	Prostaphlin
Oxytetracycline	Terramycin
Penicillin G	
Potassium	Pentids, Pfizerpen
Procaine	Wycillin
Benzathine	Bicillin
Penicillin V	Pen-Vee K, Veetids, Betapen-VK
Piperacillin	Pipracil
Piperacillin/tazobactam	Zosyn
Quinupristin/dalfopristin	Synercid
Rifampin	Rifadin, Rifamate, Rimactane
Silver sulfadiazine	Silvadine
Tetracycline	Achromycin, Sumycin
Ticarcillin	Ticar
Ticarcillin/clavulanate	Timentin
Tobramycin	Nebcin
Trimethoprim/sulfamethoxazole	Bactrim, Septra
Trovafloxacin	Trovan
Vancomycin	Vancocin

APPENDIX 3

Trade and Generic Names of Antibiotics Commonly Used in Foot Infections

TRADE	GENERIC
Achromycin	Tetracycline
Amikin	Amikacin
Amoxcil	Amoxicillin
Ancef	Cefazolin
Anspor	Cephradine
Augmentin	Amoxicillin/clavulanate
Avelox	Moxifloxacin
Azactam	Aztreonam
Bactrim	Trimethoprim/sulfamethoxazole
Bactroban	Mupirocin
Betapen-VK	Penicillin V
Biaxin	Clarithromycin
Bicillin	Benzathine penicillin
Ceclor	Cefaclor
Cedax	Ceftibuten
Cefadyl	Cephapirin
Cefizox	Ceftizoxime
Cefobid	Cefoperazone
Cefotan	Cefotetan
Ceftin	Cefuazroxime axetil
Cefzil	Cefprozil
Chloromycetin	Chloramphenicol
Cipro	Ciprofoxacin
Claforan	Cefotaxime
Cleocin	Clindamycin
Doryx	Doxycycline
Duricef	Cefadroxil
Dynapen	Dicloxicillin
E-mycin	Erythromycin
EES	Erythromycin ethyl succinate
Eryc	Erythromycin
Erythrocin	Erythromycin lactobionate
Flagyl	Metronidazole
Fortaz	Ceftazidime
Garamycin	Gentamicin
Geocillin	Carbenicillin (oral)
Geopen	Carbenicillin
Ilosone	Erythromycin estolate
Invanz	Ertapenem

Continued

APPENDIX 3

Trade and Generic Names of Antibiotics Commonly Used in Foot Infections—cont'd

TRADE	GENERIC
Kantrex	Kanamycin
Keflet	Cephalexin
Keflex	Cephalexin
Keflin	Cephalothin
Keftab	Cefalexin hydrochloride
Kefzol	Cefazolin
Levaquin	Levofloxacin
Lincocin	Lincomycin
Mandol	Cefamandole
Maxipime	Cefepime
Mefoxin	Cefoxitin
Merrem	Meropenem
Mezlin	Mezlocillin
Minocin	Minocycline
Nafcil	Nafcillin
Nebcin	Tobramycin
Omipen	Ampicillin
Omnicef	Cefdinir
Pathocil	Dicloxicillin
Pentids	Penicillin G
Pen-Vee K	Penicillin V
Pfizerpen	Penicillin G
Pipracil	Piperacilin
Polycillin	Ampicillin
Polymox	Amoxicillin
Primaxin	Imipenem/cilastatin
Prostaphlin	Oxacillin
Protostat	Metronidazole
Rifadin	Rifampin
Rifamate	Rifampin
Rimactane	Rifampin
Rocephin	Ceftriaxone
Silvadene	Silver sulfadiazine
Septra	Trimethoprim/sulfamethoxazole
Staphcillin	Methicillin
Sumycin	Tetracycline
Suprax	Cefixime
Synercid	Quinupristin/dalfopristin

APPENDIX 3

Trade and Generic Names of Antibiotics Commonly Used in Foot Infections—cont'd

TRADE	GENERIC
Tazicef	Ceftazidime
Tazidime	Ceftazidime
Tegopen	Cloxacillin
Tequin	Gatifloxacin
Terramycin	Oxytetracycline
Ticar	Ticarcillin
Timentin	Ticarcillin/clavulanate
Trimox	Amoxicillin
Trovan	Trovafloxacin
Ultracef	Cefadroxil
Unasyn	Ampicillin/sulfactam
Unipen	Nafcillin
Vancocin	Vancomycin
Velocef	Cephradine
Vibramycin	Doxycycline
Vibratab	Doxycycline
Wycillin	Procaine penicillin G
Wymox	Amoxicillin
Zinacef	Cefuroxime
Zithromax	Azithromycin
Zosyn	Piperacillin/tazobactam
Zyvox	Linezolid

APPENDIX 4

Antibiotic Therapy of Pseudomonas aeruginosa Infections

Aminoglycosides*
    Tobramycin
    Amikacin
    Gentamicin
Antipseudomonal Penicillins[†]
    Piperacillin[‡]
    Mezlocillin
    Ticarcillin[†]
Cephalosporins
    Ceftazidime
    Cefepime
    Cefoperazone

Monobactams
    Aztreonam
Carbapenems
    Imipenem/Cilastatin
    Meropenem
Quinolones (Only Oral Agents)
    Ciprofloxacin
    Levofloxacin
    Moxifloxacin
    Trovafloxacin

*Aminoglycosides should be used rarely. If used, they should be combined with a penicillin for synergy.
†Penicillins should not be used as single agents because of resistance development. All other drugs on this list have been used effectively as single agents.
‡Ticarcillin/clavulanic acid and Piperacillin/tazobactam can not be used as a single agent. They are no more effective against *Pseudomonas* than the uncombined penicillin.

APPENDIX 5

Select Internet Sites of Interest

Site Name	Address
American Medical Association (AMA)	www.ama-assn.org
American Society for Microbiology Home Page and Journal Search	www.asmusa.org
Centers for Disease Control and Prevention	www.cdc.gov
Infectious Diseases Society of America (IDSA)	www.idsociety.org
IDSA Journal Search (Journal of Infectious Diseases and Clinical Infectious Diseases)	www.journals.uchicago.edu
Johns Hopkins Antibiotic Guide	http://hopkins-abxguide.org
Link to OSHA Bloodborne Pathogen Guidelines	www.osha.gov
Lyme Disease Network	www.lymenet.org
Medline	www.ncbi.nlm.nih.gov/ PubMed/
Medscape Infectious Disease Page	http://id.medscape.com/ Home/Topics/ID/ InfectiousDiseases.html
Mosby's Drug Consult	www.harcourthealth.com/ Mosby/PhyGenRx/ genrxhome.html
Musculoskeletal Infection Society of North America	www.msisna.org
Physicians' Desk Reference On-Line	http://physician.pdr.net/ physician/index.htm

APPENDIX 6

Drugs for Bugs

ORGANISM	FIRST CHOICE	ALTERNATIVE
Gram-Positives		
Staphylococcus-methicillin sensitive	ASOC* (O) Cefazolin (IV)	Clindamycin (O) Vancomycin (IV) Azithromycin Dicloxacillin Nafcillin (IV)
Streptococcus	ASOC* (O) Cefazolin (IV)	Penicillin (IV/O) Clindamycin (O) Vancomycin (IV)
Staphylococcus-methicillin resistant	Vancomycin (IV) Linezolid (IV/O)	Minocycline (O) TMP/SMX (O)
Enterococcus	Amoxicillin (O) Vancomycin (IV) VRE	Amox/Clav (O) Linezolid (IV/O) Linezolid/ Dalfopristin-Quinupristin
Gram-Negatives		
E. coli/Proteus	ASOC* (O) Cefazolin (IV)	Quinolone (O)
E/C/S/M Group	Quinolone (O)	Third-generation cephalosporin Aztreonam (IV) TMP/SMX (O)
P. aeruginosa	Ciproflox (O)	Ceftazidime (IV) Aztreonam (IV) +/- Aminoglycoside
Bacteroides (Anaerobes)-diabetic foot	Zosyn (IV) Augmentin (O) Timentin (IV) Unasyn (IV)	Metronidazole Clindamycin Cefoxitin (IV) –Penem (IV)

*Antistaphylococcal oral cephalosporin (i.e., Cephalexin, Cefdinir, Cefuroxime axetil, Cefprozil).

APPENDIX **6**

Drugs for Bugs—cont'd

ORGANISM	FIRST CHOICE	ALTERNATIVE
Less Common Organisms		
Stenotrophomonas	TMP/SMX (IV/O)	Minocycline (O)
		- Penems
Burkholderia	TMP/SMX (IV/O)	Ceftazidime (IV)
Aeromonas	Quinolones (O)	TMP/SMX (IV)
		Penems
		Third-/fourth-generation cephalosporin
Diphtheroids	Vancomycin (IV)	
Borrelia (Lyme)	Doxycycline (O)	Amoxicillin (O)
	Ceftriaxone (IV)	

APPENDIX 7

Antibiotic Pharmacokinetics and Dosing

Pharmacology: Penicillins

Drug (% oral absorption)	Dose (g)	Serum (peak)	Oral	Parenteral	Oral	Parenteral
		DRUG CONCENTRATIONS ACHIEVED WITH SPECIFIC DOSES — MEASURED LEVELS (μg/ml)	ADULTS		CHILDREN	
Amoxicillin* (74-92)	0.25 PO† 0.5 PO†	3.5-5.0 5.5-11.0	0.25-0.5 g q8h		6.7-13.3 mg/kg q8h[c]	
Amoxicillin clavulanate	0.25 PO 0.5 PO	3.7-4.8 6.0-9.7	0.25-0.5 g q8h		6.6-13.3 mg/kg q8h[d]	
Ampicillin* (30-55)	0.25 PO† 0.5 PO† 2.0 IV	1.8-2.9 3-6 47.6	0.25-0.5 g q6h	0.5-2 g q4-6h	6.25-25 mg/kg q6h[e]	6.25-25 mg/kg q6h[f]
Ampicillin/ sulbactam	1.5 IV 3.0 IV	40-71 109-150		1.5-3.0 g q6h		25-50 mg/kg q6h
Azlocillin (minimal)	2 IV[g] 3 IV[g]	165 214		2-4 g q4-6h		75 mg/kg q6h (not approved)[f]
Carbenicillin	1 IV 3 IV[i]	45-71 278		5-6 g q4h		25-100 mg/kg q4-6h
Carbenicillin indanyl sodium (30-40)	0.382 PO	6.5	0.382-0.764 g q6h			
Cloxacillin * (37-60)	0.5 PO	6.9-15	0.25-1.0 g q6h		12.5-25 mg/kg q6h	
Dicloxacillin* (35-76)	0.5 PO	10-18	0.125-0.5 g q6h		3.125-6.25[e] mg/kg q6h	
Mezlocillin	1 IV[j] 2 IV[j] 5 IV[j]	64-143 161-364 199-597		3-4 g q4-6h		50-75 mg/kg q4h
Nafcillin* (36)	1 PO 1 IM 0.5 IV[j]	7.7 7.6 40	0.5-1 g q6h	0.5-2 g q4-6h	12.5-25 mg/kg q6h[e]	12.5-25 mg/kg q6h[e]
Oxacillin* (30-35)	0.25 PO 0.5 PO 0.5 IV	1.65 2.6-3.9 52-63	0.5-1 g q4-6h	0.5-2 g q4-6h	12.5-25 mg/kg q6h[e]	12.5-50 mg/kg q6h[e]
Penicillin G* (15-30)	400,000 U PO 2 mU q2h IV	0.5 U/ml[p] 20	0.5-1 g qh6	1-4 mU q4-6h	25,000-90,000 U/kg/d in 3-6 doses	25,000-400,000 U/kg/d q4-6h[q]
Penicillin G benzathine	1.2 mU IM	0.15 U/ml		0.6-1.2 mU IM q12h		0.6 mU IM × 1[c]
Penicillin G procaine	0.6 mU IM 1.2 mU IM	1.6 1.95		0.6-1.2 mU IM q12h		25,000-50,000 U/kg/d IM[q]
Penicillin V* potassium (60-73)	0.25 PO 0.5 PO	2.3-2.7 4.9-6.3	0.25-0.5 g q6h		25,000-100,000 U/kg/d in 3-6 doses	
Piperacillin	2 IV[j] 4 IV[j] 6 IV[j]	159-615 389-484 695-849		3-4 g q4-6h		50 mg/kg q4h[q]
Piperacillin/ tazobactam	3.375 IV[g] 4.5 IV[g]	209 224		3.375-4.5 g q6-8h		
Ticarcillin	1 IV[j] 2 IV[j] 3 IV[j]	70-100 200-218 257		3 g q4-6h		200-300 mg/kg/d q4-6h[e]
Ticarcillin/ clavulanate	3.1 IV	324		3.1 g q4-8h		50 mg/kg q4-6h

* Decreased rate and/or extent of absorption when given with food.
† Fasting.
[a] Specified dose is supplemental to that after hemodialysis.
[b] Inflamed meninges.
[c] Children <20-27 kg.

[d] Children <40 kg should not receive the 250-mg film-coated tablet.
[e] Children <40-50 kg.
[f] 16.7-33.3 mg/kg q4h for meningitis.
[g] Infusion over 15-30 min.
[h] Mean concentration.

SERUM HALF-LIFE (h) WITH NORMAL AND ANURIC Cl_{Cr} VALUES (ml/min)		STANDARD DOSE WITH DOSING INTERVALS IN RENAL IMPAIRMENT					DOSAGE WITH DIALYSIS	
			FOR Cl_{Cr} RANGES (ml/min)					
>80	<10	Usual Adult Dose	>80	80-50	50-10	<10 (anuric)	After HD[a]	During PD (daily dose)
0.7-1.4	7.4-21	0.25-0.5 g	8h	8h	8-12h	12-16h	0.25-0.5 g	
1.1-1.3	7.5	0.25-0.5 g	8h	8h	12h	12-24h	0.25 g	
0.7-1.4	7.4-21	0.5-2 g	4-6h	4-6h	8h	12h	0.5-2 g	1-4 g
1	9	1.5-3.0 g	6-8h	6-8h	8-12h	24h		
1	5	2-4 g	4-6h	4-6h	8h	12h	3 g	
0.78-1	9.4-23.4	5-6 g	4h	4h	2-3 g q6h	Avoid	0.75-2 g	2 g q6-12h
0.78-1	9.4-23.4							
0.4-0.8	0.8-2.3	0.5-1 g	6h	6g	6h	6h	Usual regimen	Usual regimen
0.6-0.8	1-2.2	0.125-0.5 g	6h	6h	6h	6h	Usual regimen	Usual regimen
0.71-1.3	1.6-14	3-4 g	4-6h	4-6h	8h	2 g q8h	2-3 g	3 g q12h
0.5-1.5	1.8-2.8	0.5-2 g	4-6h	4-6h	4-6h	4-6h	Usual regimen	Usual regimen
0.3-0.8	0.5-2	0.5-2 g	4-6h	4-6h	4-6h	4-6h	Usual regimen	Usual regimen
0.4-0.9	6-20	1-4 mU	4-6h	4-6h	4-6h	0.5-2 mU q4-6h	500,000 U	
days								
24		0.6-1.2 mU	12h	12h	12h	12h		
0.5	7-10	0.25-0.5 g	6h	6h	6h	6h	0.25 g	
0.6-1.3	2.1-6	3-4 g	4-6h	4-6h	8h	12h	1 g, then 2 g q8h	
0.7-1.1	1.9-3.5	2.5-4.5 g	6-8h	6-8h				
0.93-1.3	13.5-16.2	3 g	4-6h	4-6h	6-8h	2 g q12h	3 g, then 2 g q12h	3 g q12h
1.1-1.5	8.5	3.1 g	4-6h	4-6h	2-3.1 g q6-8h	2 g q12h	3.1 g	3.1 g q12h

[i] 100% of bacampicillin is metabolized to ampicillin.

[j] IV push (over 2-10 min).

[k] Over 3 hours.

[l] Hetacillin is rapidly converted to ampicillin.

[m] Depending on severity of infection.

[n] q6h if >2 kg; q8h if <2 kg.

[o] q8h if >2 kg; q12h if <2 kg.

[p] Higher when given with probenecid.

[q] Dosage should not exceed adult dosage.

Abbreviations: Cl_{Cr}, Creatinine clearance; CSF, cerebrospinal fluid; HD, hemodialysis; PD, peritoneal dialysis.

Antibiotic Pharmacokinetics and Dosing—cont'd

Pharmacology: Cephalosporins

Drug (% oral absorption)	Dose (g)	DRUG CONCENTRATIONS ACHIEVED WITH SPECIFIC DOSES — MEASURED LEVELS (µg/ml) Serum (peak)	DOSAGE RECOMMENDATIONS — ADULTS Oral	ADULTS Parenteral	CHILDREN Oral	CHILDREN Parenteral
First-Generation Agents						
Cefadroxil (100)	0.5 PO	10-18	0.5-1 g q12-24h		30 mg/kg/d q21h	
	1 PO	24-35				
Cefazolin	1 IV	188		0.5-2 g q8h		25-100 mg/kg/d q6-8h
	1 IM	64-76				
Cephalexin (100)	0.25 PO	9	0.25-1 g q6h		25-100 mg/kg/d in 4 doses	
	0.5 PO	15-18				
Cephalothin	1 IM	15-21		0.5-2 g q4-6 h		80-160 mg/kg/d q6 h
	1 IV	30				
Second-Generation Agents						
Cefaclor* (≥52)	0.25 PO	5-7	0.25-0.5 g q8h		20-40 mg/kg/d q8h^c	
	0.5 PO	13-15				
Cefamandole	1 IV^d	139		0.5-2 g q4-8 h		50-150 mg/kg/d q4-8h^e
	2 IV^d	214				
	3 IV^d	534				
Cefmetazole				2 g q6-12h		
Cefonicid	7.5 mg/kg IV^d	95-156		0.5-2 g q24 h		
	0.5 IV	91				
	1 IV	221				
Cefotetan	1 IV^d	142-179.6		1-2 g q12h		40-60 mg/kg/d q12h
	2 IV^d	237				
Cefoxitin	1 IM	22-24		1-2 g q6-8 h		80-160 mg/kg/d q4-8h^f
	1 IV^a	110-125				
	2 IV^d	221				
Cefprozil (95)	0.25 PO	5.6-6.8	0.25-0.5 g q12-24h		15 mg/kg q12h	
	0.5 PO	8.2-10.4				
	1 PO	15.5-19.9				
Cefuroxime (37-52)^g	0.5 PO	7	0.125-0.5 g q12 h	0.75-1.5 g q8 h	0.125-0.25 g q12 h^i	50-100 mg/kg/d q6-8 h^j
	0.75 IV^h	51.1				
Third-Generation Agents						
Cefdinir* (36)	0.2 PO	0.7-1.7	0.3-0.6 g q12-24h		14 mg/kg/d	
	0.6 PO	2.4				
Cefixime* (30-50)	0.4 PO tabs	3.7	0.4 g q24 h		8 mg/kg/d q24 h	
	0.4 PO susp	4.6				
Cefoperazone	1 IV^h	153		1-2 g q6-12h		25-100 mg/kg q12h (not approved)
	2 IV^h	253				
Cefotaxime	0.5 IM	11.7-11.9		0.5-2 g q8-12 h		50-200 mg/kg/d q4-8 h
	1 IV^d	102.4				
	2 IV^d	214.1				
Cefpodoxime^f (50)	0.1 PO	1.4	0.1-0.4 g q12h		5 mg/kg q12h^m	
	0.2 PO	2.3				
	0.4 PO	3.9				
Ceftazidime^o	0.5 IV^h	42		1-2 g q8-12 h		25-50 mg/kg q8h
	1 IV^h	69				
	2 IV^h	159-185.5				
Ceftibuten (80)	0.4 PO	15	0.2-0.4 q12-24h		9 mg/kg/d	
Ceftizoxime	1 IV^h	84.4		1-3 g q6-8 h		33-50 mg/kg q6-8h^f
	2 IV	131.8				
	3 IV	221.1				
Ceftriaxone	1 IV^h	123.2-150.7		0.5-2 g q12-24h		50-100 mg/kg/d q12-24h
	2 IV^h	223-276				
	2 IV^q	216-281				
Moxalactam	1 IV^h	60-100		0.5-4 g q8-12 h^s		50 mg/kg q6-8 h^{s,t}
	2 IV^d	150-200				
Fourth-Generation Agent						
Cefepine	1 IV	81.7		0.5-2 g q8-12h		50 mg/kg q8-12h
	2 IV	163.9				

* Decreased rate and/or extent of absorption when given with food.
^{a} Specified dose is supplemental to that after hemodialysis.
^{b} Inflamed meninges.
^{c} Should not exceed 1 g.
^{d} IV push (over 2-10 min).
^{e} Dosage should not exceed adult dosage.
^{f} Should not exceed 12 g.

^{g} 52% after food.
^{h} Infusion over 15-30 min.
^{i} 0.125 g q12 h for children <2 yr.
^{j} 200-240 mg/kg/d q6-8 h for meningitis.
^{k} Microbiologic activity in hepatic bile/microbiologic activity in serum.
^{l} Should be given with food to increase absorption.

SERUM HALF-LIFE (h) WITH NORMAL AND ANURIC Cl_{Cr} VALUES (ml/min)		STANDARD DOSE WITH DOSING INTERVALS IN RENAL IMPAIRMENT					DOSAGE WITH DIALYSIS	
		Usual Adult Dose	FOR Cl_{Cr} RANGES (ml/min)				After HD[a]	During PD (daily dose)
>80	<10		>80	80-50	50-10	<10 (anuric)		
1.1-2	20-25	0.5-1 g	12-24h	12-24h	0.5 g q12-24h	0.5 g q36h	0.5-1 g	
1.2-2.2	18-36	0.5-2 g	8h	8h	0.5-1 g q8-12h	0.5-1 g q18-24h	0.25-0.5 g	
0.5-1.2	5-30	0.25-1 g	6h	6h	8-12h	24-48h	0.25-1 g	
0.5-0.9	3-8	0.5-2 g	4-6h	4-6h	1-1.5 g q6h	0.5 g q8h	0.5-2 g	≤6 mg/L of dialysate
0.5-1	2.8	0.25-0.5 g	8h	8h	8h	8h	0.25-0.5 g	
0.5-2.1	12.3-18	0.5-2 g	4-8h	6h	8h	0.5-1 g q12h	0.5-1 g	
1.2		1-2 g	6-12h	12h	16-24h	48h	1-2 g	
3.5-5.8	50-60	0.5-2 g	24h	8-25 mg/kg q24h	4-15 mg/kg q24-48h	3-15 mg/kg q3-5 d	None	
2.8-4.6	12-30	1-2 g	12h	12h	24h	48h	25% on non dialysis days, 50% on dialysis days	
0.7-1.1	13-22	1-2 g	6-8h	8-12h	12-24h	0.5-1 g q12-48h	1-2 g	
0.9-1.5	5.9	0.25-0.5 g	12-24h	12-24h	50% q12-24h	50% q12-24h		
1-2	20	0.125-0.5 g PO; 0.75-1.5 g IV	12h; 8h	12h; 8h	12h; 8-12h	0.25 g q24h; 0.75 g q24h	0.75 g	15 mg/kg after dialysis
1.1-4.4		0.3-0.6 g	12-24h					
2.4-4	11.5	0.4 g	24h	24h	0.3 g q24h	48h	None	
1.6-2.6	2-2.5	1-2 g	6-12h	6-12h	6-12h	6-12h	Dose after dialysis	
0.9-1.7		0.5-2 g	8-12h	8-12	12-24h	24h	0.5-2 g	
1.9-3.2	9.8	0.1-0.4 g	12h	12h	24h[n]	24h	Usual dose 3 × wk	
1.4-2	11.9-35	1-2 g	8-12h	8-12h	12-24h	0.5 g q24-48h	1 g load then 1 g after dialysis	0.5 g q24h or 250 mg/2L of dialysate
1.5-2.9	18-29	0.2-0.4 g	12-24h	12-24h	24h	0.1 g q24h	0.4 g	0.2 g q24h
1.4-1.8	25-35	1-3 g	6-8h	0.5-1.5 g q8h	0.25-1 g q12h	0.5 g q12h	Dose after dialysis	3 g q48h
5.4-10.9	12.2-18.2	0.5-2 g	12-24h	12-24h	12-24h	12-24h	None	
2	20	0.5-4 g	8-12h	3 g q8h	2-3 g q12h	1 g q12-24h	1-2 g	0.5 g q18-24h
2	13.5	0.5-2g	8-12h	12-24h	24h	0.25-0.5 g q24h	0.25 g	1-2 g q48h

m No more than 400 mg/d for otitis or 100 mg/d for pharyngitis/tonsillitis.
n Cl_{Cr} <30 ml/min.
o Arginine component not approved for children <12 yr.
p 30-50 mg/kg q12h for <2 kg; 30 mg/kg q8h for >2 kg.
q 2 g q24h at steady state.
r 50 mg/kg/d for <2 kg; 50-75 mg/kg/d for >2 kg.

s Bleeding time should be monitored in patients receiving more than 4 g/d for more than 3 d. Prophylactic vitamin K, 10 mg/wk, should be given to patients receiving moxalactam.
t For meningitis due to gram-negative organisms in children, the manufacturer recommends an initial loading dose of 100 mg/kg.
Abbreviations: Cl_{Cr}, Creatinine clearance; CSF, cerebrospinal fluid; HD, hemodialysis; PD, peritoneal dialysis.

APPENDIX 7

Antibiotic Pharmacokinetics and Dosing—cont'd

Pharmacology: Additional β-Lactams

Drug (% oral absorption)	Dose (g)	DRUG CONCENTRATIONS ACHIEVED WITH SPECIFIC DOSES MEASURED LEVELS (µg/ml) Serum (peak)	DOSAGE RECOMMENDATIONS ADULTS Oral	Parenteral	CHILDREN Oral	Parenteral
Aztreonam	1 IV[c] 2 IV[c]	90–164 204–255		1–2 g q6h		30–50 mg/kg q6–12h (not approved)
Imipenem	0.25 IV[c] 0.5 IV[c] 1 IV[c]	14–24 21–58 41–83		0.5–1 g q6h		15–25 mg/kg q6h (not approved)
Meropenem	0.5 IV[c] 1.0 IV[c]	26 55–62		0.5–2 g q8–12h		20–40 mg/kg q8h
Loracarbef* (90)	0.2 PO cap 0.4 PO cap 0.4 PO	8 14 17	0.2–4 g q12–24h			15–30 mg/kg/d q12h

*Decreased rate and/or extent of absorption when given with food.
[a] Specified dose is supplemental to that in hemodialysis.
[b] Inflamed meninges.
[c] IV infusion over 15–30 min.
[d] 2.7h during dialysis/7–9h between dialysis sessions.
Abbreviations: Cl_{Cr}, Creatinine clearance; *CSF*, cerebrospinal fluid; *HD*, hemodialysis; *PD*, peritoneal dialysis.

Pharmacology: Aminoglycosides

Drug (% oral absorption)	Dose (g)	DRUG CONCENTRATIONS ACHIEVED WITH SPECIFIC DOSES MEASURED LEVELS (µg/ml) Serum (peak)	DOSAGE RECOMMENDATIONS ADULTS Oral	Parenteral	CHILDREN Oral	Parenteral
Amikacin[c]	0.5 IM 7.5 mg/kg IV[d]	38 17–25		15 mg/kg/d q8–12h[c]		15 mg/kg/d q8–12h[c]
Gentamicin[g]	1 mg/kg IM 1 mg/kg IV[h]	4–7.6 4–7.6		3–5 mg/kg/d q8 h[c]		3–7.5 mg/kg/d q8 h[c]
Netilmicin[i]	2 mg/kg IV[d] 2 mg/kg IM	16.6 7		4–6.5 mg/kg/d q8–12 h[e]		3–7.5 mg/kg/d q8–12 h[e]
Tobramycin[g]	1 mg/kg IM 1 mg/kg IV[d]	4–6 4–6		3–5 mg/kg/d q8h[c] 3–5 mg/kg/d q8h[c]		3–6 mg/kg/d q8h[c]

[a] Specified dose is supplemental to that in hemodialysis.
[b] Inflamed meninges.
[c] Desired concentrations: peak 15–30 µg/ml; trough <5–10 µg/ml.
[d] Infused over 30–60 min.
[e] The dosing strategy for aminoglycosides involves the use of ideal (lean) body weight (IBW) for dosage calculation. In obese patients, this approach would result in serum aminoglycoside concentrations less than expected. Alternative dosing recommendations have been proposed that account for the change in drug distribution volume with obesity:
1. Lean body weight + 40% of excess weight, defined as total body weight (TBW) minus IBW (J Infect Dis. 1978:138:499-505).
2. IBW + 58% of excess weight (TBW - IBW) (Clin Pharmacol Ther. 1979;26:508).
3. IBW + 38% of excess weight (TBW - IBW) (Am J Hosp Pharm. 1980;37:519-522).

SERUM HALF-LIFE (h)		STANDARD DOSE WITH DOSING INTERVALS IN RENAL IMPAIRMENT					DOSAGE WITH DIALYSIS	
WITH NORMAL AND ANURIC Cl_{Cr} VALUES (ml/min)		Usual Adult Dose	FOR Cl_{Cr} RANGES (ml/min)				After HD[a]	During PD (daily dose)
>80	<10		>80	80-50	50-10	<10 (anuric)		
1.3-2.2	6-9	1-2 g	6h	8-12h	12-18h	24h	1/8 initial dose	Usual initial dose, then 1/4 usual dose at usual intervals
0.8-1	3.5	0.5-1 g	6h	0.5 g q6-8h	0.5 g q8-12h	0.25-0.5 g q12h	0.25-0.5 g after, then q12h	
0.8-1	6-20	0.5-2 g	8-14 h	8-12 h	0.5-1 g q12 h	0.5 g q24 h	0.5 g	
1	32	0.2-0.4 g	12-24h	12-24h	24-48h	3-5 d	0.2-0.4 g	

SERUM HALF-LIFE (h)		STANDARD DOSE WITH DOSING INTERVALS IN RENAL IMPAIRMENT					DOSAGE WITH DIALYSIS	
WITH NORMAL AND ANURIC Cl_{Cr} VALUES (ml/min)		Usual Adult Dose	FOR Cl_{Cr} RANGES (ml/min)				After HD[a]	During PD (daily dose)
>80	<10		>80	80-50	50-10	<10 (anuric)		
2-3	30-86	5-7.5 mg/kg	8h	8-12h	12-48h	≥48h[f]	2.5-3.75 mg/kg	2.5 mg/kg/d
2-3	24-60	1-1.7 mg/kg	8 h	8-12 h	12-48 h	≥48 h[f]	1.0-1.7 mg/kg	1 mg/2 L of dialysate removed
2-2.5	30	2-2.2 mg/kg	8 h	8-12 h	12-48 h	≥48 h[f]	2 mg/kg	
2-3	5-70	1-1.7 mg/kg	8h	8-12h	12-48h	≥48h	1 mg/kg	1 mg/2 L of dialysate removed

[f] Dosing at Cl_{Cr} ≤10 ml/minute should be assisted with serum concentrations.
[g] Desired concentrations: peal 4-10 μg/ml; trough <2 μ/ml.
[h] Infused over 2 h.
[i] q24h for infants <16 days old; q12h for those ≥16 days old.
[j] 15 mg/kg/d q12h for ≤ 2 kg; 20 mg/kg/d q12h for >2 kg.
[k] Parenteral administration of neomycin is no longer recommended.
[l] Desired concentrations: peak 6-12 μg/ml; trough <2 μg/ml.
[m] For premature or full-term infants <6 weeks of age.
[n] Desired concentrations: peak 5-25 μg/ml; trough <5 μg/ml.
Abbreviations: Cl_{Cr}, Creatinine clearance; CSF, cerebrospinal fluid; HD, hemodialysis; PD, peritoneal dialysis.

APPENDIX 7

Antibiotic Pharmacokinetics and Dosing—cont'd

Pharmacology: Tetracyclines[a]

	DRUG CONCENTRATIONS ACHIEVED WITH SPECIFIC DOSES		DOSAGE RECOMMENDATIONS			
		MEASURED LEVELS (μg/ml)	ADULTS		CHILDREN	
Drug (% oral absorption)	**Dose (g)**	**Serum (peak)**	**Oral**	**Parenteral**	**Oral**	**Parenteral**
Chlortetracycline[d] (30)	0.25 PO 0.5 PO	1.5-2.5 7	As for tetracyline		As for tetracyline	
Doxycycline (90-100)	0.1 PO 0.1 IV[f]	1.5-2.1 2.5	0.1 g q12h	0.1 g q12h	2.2 mg/kg q12-24h	2.2 mg/kg q12-24h
Minocycline (90-100)	0.2 PO	2-3.5	0.1 g q12h	0.1 g q12h	2 mg/kg q12h	2 mg/kg q12h
Oxytetracycline[d] (60)	0.25 PO 0.5 PO	1.3-1.4 4-4.2	1-2 g/d q6h	0.25 g IM q24h	25-50 mg/kg/d q6h	15-25 mg/kg/d q8-12h[g]
Tetracycline[d] (75-80)	0.25 PO 0.5 PO 0.5 PO[h]	1.5-2.2 3-4.3 2-5	0.25-0.5 g q6h		25-50 mg/kg/d q6-12h	

[a] The tetracyclines cause a brown discoloration of the teeth and may retard the growth of bone in the human fetus and children. The American Academy of Pediatrics recommends that tetracyclines be used children who are 9 years of age or older.
[b] Specified dose is supplemental in hemodialysis.
[c] Inflamed meninges.
[d] All tetracyclines should be given 1 hour before or 2 hours after meals.
[e] Patients in the convalescent stage of poliomyelitis.
[f] Infused over 60 minutes.
[g] No more than 250 mg/d.
[h] At steady-state.

SERUM HALF-LIFE (h) WITH NORMAL AND ANURIC Cl_{Cr} VALUES (ml/min)			STANDARD DOSE WITH DOSING INTERVALS IN RENAL IMPAIRMENT				DOSAGE WITH DIALYSIS	
		Usual Adult Dose	FOR Cl_{Cr} RANGES (ml/min)				After HD[a]	During PD (daily dose)
>80	<10		>80	80-50	50-10	<10 (anuric)		
5.6	6.8-11	0.25-0.5 g	6h		Not recommended			
14-24	18-30	0.1 g	12h	12h	12h	12h	0.1 g q12h	0.1 g q12h
11-26	12-30	0.1 g	12h	12h	12h	12h	0.1 g q12h	0.1 g q12h
6-10	47-66	0.25-0.5 g PO 0.25 g IM	6 h 24 h	6h 24h	Use doxycycline			
6-12	57-120	0.25-0.5 g	6h	6h	Use doxycycline			

APPENDIX **7**

Antibiotic Pharmacokinetics and Dosing—cont'd

Pharmacology: Azalides, Macrolides, Lincosamides, Chloramphenicol, and Metronidazole

Drug (% oral absorption)	DRUG CONCENTRATIONS ACHIEVED WITH SPECIFIC DOSES		DOSAGE RECOMMENDATIONS			
		MEASURED LEVELS (μg/ml)	ADULTS		CHILDREN	
	Dose (g)	Serum (peak)	Oral	Parenteral	Oral	Parenteral
Azithromycin[a] (35-40)	0.5 PO 0.5 IV	0.09-0.44 3.63	0.5 g q24h × 3 d	0.5 g q24h	5-12 mg/kg/d	10-12 mg/kg/d[d]
Clarithromycin (50-55)	0.25 PO[e] 0.5 PO[e] 0.5 PO[e]	1 2-3 1[f]	0.25-0.5 g q12h		7.5 mg/kg q12h (not approved)	
Dirithromycin[g] (6-14)	0.5 PO	0.3-0.4	0.5 g q24h		0.5 g q24h	
Erythromycin base[i,j]	0.25 PO	0.1-2	0.25-0.5 g q6h		30-50 mg/kg/d q6h	
Erythromycin stearate[j]	0.25 PO	0.1-2	0.25-0.5g q6h		30-50 mg/kg/d q6h	
Erythromycin ethyl succinate[j]	0.4 PO	0.1-2	0.4 g q6h		30-50 mg/kg/d q6h	
Erythromycin lactobionate[k,j]	0.2 IV	3-4		0.5-1 g q6h		15-20 mg/kg/d q6h
Erythromycin gluceptate[k]	0.2 IV	3-4		15-20 mg/kg/d q6h		15-20 mg/kg/d q6h
Erythromycin estolate[j]	0.25 PO	0.1-2[m]	0.25-0.5g q6h		30-50 mg/kg/d q6h	
Roxithromycin	0.15 PO 0.3 PO	6 10	0.15-0.3 g q12-24h		5-7.5 mg/kg/d q12h	
Clindamycin[i] (90)	0.15 PO 0.6 IV[h]	1.9-3.9 10	0.15-0.3 g q6h	0.3-0.9 g q6-8h	8-25 mg/kg/d q6-8h	15-40 mg/kg/d q6-8h
Chloramphenicol[a] (75-90)	1 PO 1 PO[e] 1 IV	11 18 4.9-12	0.25-0.75 g q6h	0.25-1 g q6h	50-100 mg/kg/d q6h	50-100 mg/kg/d q6h
Metronidazole[i] (80)	0.25 PO 7.5 mg/kg[u]	4.6-6.5 26	0.25-7.5 g q8h	0.5 g q6h		

[a] Specified dose is supplemental to that in hemodialysis.
[b] Inflamed meninges.
[c] Decreased extent of absorption of capsule formulation only when given with food.
[d] No studies to support; extrapolated from adult conversion.
[e] At steady state.
[f] Of 14-hydroxyclarithromycin (active metabolite).
[g] Must be given with food.
[h] Not approved for children <12 years of age.
[i] Denotes decreased rate and/or extent of absorption when given with food.
[j] Erythromycin and its derivatives have varying degrees of bioavailability (18 to 45%).
[k] Oral erythromycin therapy should replace IV therapy as soon as possible.

SERUM HALF-LIFE (h)		STANDARD DOSE WITH DOSING INTERVALS IN RENAL IMPAIRMENT					DOSAGE WITH DIALYSIS	
WITH NORMAL AND ANURIC Cl_{Cr} VALUES (ml/min)		Usual Adult Dose	FOR Cl_{Cr} RANGES (ml/min)				After HD[a]	During PD (daily dose)
>80	<10		>80	80-50	50-10	<10 (anuric)		
68	68	0.5 g	24h	24h	24h	24h	24h	24h
5-7		0.25-0.5 g	12h	12h	12-24h	24h		
20-50	20-50	0.5 g	24h	24h	24h	24h	Usual regimen	Usual regimen
1.5-2	6	0.25-0.5 g	6h	6h	6h	6h	Usual regimen	Usual regimen
1.5-2	6	0.25-0.5 g	6h	6h	6h	6h	Usual regimen	Usual regimen
1.5-2	6	0.4 g	6h	6h	6h	6h	Usual regimen	Usual regimen
1.5-2	6	0.5-1 g	6h	6h	6h	6h	Usual regimen	Usual regimen
1.5-2	6	15-20 mg/kg/d	6h	6h	6h	6h	Usual regimen	Usual regimen
1.5-2	6	0.25-0.5 g	6h	6h	6h	6h	Usual regimen	Usual regimen
12	≈12	0.15-0.3 g	12-24h	12-24h	12-24h	24-48h		
2-3	2-3.5	0.15-3 g PO 0.3-0.9 g IV	6h 6-8h	6h 6-8h	6h 6-8h	6h 6-8h	Usual regimen	Usual regimen
1.5-4.1	3.7	0.25-0.75 g PO 0.25 g IV	6h 6h	6h 6h	6h 6h	6h 6h	Schedule dose post HD	Usual regimen
6-14	8-15	0.25-0.75 g PO 0.5 g IV	8h 6h	8h 6h	8h 6h	8h 6h	Usual regimen	Usual regimen

[l] Owing to the local irritative effects, the drug must not be administered rapidly by direct IV injection (IV push).
[m] Higher serum concentrations have been reported in patients taking erythromycin estolate versus other derivatives.
[n] Over 20 min.
[o] When IV clindamycin is given to neonates and infants, organ system functions should be monitored.
[p] When given over 2 h.
[q] Chloramphenicol dosage should be administered to maintain serum concentrations of 10-25 mg/L for peak and 5-10 mg/L for trough.
[r] <2 wk.
[s] >2 wk.
Abbreviations: Cl_{Cr}, Creatinine clearance; *CSF*, cerebrospinal fluid; *HD*, hemodialysis; *PD*, peritoneal dialysis.

APPENDIX 7

Antibiotic Pharmacokinetics and Dosing—cont'd

Pharmacology: Miscellaneous Gram-Positive Agents/Fusidic Acid

| Drug (% oral absorption) | DRUG CONCENTRATIONS ACHIEVED WITH SPECIFIC DOSES | | DOSAGE RECOMMENDATIONS | | | |
| | | MEASURED LEVELS (µg/ml) | ADULTS | | CHILDREN | |
	Dose (g)	Serum (peak)	Oral	Parenteral	Oral	Parenteral
Vancomycin (minimal)	1 g IV	25	0.5-2 g/d q6-8h	1 g q12h	40 mg/kg/d q6-8h[g]	40 mg/kg/d q6-12h
Teicoplanin	3 mg/kg IV[h] 6 mg/kg IV[h]	53 112		0.2-0.4 g q24 h		10 mg/kg q24 h
Fusidic acid	0.5 g PO	14-38[i]	0.5-1 g q8h	0.58 g q8h[j]	6.6-16.6 mg/kg q8h	6.6 mg/kg q8h
Quinupristin-dalfopristin	7 mg/kg IV	5		7.5 mg/kg q8-12 h		7.5 mg/kg q8 h
SCH 27899 (Ziracin)	6 mg/kg IV	49-55		1-12 mg/kg/d[k]		
Linezolid			0.375-0.625 g q12h[k]			

[a] Specified dose is supplemental to that in hemodialysis.
[b] Inflamed meninges.
[c] Colistimethate is the sulfamethyl derivative of colistin; colistin is absorbed to some extent in infants.
[d] Of colistin.
[e] Bioavailability can be up to 10% in infants.
[f] For Cl_{Cr} of 5-20 ml/min, dose should be 7500-12,500 U/kg/d q12h.
[g] Not to exceed 2 g/d.
[h] 5-min infusion.
[i] Accumulation occurs with multiple doses of 0.5 g given q8h; a mean serum concentration of 71 µg/ml has been reported after 96 h of therapy.
[j] Diethanolamine fusidate, 580 mg, is equivalent to 500 mg sodium fusidate.
[k] Based on early phase I studies.
Abbreviations: *Cl_{Cr}* Creatinine clearance; *CSF*, cerebrospinal fluid; *HD*, hemodialysis; *PD*, peritoneal dialysis.

Pharmacology: Sulfonamides and Trimethoprim

| Drug (% oral absorption) | DRUG CONCENTRATIONS ACHIEVED WITH SPECIFIC DOSES | | DOSAGE RECOMMENDATIONS | | | |
| | | MEASURED LEVELS (µg/ml) | ADULTS | | CHILDREN | |
	Dose (g)	Serum (peak)	Oral	Parenteral	Oral	Parenteral
Trimethoprim-sulfamethoxazole* (85)	0.16/0.8 PO 0.16/0.8 IV	1-2/40-60[c] 9/105[c]	0.16/0.8 g q12-24h	3-5 mg/kg q6-8h[d]	6-12 mg/kg/d q6-12h[d]	6-12 mg/kg/d q6-12h[d]

* Decreased rate and/or extent of absorption when given with food.
[a] Specified dose is supplemental to that in hemodialysis.
[b] Inflamed meninges.
[c] At steady state.
[d] Based on the trimethoprim component.
[e] Uninflamed meninges.
[f] Amniotic fluid concentrations (µg/ml).
[g] Not approved for children <12 years of age.
[h] For malaria prophylaxis. The first dose should be given 1-2 d before departure to an endemic area and the course continued throughout the stay and 4-6 wk thereafter.

SERUM HALF-LIFE (h)		STANDARD DOSE WITH DOSING INTERVALS IN RENAL IMPAIRMENT					DOSAGE WITH DIALYSIS	
WITH NORMAL AND ANURIC Cl_{Cr} VALUES (ml/min)		Usual Adult Dose	FOR Cl_{Cr} RANGES (ml/min)				After HD[a]	During PD (daily dose)
>80	<10		>80	80-50	50-10	<10 (anuric)		
4-6	44.1-406.4	15 mg/kg	12h	See nomogram in Chapter 28			1 g/wk	0.5-1 g/wk
40-70	125	0.4 g 0.5-1 g PO	24h 8h	48h 8h	48 h 8 h	72 h 8 h		
1.3-1.5								10-20 mg/kg/d q12h
8.6		1-12 mg/kg[k]	24h	24h				
5.5		0.375-0.625 g[k]	12h	12h				

SERUM HALF-LIFE (h)		STANDARD DOSE WITH DOSING INTERVALS IN RENAL IMPAIRMENT					DOSAGE WITH DIALYSIS	
WITH NORMAL AND ANURIC Cl_{Cr} VALUES (ml/min)		Usual Adult Dose	FOR Cl_{Cr} RANGES (ml/min)				After HD[a]	During PD (daily dose)
>80	<10		>80	80-50	50-10	<10 (anuric)		
8-15/7-12	24/22-50	3-5 mg/kg IV[d]	6-12h	18h	24h	Avoid	4-5mg/kg[d]	0.16/0.8 g q48h

[i] One tablet = 500 mg sulfadoxine and 25 mg pyrimethamine.
[j] Under 4 years: ¼ tablet weekly or ½ tablet every other week; 4-8 years: ½ tablet weekly or 1 tablet every other week; 9-14 years; ¾ tablet weekly or 1½ tablets every other week.
[k] Sulfasalazine/sulfapyridine.
[l] Although doses up to 12 g have been administered, a daily dosage exceeding 4 g is associated with an increased incidence of adverse effects.
[m] Sulfapyridine.

Abbreviations: Cl_{Cr}, Creatinine clearance; *CSF*, cerebrospinal fluid; *HD*, hemodialysis; *PD*, peritoneal dialysis.

APPENDIX 7

Antibiotic Pharmacokinetics and Dosing—cont'd

Pharmacology: Quinolones

| Drug (% oral absorption) | DRUG CONCENTRATIONS ACHIEVED WITH SPECIFIC DOSES | | DOSAGE RECOMMENDATIONS | | | |
| | | | ADULTS | | CHILDREN | |
	Dose (g)	MEASURED LEVELS (μg/ml) Serum (peak)	Oral	Parenteral	Oral	Parenteral
Quinolones						
Ciprofloxacin* (50-85)	0.5 PO 0.75 PO 0.4 IV[f]	1.6-2.9 2.5-4.3 4.6	0.25-0.75 g q12h	0.2-0.4 g q8-12h	25 mg/kg/d q12h	3.2-12.5 mg/kg/d q12h
Gatifloxacin	0.4 PO 0.6 PO	4.2 5.7	0.4-0.6 g q24h			
Levofloxacin (99)	0.5 PO 0.5 IV[f]	5.7 6.2	0.25-0.5 g q24h	0.25-0.5 g q24h		
Ofloxacin* (85-100)	0.4 PO 0.2 PO 0.4 IV[f]	2.9-5.6 1.5-2.7 4	0.2-0.4 g q12h	0.2-0.4 g q12h		
Pefloxacin (98)	0.4 PO 0.4 IV[f]	3.8-5.6 5.8	0.4 q12-24h			
Trovafloxacin (88-90)	0.2 PO 0.3 PO 0.3 IV[f]	2.3 2.9 3.6	0.1-0.2 g q24h	0.2-0.3 g q24h	3 mg/kg q24h	3 mg/kg q24h

* Decreased rate and/or extent of absorption when given with food.
[a] Specified dose is supplemental to that in bemodialysis.
[b] Inflamed meninges.
[c] Use primarily for the treatment of urinary tract infections.
[d] Use during pregnancy not recommended.
[e] Animal pharmacology studies indicate the presence of drug in the milk of lactating rats receiving oral doses of cinoxacin. Human data are not currently available.
[f] Infused over 60 min.
[g] 3.2h during dialysis/5.8h in between sessions.
[h] Case report.
[i] For Cl_{Cr} of <30 ml/min; for >30 ml/min, use normal dose.

SERUM HALF-LIFE (h) WITH NORMAL AND ANURIC Cl$_{Cr}$ VALUES (ml/min)		Usual Adult Dose	STANDARD DOSE WITH DOSING INTERVALS IN RENAL IMPAIRMENT FOR Cl$_{Cr}$ RANGES (ml/min)				DOSAGE WITH DIALYSIS	During PD (daily dose)
>80	<10		>80	80-50	50-10	<10 (anuric)	After HD[a]	
3-5	5-10	0.25-0.75 g PO 0.2-0.4 g IV	12h 8-12h	12h 8-12h	0.25-0.5 q12h 12-24	0.25-0.5 q18h 0.2-0.4 q18-24h	0.25-0.5 g q24h	0.25-0.5 g q24h
7								
6-8		0.25-0.5 g	24h	24h	24-48h	48h	0.25 q48h	0.25 g q48h
4-8	16.9-28.4	0.2-0.4 g PO/IV	12h	12h	24h	0.1-0.2 g q24h	0.2 g load, then 0.1 g q24h	
8-12	11-15							
9-13	9-13	0.1-0.3 g	24h	24h	24h	24h		

[j] 12-24 h after dose.

[k] Ineffective urinary concentrations expected with compromised renal function.

[l] 8-12 h during dialysis/13-48 h in between sessions.

[m] Usually coadministered with an acidifying agent to convert the methenamine salts in urine to ammonia and bactericidal formaldehyde (pH ≤5.5). Mandelic acid and hippuric acid are mildly antiseptic and contribute to urine acidification.

[n] Methenamine penetrates a number of body fluids, including bile and CSF. This penetration proves clinically inconsequential because negligible amounts of formaldehyde are generated at physiologic pH.

[o] Nitrofurantoin accumulates in the serum of patients with a Cl$_{Cr}$ of <60 ml/min, which leads to systemic toxicity.

[p] Although only small amounts of nitrofurantion have been detected in breast milk, the drug could cause hemolytic anemia in a G-6-PD-deficient infant exposed in this manner.

Abbreviations: *Cl$_{Cr}$*, Creatinine clearance; *CSF*, cerebrospinal fluid; *HD*, hemodialysis; *PD*, peritoneal dialysis.

Antibiotic Pharmacokinetics and Dosing—cont'd

Pharmacology: Antimycobacterial Agents

| Drug (% oral absorption) | DRUG CONCENTRATIONS ACHIEVED WITH SPECIFIC DOSES | | DOSAGE RECOMMENDATIONS | | | |
| | | MEASURED LEVELS (μg/ml) | ADULTS | | CHILDREN | |
	Dose (g)	Serum (peak)	Oral	Parenteral	Oral	Parenteral
Ethambutol (75-80)	25 mg/kg PO	2-5	15 mg/kg q24h		10-15 mg/kg q24h (not recommended)	
Isoniazid†ʲ	7 mg/kg PO	4.5/lᵏ	0.3 g q24h	0.3 g IM q24h	10-20 mg/kg/d q12-24h	10-20 mg/kg/d q12-24h
Pyrazinamide	0.5 PO	9-12	15-30 mg/kg q24h		30 mg/kg/d q12-24h (not approved)	
Rifampin (100)	0.6 PO 0.6 IVᵐ	7 17.5	0.6 g q24h	0.6 g q24h	10-20 mg/kg/d q12-24h	

* Should be taken with food.
† Decreased rate and/or extent of absorption when given with food.
ᵃ Specified dose is supplemental to that in hemodialysis.
ᵇ Inflamed meninges.
ᶜ Pharmacokinetics similar to those of streptomycin.
ᵈ Administer for 60-120 d followed by 1 g q2-3 ×/wk.
ᵉ In leprosy patients.
ᶠ At steady state.
ᵍ g-d serum half-life/70-d tissue half/life.
ʰ Dosage should be adjusted to maintain plasma concentrations <30 μg/ml.

SERUM HALF-LIFE (h)		STANDARD DOSE WITH DOSING INTERVALS IN RENAL IMPAIRMENT					DOSAGE WITH DIALYSIS	
WITH NORMAL AND ANURIC Cl_{Cr} VALUES (ml/min)		Usual Adult Dose	FOR Cl_{Cr} RANGES (ml/min)				After HD[a]	During PD (daily dose)
>80	<10		>80	80-50	50-10	<10 (anuric)		
3.3	≥7	15-25 mg/kg	24h	15 mg/kg q24h	15 mg/kg q24-36h	15 mg/kg q48h	15 mg/kg/d	15 mg/kg/d
0.5-4	2-10	0.3 g PO/IM	24h	24h	24h	½ dose in slow acetylators	5 mg/kg	Daily dose after dialysis
10-16		15-30 mg/kg	24h	24h	24h	12-20 mg/kg q24h		
2-5	2-5	0.6 g	24h	24h	24h	24h		

[i] Limited evidence suggests that 20 mg/kg daily given as a single dose in children is more likely to produce CSF concentrations exceeding the MIC of 2.5 µg/ml for *Mycobacterium tuberculosis*.

[j] To minimize the risk of polyneuritis from isoniazid-induced pyridoxine deficiency, pyridoxine (15-50 mg) is often given concurrently.

[k] 4.5 µg/ml in slow inactivators/1.0 µg/ml in rapid inactivators.

[l] Should not exceed the adult dose.

[m] Infused over 30 min.

[n] Desirable serum concentrations; peak 5-25 µg/ml; trough <5 µg/ml.

Abbreviations: Cl_{Cr}, Creatinine clearance; *CSF*, cerebrospinal fluid; *HD*, hemodialysis; *MIC*, minimal inhibitory concentration; *PD*, peritoneal dialysis.

APPENDIX 7

Antibiotic Pharmacokinetics and Dosing—cont'd

Pharmacology: Antifungal Agents

| Drug (% oral absorption) | DRUG CONCENTRATIONS ACHIEVED WITH SPECIFIC DOSES | | DOSAGE RECOMMENDATIONS | | | |
| | | | ADULTS | | CHILDREN | |
	Dose (g)	MEASURED LEVELS (μg/ml) Serum (peak)	Oral	Parenteral	Oral	Parenteral
Amphotericin B (poor)	0.03 IV[c] 0.05 IV[c]	1 2		0.25–1 mg/kg q24h[d, e]		0.25–1 mg/kg q24–48h[d]
Fluconazole (≥90)	0.4 PO 0.1 IV[g]	6.72 3.86–4.96	0.05–0.4 g q24h	0.05–0.4 g q24h		
Griseofulvin (50/>50)[i]	0.5/0.25 PO[i]	0.4-2/0.4-2	0.5-1 g q24h/ 0.33-0.66 g q24h		15 mg/kg/d q24h	
Itraconazole (99.8)[j, k]	0.2 PO[i]	2.3/3.5[m]	0.2–0.4 g q24h			
Ketoconazole[h]	0.2 PO	4.2	0.2-0.4 g q12-24h		5-10 mg/kg/d q12-24h	
Miconazole (50)	0.522 IV[o]	6		0.4–1.2 q8h		20–40 mg/kg/d q8h
Nystatin (minimal)	All doses	Not detectable	0.4-1 mU q8h		0.4-0.6 mU q6h	
Terbinafine (80)			0.125–0.5 g q12–24h			

* Decreased rate and/or extent of absorption when given with food.

[c] Infused over several hours

[d] A test dose of 1 mg infused over 15 minutes is often given to assess febrile reactions prior to proceeding to higher doses

[e] Should be administered by slow infusion; rapid IV infusion should be avoided since potentially serious adverse effects (e.g., hypotension, hypokalemia, arrhythmias, shock) may occur

[f] Or 1.5 mg/kg every other day

[g] Infused over 30 minutes; ascertained on day 6-7

[h] Peak concentration should be above 25 μg/ml to avoid development of resistance but should not exceed 100-120 μg/ml to avoid side effects

From Mandell GE, Bennett JE, Dolin R, editors: *Principles and practice of infectious diseases,* ed 5, Philadelphia, 2000, Churchill Livingstone.

SERUM HALF-LIFE (h)		STANDARD DOSE WITH DOSING INTERVALS IN RENAL IMPAIRMENT					DOSAGE WITH DIALYSIS	
WITH NORMAL AND ANURIC Cl_{cr} VALUES (ml/min)		Usual Adult Dose	FOR Cl_{cr} RANGES (ml/min)				After HD[a]	During PD (daily dose)
>80	<10		>80	80-50	50-10	<10 (anuric)		
24 or more	24 or more	0.25-1 mg/kg	24h	24h	24h	24h	Usual regimen	Usual regimen
20-50	48	0.05-0.4 g	24h	24h	50% of dose	25% of dose		
24	24	0.5-1 g/ 0.33-0.66 g	24h/24h	24h/24h	24h/24h	24h/24h		
21-60[n]		0.2-0.4 g	24h	24h				
8	8	0.2-0.4 g	12-24h	12-24h	12-24h	12-24h	Usual regimen	Usual regimen
0.4-24.1[p]	0.4-24.1[p]	0.4-1.2 g	8h	8h	8h	8h		<3-48
		0.4-1 mU	8h	8h	8h	8h		
22-30		0.125-0.25 g	12-24h	12-24h				

[i] Microsize/ultramicrosize
[j] When given with meals
[k] Gastric acid suppressing agents decrease bioavailability to <5%
[l] Taken 2 × day for 15 days
[m] Parent drug/active metabolite (hydroxyitraconazole)
[n] Half-life extends as dosing continues
[o] Infused over 15 minutes
[p] Triphasic elimination: alpha = 0.4h; beta = 2.1h; gamma = 24.1h

INDEX

Page numbers followed by *f* indicate figures; *t*, tables; *b*, boxes.

A

Abscess
  bacteremia due to, 24
  in bite wound, 92
  bone scan differentiation of, 63
  C. minutissimum in, 287
  C. perfringens in, 286
  in cellulitis, 31
  CT scan to locate, 65
  culture specimen from, 23–24
  in dorsal space infections, 124
  endocarditis prophylaxis for, 144
  in injection site, 38–39
  in osteomyelitis, 61
  in plantar space infections, 123
Absolute neutrophil count (ANC), 15
Acetic acid for wound care, 83
Acid-fast smears, diagnostic
  in hematogenous osteomyelitis, 72
  in lower extremity infections,
      22–23
  in osteomyelitis, 60
Acinetobacter, 296
  ciprofloxacin's susceptibility to, 265
  imipenem/cilastatin against, 247
  resistant to aztreonam, 248
  resistant to cephalosporins, 232
Acinetobacter baumanii
  aminoglycosides against, 249
  imipenem/cilastatin against, 246
  resistance of, 296
Acquired immune deficiency
      syndrome (AIDS), 195, 270
Actinomadura madurae
  Madura foot due to, 51
  tetracyclines against, 274
Acute hematogenous osteomyelitis.
      See Hematogenous
      osteomyelitis, acute.
Additive effect of drug
      combinations, 196
Aerobic gram-negative rods,
      296–301. *See also*
      Enterobacteriaceae.

Aerobic organisms
  aztreonam against, 248
  in bite wound infections, 92
  in diabetic foot infections, 111
  imipenem/cilastatin against, 246
  in moderate to severely infected
      ulcerations, 119–120
  piperacillin/tazobactam against,
      228
  in plantar space infections, 124
  tissue gas due to, 110
Aeromonas hydrophilia, 296–297
  in marine puncture wounds, 90,
      296
  myonecrosis due to, 45
  vs. *Vibrio*, 296
Age
  aminoglycoside toxicity and, 250
  antibiotic selection and,
      193–194
  immune status and, 195
  surgical site infections and,
      133–134
Agglutination in diagnosis of
      infection, 25
Agranulocytosis, 206
Air ventilation, 135
Albendazole, 52
Alcaligenes, 297
Alcohol usage
  and agents with MTT sidechain,
      208, 236
  and antibiotic selection, 195
  in diagnosis of lower extremity
      infections, 7
  and *klebsiella* infections, 293
Allergic reactions
  vs. anaphylactoid reaction, 208
  types of, 210–212
Allergies
  and antibiotic selection, 209
  in diagnosis of lower extremity
      infections, 7
Allylamine antifungals, 155, 157

Alternative therapy
  history of, for diagnosis, 6–7
  onychomycosis and, 167
  tinea pedis and, 155
  wound care and, 83
American College of Chest
    Physicians, 13–14
American Diabetes Association, 103
American Heart Association, 144
American Medical Association
    (AMA) Internet site, 311t
American Society for Microbiology
    Internet site, 311t
American Society of Anesthesiology,
    129
Americans with Disabilities Act
    (ADA), 7
Amikacin (Amikin), 249
  daily doses of, 252, 254
  for marine puncture wounds, 90, 91
  for mycobacteria infections, 302
  normal blood levels of, 253
Aminoglycosides, 249–255
  combinations of agents using, 255
  dosing of, 251–254
  mezlocillin and, 224
  monitoring serum levels of, 209
  nephrotoxicity from use of, 203, 250
  neuromuscular blockade from,
    201, 251
  open fracture infections and, 100
  ototoxicity from use of, 201,
    250–251
  penicillin with, 198, 253, 283
  risk factors for adverse reactions
    to, 250
  ticarcillin with, 223
  vancomycin and, 250
Aminoglycosides, drug activity of,
    249–250
  against *Acinetobacter*, 296
  against *Aeromonas*, 297
  against *Alcaligenes*, 297
  against *Citrobacter, Morganella,
    Serratia*, 291, 293, 295
  against *E. coli* and *Klebsiella*, 292,
    293
  against *Kingella kingae*, 289
  against *P. aeruginosa*, 299
  against *P. vulgaris* and *Providencia*,
    294

Aminopenicillins, 218–220
  list of agents in, 215b
  spectrum of activity by, 215
Amoebae, 255
Amorolfine (non-FDA approved), 167
Amoxicillin, 220
  for Lyme disease, 49, 50
  rash due to, 211
Amoxicillin/clavulanic acid
    (Augmentin), 226–227
  for bite wound infections, 93
  against *E. corrodens*, 298
  against enterococci, 284
  to fill "therapeutic holes", 197
  for mildly infected ulcerations, 118
  for puncture wound infections, 89
Ampicillin, 218–219
  aminoglycoside with, 218, 255
  amoxicillin vs., 220
  against *C. diversus*, 291
  against enterococci, 284
  H. influenza resistant to, 298
  interstitial nephritis due to, 203
  P. mirabilis resistant to, 294
  against *P. multocida*, 299
  penicillins vs., 217, 218
  piperacillin vs., 224
  platelet dysfunction due to, 207
  rash due to, 211
  seizures due to, 201
Ampicillin/sulbactam (Unasyn),
    227–228
  against *Acinetobacter*, 296
  for bite wound infections, 93
  against enterococci, 284
  for infected vascular gangrene, 46
  for moderate to severely infected
    ulcerations, 121
  for nonclostridial cellulitis, 41
  for puncture wound infections, 89
Amputation, limb
  for clostridial myonecrosis, 44
  incidence of, 103
  for Madura foot, 51
  in necrotizing infections, 40
  rate of infection after, 126–127
  for synergistic necrotizing
    cellulitis, 43
Anaerobic culture, 60
Anaerobic gram-negative rods,
    289–290

Anaerobic organisms
  in bite wound infections, 92
  culture and sensitivity for, 23–24
  in diabetic foot infections, 109,
      110, 111
  ecthyma due to, 39
  ertapenem for infections with,
      248
  gram staining and, 21
  hematogenous osteomyelitis due
      to, 72
  infected vascular gangrene due to,
      46
  in moderate to severely infected
      ulcerations, 120
  myonecrosis due to, 45
  necrotizing fasciitis due to, 42
  nonclostridial cellulitis due to, 41
  in plantar space infections, 124
  secondary osteomyelitis due to, 75
  synergistic necrotizing cellulitis
      due to, 43
  in trauma wound infections, 81t
Anaerobic organisms (drug activity in)
  agents against, 255–258, 290
  aminoglycosides ineffective
      against, 250
  amoxicillin/clavulanic acid
      against, 226
  ampicillin/sulbactam against, 228
  antianaerobic agents against,
      255–258
  cefazolin against, 233
  cefotaxime against, 240
  cefotetan against, 236
  cefoxitin against, 235, 236
  cefuroxime axetil against, 238
  clindamycin against, 256, 257
  ertapenem vs. imipenem against,
      247
  erythromycin against some, 271
  first-generation cephalosporins
      against, 231
  imipenem/cilastatin against, 246
  metronidazole against, 255–256
  penicillin G against, 217
  piperacillin/tazobactam against,
      228
  resistance of, to ciprofloxacin, 265
  second-generation cephalosporins
      against, 232

    tetracyclines against some, 274
    third-generation cephalosporins
        against, 232
    ticarcillin against, 222
    ticarcillin/clavulanic acid against,
        225, 226
    vancomycin against, 259
Anaerobic streptococcal
    myonecrosis, 45
Anaphylactoid reaction, 208
Anaphylaxis reaction, 210
    from cephalosporins, 233
    due to sulfonamide, 269
Ancef. *See* Cefazolin.
Ancylostoma brazilienses, 52
Anderson JT, 100
Anesthesia intubation, 144
Angiograms, 122
Angioplasty, 122
Animal bite wound infections. *See
    also specific animal.*
    P. multocida in, 299
    septic arthritis from, 76
    variables resulting in, 91–92
Animal feed, antibiotics in, 295
Antabuse reaction
    antibiotic therapy and, 7
    antibiotic usage and, 208
    due to cefoperazone, 242
    due to metronidazole, 256
Antacids, 265
Antagonism effect of drug
    combinations, 196, 198
Anthropophilic organisms, 148, 149
Antianaerobic agents, 255–258, 290
Antibiogram, 134, 184
Antibiotic agents, 213–275. *See also
    specific agent.*
    bactericidal vs. bacteriostatic, 188
    cost of, 192
    dosage and administration of,
        251–255
    generic and trade names of,
        305t–309t
    killing effects of, 192–193
    pharmacokinetics of, 191–192
    for prophylaxis, 141–143
    resistance of organisms to,
        190–191
    spectrum of activity by, 189–190
Antibiotic breakpoints, 186–187

Antibiotic combinations. *See also specific combination.*
  contraindications for, 198
  indications for, 196–197
Antibiotic prophylaxis, 135–145
  adverse effects and failures of, 145
  after bite wound infection, 93
  ciprofloxacin not indicated for, 267
  definition of, 136
  indications for, 137
  puncture wound trauma and, 86
  review of literature in, 135–136
  risk of endocarditis and, 143–145
  rules for use of, 136–137
  selection and administration of agents for, 140–141
  specific antibiotics for, 141–143
  surgical cases indicating, 138–140
  traumatic wounds indicating, 138
Antibiotic resistance, 190–191. *See also* Methicillin resistance; Penicillin resistance; *specific antibiotic; specific organism.*
  aminoglycosides and, 249–250, 255
  anti-gram-positive antibiotics and, 258
  carbapenems for, 245
  cephalosporins and, 229, 231
  ciprofloxacin and, 265, 266
  penicillins and, 213–214
  prevention of, 197
  quinolones and, 264
  surgical prophylaxis and, 134, 145
  susceptibility patterns and, 183–184
Antibiotic selection, 180–200
  agent combinations for, 196–198
  cost to determine, 192. *See also* Costs and cost analysis.
  drug activity to determine, 189–190
  drug of choice for, 180–181
  drug resistance to determine, 190–191
  "drugs for bugs" list for, 312t–313t
  host factors in, 193–196
  identity of organism for, 182–183
  killing effects of agent to determine, 192–193
  laboratory tests to determine, 184–189
  pharmacokinetics to determine dosage of, 191–192

  for prophylaxis, 140–141
  requirements for home IV, 198–200
  susceptibility of organism for, 183–184
Antibiotic serum/blood levels
  guidelines for determining, 253
  monitoring, 209, 254
Antibiotic therapy. *See also specific agent.*
  arterial ulcerations and, 122
  for bite wound infections, 93
  for burn wound infections, 97
  for carbuncles, 36
  for contiguous focus osteomyelitis, 74
  culture and sensitivity during, 23, 59
  definition of empiric, 181
  diagnosis of lower extremity infections and, 5–6, 15
  fever of unknown origin (FUO) and, 13
  folliculitis and, 36
  for hematogenous osteomyelitis, 72–73
  history of, 126
  home intravenous, 198–200
  impaired immune system and, 107
  ingress-egress drainage for, 70
  for moderate to severely infected ulcerations, 120–121
  noninfected mal perforans and, 114, 115, 117
  open fracture infections and, 97, 100
  for osteomyelitis, 66–67
  paronychia and, 33
  for plantar space infections, 124
  for post-puncture-wound osteomyelitis, 89
  for secondary osteomyelitis, 75
  for septic arthritis, 79
  stingray envenomation and, 91
  synergistic necrotizing cellulitis and, 43
  usual dosages for oral, 303t
  wound irrigation and, 82–83
Antibiotic therapy, non-prescribed
  in diagnosis of lower extremity infections, 5–6
  and injection site infections, 39

Antibiotic usage
    allergic reactions from, 209–212
    monitoring blood levels during,
        209, 253
    principles for selecting agents for,
        180–200
    side effects from, 203–209
    side effects from multiple, 198
    side effects from prophylactic, 145
    toxicities from, 200–203, 250–251
Antibiotic-associated diarrhea
    (AAD), 203–204, 205
Antibiotic-impregnated beads/fillers,
    69
Antibiotic-killing effects, 192
Antibiotics, topical
    for burn wound, 96
    against *C. minutissimum*, 287
    for folliculitis, 36
    gentamicin as, 251
    for impetigo, 37
    for mildly infected ulcerations, 119
    for noninfected mal perforans, 117
    for wound care, 98t
Antibody detection, 25
Antidiarrheal agents for CDAD, 205
Antifungal agents, oral
    for onychomycosis, 164
    for tinea pedis, 155
Antifungal agents, topical
    allylamines class of, 155, 157
    azoles class of, 157–158
    dosages for, 156t
    FDA approval of, 167
    forms of, 154–155
    hydroxypyridone class of, 158
    for onychomycosis, 164, 167–168
Antifungal therapy
    discussion of oral, 169–171
    for donor-leg cellulitis, 32
    and lateral subungual
        onychomycosis, 162
    monitoring, 171–172
    pros and cons of topical, 167–168
Anti-gram-positive antibiotics,
    258–263
    new developments in, 263
Antihistamines, 211, 259–260
Anti-inflammatory drugs (NSAIDs),
    11
Antipseudomonal penicillins, 215t

Antipyretic therapy and diagnosis of
    infection, 12
Antistreptolysin O titer (ASO), 16
Aplastic anemia, 206
Aqueous penicillin, 31, 216, 217
Arterial occlusive disease, 107
Arterial ulcerations, 121–122
Arteriosclerosis, 74
Arthralgias, 261
Arthritis. *See* Gouty arthritis;
        Migratory arthritis; Septic
        arthritis (SA).
Arthroscopic examination, 79
Asepsis, 21, 24
Aspergillus species, 160, 174
Aspirin, 11
Atelectasis, 12
Athlete's foot, 148
Atypical mycobacterium, 301
Augmentin. *See* Amoxicillin/
        clavulanic acid.
Autonomic neuropathy, 105
Avelox. *See* Moxifloxacin.
Azithromycin (Zithromax), 271–272
    against *B. henselae*, 297
    for bite wound infections, 94
    for cellulitis, 31
    vs. clarithromycin, 272, 273
    vs. dirithromycin, 273
    for erythrasma, 35
    for gonococcal infection, 288
    against *H. influenza*, 299
    for Lyme disease, 49
Azlocillin, 224
Azole antifungals, 157–158
Aztreonam (Azactam), 248–249
    against *Citrobacter, Morganella,
        Serratia*, 291, 293, 295
    against *E. coli* and *Klebsiella*, 292, 293
    for infected vascular gangrene, 46
    for nonclostridial cellulitis, 42
    against *P. vulgaris* and *Providencia*,
        294
    and penicillin, 212

B

Babesia microti, 50
Babesiosis, 50
Bacteremia, 24. *See also* Septicemia;
        Toxemia.
    ecthyma with, 38

Bacteremia, (*Continued*)
  endocarditis prophylaxis and, 144
  furuncle and carbuncle with, 36
  hematogenous osteomyelitis with, 71
  nosocomial fever with, 12
  septic arthritis with, 76
Bacterial pathogens. *See also specific organism.*
  in common lower extremity infections, 4, 25–26
  identification of, 182–183
  infections caused by "higher", 51–52
  list of antibiotics against, 312t–313t
  number of, to cause infection, 22, 82
  resistance patterns of, 112, 134–135, 145
  in site infections, 2
  susceptibility of, 183–184
  suspicion of anaerobic, 21
  virulence of, 134
Bacteriologic techniques for diagnosis of infections, 18–26
Bacteroides, 289–290
  in bite wound infections, 92
  in diabetic foot infections, 111
  glycocalyx formation by, 134
  in moderate to severely infected ulcerations, 120
  nonclostridial cellulitis due to, 41
  pathogenicity of, 112
  synergistic necrotizing cellulitis due to, 43
  in trauma wound infections, 81t
Bacteroides (drug activity in)
  cefazolin ineffective against, 233
  cefotaxime against, 240
  cefotetan and, 236
  cefoxitin against, 235
  ceftizoxime and, 240
  cephalosporins against, 232
  clindamycin against, 257
  imipenem/cilastatin against, 246
  mezlocillin against, 223
  penicillin G and, 217
Bacteroides asaccharolyticus. See
  Porphyromonas asaccharolytica.
Bacteroides fragilis, 289
  amoxicillin/clavulanic acid against, 226
  cefazolin ineffective against, 233

in diabetic foot infections, 111
erythromycin not against, 271
incidence of diabetic foot infections due to, 112
infected vascular gangrene due to, 46
metronidazole against, 255
in moderate to severely infected ulcerations, 120
ticarcillin/clavulanic acid against, 225
in trauma wound infections, 81t
Bacteroides melaninogenicus. See Prevotella melaninogenica.
Bacteroides thetaiotaomicron, 289
Bacteroides vulgatus, 289
Bactrim, 269–270
Bactroban (mupirocin), 117
Balance impairment, 251
Bartonella henselae, 81t, 93, 297–298
Bell's palsy, 48, 49
Benzathine penicillin, 216, 217
Betadine (povidone iodine), 117
Beta-lactam antibiotics, 245–249
  aminoglycosides with, 250, 255
  effect of combining, 198
  neutropenia due to, 206
  platelet dysfunction due to, 206–207
Beta-lactamase inhibitor combinations, 224–228
  against *Alcaligenes*, 297
  against anaerobic gram-positive cocci, 285
  against *Bacteroides*, 290
  against *C. canimorsus*, 298
  against *C. perfringens*, 286
  vs. cefoxitin, 236
  against *Citrobacter, Morganella, Serratia*, 291, 293, 295
  against *E. coli* and *Klebsiella*, 292, 293
  against enterococci, 284
  against *H. influenzae*, 299
  list of agents in, 215b
  vs. metronidazole, 256
  against *P. mirabilis*, 294
  against *P. multocida*, 299
  against *P. vulgaris* and *Providencia*, 294
  rule for use of, 225
  spectrum of activity by, 215–216

Beta-lactamase production
amoxicillin/clavulanic acid and, 226
ampicillin and, 218
antibiotic development due to, 213
carbapenem agents resistant to, 245
chromosomal. *See* Richmond-Sykes I beta-lactamase.
ciprofloxacin resistant to, 264
by *Enterobacter*, 292
imipenem/cilastatin resistant to, 246
methicillin resistance due to, 279
by *Morganella*, 293
penicillin G and, 217
penicillins' action and, 214
by *Serratia*, 295
third-generation cephalosporins and, 232
ticarcillin and, 222
ticarcillin/clavulanic acid and, 225
Beta-lactam/beta-lactamase inhibitor compounds
for bite wound infections, 93
for moderate to severely infected ulcerations, 121
resistance to, 191
Betamethasone dipropionate and clotrimazole (Lotrisone), 156t, 157
Bifonazole (non-FDA approved), 167
Biliary elimination
of cefoperazone, 243
of ceftriaxone, 241
Bioavailability, drug, 191
Biopsy, skin
of cutaneous larva migrans (CLM), 52
for diagnosis of Lyme disease, 49
following burn trauma, 95
Bite wound infections
amoxicillin/clavulanic acid for, 227
ampicillin/sulbactam for, 228
anaerobic gram-negative rods in, 290
antibiotic prophylaxis preventing, 138
B. henselae in, 297
C. canimorsus in, 298
clinical presentation of, 92
E. corrodens in, 298

laboratory findings and etiology of, 92–93
organisms causing, 81t
P. multocida in, 299
pet owners and, 8
piperacillin/tazobactam for, 228
septic arthritis due to, 78
ticarcillin/clavulanic acid for, 226
treatment for, 93–94
variables resulting in, 91–92
Bleeding
due to antibiotic usage, 206–207
due to cefoperazone, 242
due to cefotetan, 236
due to cephalosporins, 233
due to penicillins, 216
due to ticarcillin, 222
and mezlocillin, 223
in plantar space infections, 124
Blood
as alternative therapy for wound care, 83
with infection drainage vs. hematoma, 129
Salmonella in, 295
V. vulnificus in, 301
Blood chemistry in diagnosis of infection, 17–18
Blood culture, 24–25
for cellulitis, 30
for clostridial myonecrosis, 44
for contiguous focus osteomyelitis, 74
for ecthyma, 38
for hematogenous osteomyelitis, 71
for Lyme disease, 49
for moderate to severely infected ulcerations, 119
for necrotizing fasciitis, 42
for nosocomial fever, 12
for osteomyelitis, 58
for scalded skin syndrome, 36
for septic arthritis, 77
for synergistic necrotizing cellulitis, 43
Blood urea nitrogen (BUN) levels
in diagnosis of lower extremity infections, 17
in moderate to severely infected ulcerations, 119
in plantar space infections, 124

Bloodborne Pathogen link on OSHA
Internet site, 311t
Body fluid discoloration, 262
Body response to site infections, 2–3
Bone biopsy
in Charcot's joint, 106
in osteomyelitis, 59
Bone culture
contamination of, 60, 66
in diagnosis of bone and joint
infections, 59–60
of hematogenous osteomyelitis, 72
of moderate to severely infected
ulcerations, 119
after puncture wound trauma, 88
Bone fractures and osteomyelitis
(CFO), 73
Bone graft, 69
Bone infections, 54–79
ceftazidime for, 242
P. aeruginosa in, 300
Bone penetration studies in
osteomyelitis, 67
Bone scans, 62–64, 73
Bones, staining of, 274
Borrelia burgdorferi
Lyme disease due to, 47, 49
septic arthritis due to, 78
tetracyclines against, 274
travelers infected with, 8
Brodie's abscess, 61
Broth tube dilution technique,
185–186
Brotzu G, 228
Brucella, 25
Bullae, 36, 44
Burgdorfer W, 47
Burke ??, 137
Burkholderia cepacia, 300
resistant to aztreonam, 248
resistant to ciprofloxacin, 265
resistant to imipenem/cilastatin,
246
trimethoprim/sulfamethoxazole
against, 269, 270
Burn centers, 96
Burn wound infections
bacterial etiology of, 96
classification of, 94–95
clinical signs of, 95
factors leading to, 94

laboratory findings of, 95
organisms causing, 81t
topical agents for, 98t–99t
treatment for, 96–97
Butenafine (Mentax), 155, 156t

C

Caffeine with antibiotic usage, 265
Calf muscles, pyomyositis in, 46–47
Calf tenderness, 32
Cancellous bone graft, 69
Candida
itraconazole (Sporanox) for, 174
onychomycosis and, 160
paronychia due to, 33
resistance of, 153
Candida albicans, 149
Candida parapsilosis, 149
Capnocytophaga canimorsus, 81t, 298
Carbacephem, 239
Carbapenem antibiotics, 245–248
against *Alcaligenes*, 297
against *Bacteroides*, 290
against *Citrobacter, Morganella,*
Serratia, 291, 293, 295
against *E. coli* and *Klebsiella*, 292, 293
against *P. vulgaris* and *Providencia*,
294
against *S. maltophilia* and *B.*
Cepacia, 300
Carbenicillin, 222
Carboxypenicillins, 215t
Carbuncles, 35, 36
Carcinogenic effects, 256
Cartilage degeneration, 265
Casting, wound care, 116, 120
Cat bite wound infection
B. henselae in, 297
organisms causing, 81t
P. multocida in, 299
septic arthritis from, 78
variables resulting in, 91–92
Cat parasites, 52
Cat scratch disease, 81t, 93, 297
Catheters, nosocomial fever with
indwelling, 12
Cedax (ceftibuten), 244
Cefaclor (Ceclor), 238, 239
Cefadroxil (Duricef), 235
Cefamandole nafate (Mandol), 207,
237–238

Cefazolin (Ancef, Kefzol), 233–234
  for cellulitis, 31
  for open fracture infections, 100
  for puncture wound infections, 89
  for pyomyositis, 47
  for scalded skin syndrome, 37
  for surgical prophylaxis, 142
Cefdinir (Omnicef), 31, 243–244
Cefepime (Maxipime), 90, 244–245
Cefixime (Suprax), 244
Cefmetazole, 207
Cefoperazone (Cefobid), 242–243
  in hepatic dysfunction, 195
  Vitamin K metabolism disorders
    due to, 207
Cefotaxime (Claforan), 239–240
  vs. cefoperazone, 242
  vs. ceftizoxime, 240
  against *V. vulnificus*, 301
Cefotetan (Cefotan), 236–237
  against *Bacteroides*, 290
  Vitamin K metabolism disorders
    due to, 207
Cefoxitin (Mefoxin), 235
  against *Bacteroides*, 290
  for moderate to severely infected
    ulcerations, 121
  for mycobacteria infections, 302
Cefpodoxime proxetil (Vantin), 244
Cefprozil (Cefzil), 239
Ceftazidime (Fortaz, Tazicef,
    Tazidime), 242
  against *B. cepacia*, 300
  vs. cefepime, 245
  vs. cefoperazone, 242, 243
  vs. cefotaxime, 242
  for post-puncture-wound
    osteomyelitis, 90
  against *V. vulnificus*, 301
Ceftibuten (Cedax), 244
Ceftizoxime (Cefizox), 240–241
Ceftriaxone (Rocephin), 241–242
  for gonococcal infection, 288
  for *Kingella kingae* infection, 289
  for Lyme disease, 49
  for surgical prophylaxis, 142
  for systemic *N. meningitidis*
    infection, 288
Cefuroxime axetil (Ceftin), 238–239
  for bite wound infections, 94
  for cellulitis, 31

  for Lyme disease, 49
Cefuroxime (Zinacef), 142, 237
Cellulitis, 30–31. *See also* Clostridial
    cellulitis; Donor-leg cellulitis;
    Nonclostridial anaerobic
    cellulitis; Synergistic necrotizing
    cellulitis.
  after bite wound trauma, 92
  with burn wound, 95
  cardinal signs of, 9
  clinical presentation of, 30
  conditions mimicking, 9
  culture from site of, 23
  in diagnosis of lower extremity
    infections, 8–10
  documenting, 10
  due to *S. aureus*, 279
  erysipelas form of, 39
  with erythrasma, 35
  etiology of, 31
  H. influenza in, 298
  with impetigo, 37
  with injection site abscess, 38
  in mildly infected ulcerations, 117
  in moderate to severely infected
    ulcerations, 119
  with necrotizing fasciitis, 42
  with paronychia, 32
  penicillin G for superficial, 217
  in plantar space infections, 123
  with puncture wounds, 81t, 82
  treatment for, 31
Celsus, cardinal signs of, 9
Centers for Disease Control and
    Prevention
  Internet site for, 311t
  vancomycin guidelines by, 259
  wound classification by, 129
Central fever, 13
Cephalexin (Keflex, Keftab), 234
  vs. cefdinir, 243
  for cellulitis, 31
  for mildly infected ulcerations,
    118
  for puncture wound infections, 89
Cephalosporins, 228–245
  first-generation agents of, 233–235
  second-generation agents of,
    235–239
  third-generation agents of,
    239–244

Cephalosporins, (*Continued*)
  fourth-generation agents of,
      244–245
  adverse reactions to, 232–233
  ciprofloxacin vs., 267
  classification of, 230–231
  dosages of, 303t
  history of, 228–229
  list of agents in, 230b
Cephalosporins, drug activity of,
      231–232
  against *Aeromonas*, 297
  against *Alcaligenes*, 297
  Bacteroides resistant to, 289
  against *C. canimorsus*, 298
  against *C. perfringens*, 286
  against *Citrobacter, Morganella,*
      Serratia, 291, 293, 295
  against *E. coli* and *Klebsiella,* 292, 293
  against *E. corrodens,* 298
  against *H. influenza,* 299
  against *Kingella kingae,* 289
  mechanism of action in, 229
  against N. meningitidis, 288
  against *P. mirabilis,* 294
  against *P. multocida,* 299
  against *P. vulgaris* and *Providencia,*
      294
  resistance to, 280
  against *S. aureus,* 280
  S. maltophilia and *B. Cepacia*
      resistant to, 300
  against *Salmonella,* 295
  and streptococci sensitivity, 283, 284
Cephalosporins, therapy with
  for bite wound infections, 94
  CDAD due to, 204
  for endocarditis prophylaxis, 144
  for gonococcal infection, 288
  hematologic reactions due to, 207
  for impetigo, 37
  for infected vascular gangrene, 46
  for marine puncture wounds, 90
  nephrotoxicity due to, 203
  neutropenia due to, 206
  for nonclostridial cellulitis, 42
  and open fracture infections, 100
  and penicillin, 211–212
  during pregnancy, 195
Cephamycin, 235, 236
Cephradine, 234–235

Cerebrospinal fluid (CSF) and Lyme
    disease, 49
Charcot's joint
  cellulitis vs., 9
  etiology of, 106
  osteomyelitis vs., 59, 62, 106
Chemical debridement, 82–83, 122
Chemotherapy, 15, 204
Children
  antibiotic selection for, 194
  ciprofloxacin and, 265
  H. influenza in, 298
  hematogenous osteomyelitis in,
      70, 71
  Kingella kingae infections in, 288
  septic arthritis in, 78
Chloramphenicol, 275
  against *Bacteroides,* 290
  for clostridial myonecrosis, 44
  hematologic reactions due to, 206,
      207
  in hepatic dysfunction, 195
Chronic indurated cellulitis, 9
Ciclopirox (Loprox)
  for distal subungual
      onychomycosis (DSO), 162
  dosage of, 156t
  for onychomycosis, 164
  for tinea pedis, 158
Ciclopirox nail lacquer (Penlac)
  for onychomycosis, 147
  pros and cons of, 167–168
Cierny, G, 55
Cilastatin, 245
Ciprofloxacin (Cipro), 264–267
  vs. cefepime, 245
  contraindications for use of,
      266–267
  for ecthyma, 39
  vs. levofloxacin, 267, 268
  for marine puncture wounds, 90
  vs. moxifloxacin, 268
  and rifampin, 265
  S. maltophilia and *B. Cepacia*
      resistant to, 300
  for surgical prophylaxis, 143
  against *V. vulnificus,* 301
Circulatory problems
  antibiotic selection and, 196
  antibiotics in patients with, 67
  paronychia with, 34

Citrobacter, 291
  beta-lactamase by, 225
  ciprofloxacin against, 264
  in diabetic foot infections, 111
  diversus species of, 291
  freundii species of, 291
Clarithromycin (Biaxin), 272–273
  vs. azithromycin, 272, 273
  against *B. henselae*, 297
  for cellulitis, 31
  for erythrasma, 35
  against *H. influenza*, 299
  against *M. marinum*, 301
  for marine puncture wounds, 91
  for mycobacteria infections, 302
Clindamycin (Cleocin), 257–258
  with aztreonam, 249
  for babesiosis, 50
  CDAD due to, 204
  with cefotaxime, 240
  for cellulitis, 31
  with ciprofloxacin, 266
  for clostridial myonecrosis, 44
  combinations of agents using, 223
  dosage of, 304t
  for ecthyma, 39
  for folliculitis, 36
  in hepatic dysfunction, 195
  for impetigo, 37
  for infected vascular gangrene, 46
  for mildly infected ulcerations,
    118
  for moderate to severely infected
    ulcerations, 121
  for nonclostridial cellulitis, 42
  for osteomyelitis, 67
  for puncture wound infections, 89
  for pyomyositis, 47
  for surgical prophylaxis, 143
Clindamycin (Cleocin), drug activity
    of
  against anaerobic gram-positive
    cocci, 285
  against *Bacteroides*, 290
  against beta-hemolytic
    streptococci, 283
  against *C. canimorsus*, 298
  against *C. minutissimum*, 287
  against *C. perfringens*, 286
  against *S. aureus*, 280
Clindamycin solution, 35

Clinical diagnosis. *See also specific*
    infection.
  bacteriologic techniques for,
    18–26
  common organisms in, 25–26
  definition of infection for, 2–3
  etiologies in, 3–4
  hospitalization and, 26–27
  laboratory tests for, 14–18
  patient history in, 3–8
  physical examination in, 8–14
Clinical Infectious Diseases, electronic
    edition, 311t
Clostridia
  appearance of, 20t
  clindamycin moderately against,
    257
  imipenem/cilastatin against, 246
  penicillin G and, 217
  vancomycin against, 259
Clostridial cellulitis, 40–41, 218
Clostridial myonecrosis, 43–44, 286
Clostridium difficile
  cephalosporins ineffective against,
    232
  clindamycin ineffective against,
    257
  imipenem/cilastatin ineffective
    against, 246
  metronidazole against, 256
Clostridium difficile-associated
    diarrhea (CDAD), 204–205
Clostridium difficile colitis, 257, 260
Clostridium perfringens, 286
  clostridial cellulitis due to, 41
  clostridial myonecrosis due to, 44
  diabetic foot infections and,
    111–112
  infections with, 5
  tissue gas and, 110
Clostridium tetani, 285–286
Clotrimazole (Lotrimin AF), 156t,
    157
Cloxacillin, 31, 221
Cockcroft DW, 17
"Cold steel" debridement, 83, 122
Colistin, 275
Colitis. *See Clostridium difficile* colitis.
Complete bed rest, 27
Complete blood count (CBC) with
    differential, 14–15

Compresses, warm, 36. *See also* Soaks, foot.
Computed tomography, 65
"Concentration-dependent killing", 254
Congenital abnormalities, onychomycosis vs., 163
Connective tissue toxicity, 265
Contact lenses, discoloration of, 262
Contamination. *See also* Fecal contamination.
  asepsis to lessen, 21–22
  of blood cultures, 24–25
  of burn wound, 96
  by *Corynebacterium*, 287
  of diabetic foot infections, 111
  by enterococci, 284
  of fish tanks, 301
  vs. infection, 20, 281–282, 295
  by mycobacteria, 302
  of nail cultures, 160
  and noninfected mal perforans, 114–115, 116
  with *P. aeruginosa*, 299
  with *Proteus*, 293
  of raw oysters, 301
  of surgical site, 128–129
Contiguous-focus osteomyelitis (CFO), 54, 73–74
Continuous bacteremia, 24
Continuous fever, 11
Corticosteroids, 76, 158, 195
Corynebacteria, 259
Corynebacterium jeikeium, 286–287
Corynebacterium minutissimum, 35, 287
Corynebacterium organism
  appearance of, 20t
  contamination by, 25
  diphtheroids in, 286–287
Costs and cost analysis
  of aminoglycoside usage, 254
  of amoxicillin/clavulanic acid, 227
  of antibiotic selection, 181, 192
  of cefazolin vs. penicillin, 234
  of ceftriaxone, 142, 242
  of cefuroxime axetil vs. others in class, 239
  of cefuroxime vs. cefazolin, 142
  of cefuroxime vs. others in class, 237
  of cephalexin and cephradine, 235
  of cloxacillin and dicloxacillin, 221

  of combining antibiotics, 198
  of imipenem/cilastatin, 245
  of linezolid, 262
  of metronidazole, 256
  of nafcillin, 221
  of onychomycosis, 159
  of oral antifungals, 170
  of piperacillin/tazobactam, 228
  of postoperative infections, 127
  of quinupristin/dalfopristin, 261, 285
  of surgical site infections, 126
  of vancomycin, 259
C-reactive protein (CRP), 16, 58
Creatinine clearance
  aminoglycosides dosage and, 252
  ampicillin dosage and, 219
  equation for calculating, 17, 252
  mezlocillin dosage and, 223
  normal, defined, 252–253
  penicillin G dosage and, 217
  ticarcillin dosage and, 222
Creatinine levels, serum
  in diagnosis of lower extremity infections, 17
  in moderate to severely infected ulcerations, 119
  in plantar space infections, 124
  "Creeping eruption", 52
Crepitant cellulitis, 41–42
"Crossover allergy", 211–212
Cross-reactivity, 211–212
  between aminoglycosides and loop diuretics, 250
  between aztreonam and penicillins or cephalosporins, 248
  between cephalosporins and beta-lactams, 233
  between imipenem and penicillin, 246
Crystalluria and sulfonamide usage, 270
Culture and sensitivity
  and arterial ulcerations, 122
  of bite wound, 93
  of burn wound, 95, 97
  of cellulitis exudate, 30–31
  and contiguous focus osteomyelitis, 74
  of *Corynebacterium* infection, 287
  for detection of VISA, 280

and diagnosis of lower extremity
infections, 21
and diagnosis of Lyme disease, 49
of erythrasma, 35
of folliculitis, 35
of impetigo, 37
of mildly infected ulcerations, 118
and paronychia, 33
after puncture wound trauma, 88
and septic arthritis, 77
"therapeutic holes" in, 197
for wound closure, 84
Culture and sensitivity technique,
21–25
absence of exudate for, 23, 30–31
amount of specimen for, 22
broth tube dilution method of,
185–186
collecting specimen for, 22,
181–182
collection site for, 21
disc-diffusion method of, 184–185
order of specimens for, 23–24
time required for report of, 183
transportation of specimens for, 23
Culture foris *C. difficile*, 205
Cutaneous larva migrans (CLM), 8,
52
Cytochrome P450 isoenzyme 3A4, 175
Cytomegalovirus, 211, 219

D

Dakin's solution (sodium
hypochlorite), 83, 117
Daptomycin (non-FDA approved),
263
Daptomycin (non-FDA approved)
against VISA, 281
Darier's disease, 163
Deafness due to antibiotic usage,
200–201
Debilitated patients, *Enterobacter*
infection in, 291
Debridement. *See* "Cold steel"
debridement; Chemical
debridement; Manual toenail
debridement; Mechanical
debridement; Surgical
debridement.
Decompression for clostridial
myonecrosis, 44

Deep vein thrombophlebitis (DVT),
6, 9
DEET for prevention of Lyme
disease, 50
Dental procedures after joint
implants, 144
Dermatological reactions, 208–209,
210
Dermatophyte test media (DTM),
152
Dermatophytes
infections due to, 123
onychomycosis due to, 159, 160
tinea pedis due to, 148–149
Dermatophytosis complex/simplex
tinea pedis, 150–151
Desacetyl cefotaxime, 240
Devastating results, antibiotic
prophylaxis and, 140
Devitalized tissue
in bite wound infections, 92
in clostridial cellulitis, 40
in infections following trauma, 82
Diabetes Control and Complications
Trial, 104
Diabetes mellitus
antibiotic selection and, 194, 195
Enterobacter infection in, 291
hospitalization for, 27
infected vascular gangrene in, 46
MRI differentiation of, 64–65
nonclostridial cellulitis in, 41
onychomycosis in, 158
osteomyelitis in, 58
osteomyelitis secondary to, 74
site infections with, 6
surgical prophylaxis for, 139
synergistic necrotizing cellulitis in,
43
triple-agent combinations and, 255
Diabetic angiopathy, 107–108
Diabetic foot infections, 103–125
anaerobic gram-negative rods in,
290
anaerobic gram-positive cocci in,
285
Bacteroides in, 289
beta-hemolytic streptococci in, 282
microbiology of, 109–112
miscellaneous infections in,
123–125

Diabetic foot infections, (*Continued*)
  pathogenesis of, 104–109
  S. aureus major cause of, 279
  statistical data about, 103–104
  streptococci in, 284
  ulceration in, 112–122
Diabetic foot infections, treatment of
  amoxicillin/clavulanic acid for, 227
  ampicillin/sulbactam for, 228
  cefotaxime for, 240
  cefoxitin for, 236
  cefoxitin vs. beta-lactamase
    inhibitors for, 236
  ciprofloxacin plus other drugs for,
    266
  clindamycin and quinolone for,
    257
  clinical trials using linezolid for,
    262
  ertapenem vs. piperacillin/
    tazobactam for, 248
  home IV antibiotic therapy for, 199
  imipenem/cilastatin for, 246
  levofloxacin for, 267
  metronidazole plus other drugs
    for, 256
  moxifloxacin and, 268
  piperacillin/tazobactam for, 228
  ticarcillin/clavulanic acid for, 226
  triple-agent combinations for, 255
Diabetic immunopathy, 106–107
Diabetic neuroarthropathy. *See*
    Charcot's joint.
Diabetic neuropathy, 104–106
Diabetic ulceration, 73, 257
Diagnosis of lower extremity
    infections. *See* Clinical
    diagnosis.
Diagnosis-related groups (DRGs),
    199
Dialysis, 202, 280
Diarrhea
  due to amoxicillin/clavulanic acid,
    226
  due to ampicillin, 219
  due to antibiotic usage, 203–206
  due to cefoperazone, 243
  due to ceftriaxone, 241
  due to cephalosporins, 233
  due to clindamycin, 257
  due to penicillin, 216

Dicloxacillin, 221
  for cellulitis, 31
  for impetigo, 37
Diflucan (fluconazole), 173–174
Digital plethysmography, 122
Diphtheroids, 286–287
Direct extension osteomyelitis. *See*
    Contiguous-focus osteomyelitis
    (CFO).
Direct extension septic arthritis, 76
Dirithromycin (Dynabac), 273
Disc-diffusion method, 184–185
Discharge planning, 198–199
"Dishwater" pus, 43
Disinfectants, topical, 117
Disseminated gonococcal infection
    (DGI), 287–288
Distal subungual onychomycosis
    (DSO), 160–161, 162
Disulfiram-like reaction. *See*
    Antabuse reaction.
Dizziness. *See* Vertigo.
Dog bite wound infections
    C. canimorsus causing, 298
    organisms causing, 81t
    variables resulting in, 91–92
Dog hookworm, 52
Donor-leg cellulitis, 31–32
Dorsal space infections, 124–125
Dosing nomogram, 252
Dosing schedules
  aminoglycosides and, 249
  creatinine clearance equation for,
    17, 252
  of oral antifungals, 170
  types of, 252–254
Doxycycline, 273–275
  against *B. henselae*, 297
  dosage of, 304t
  for ehrlichiosis, 50
  for Lyme disease, 49
  against *M. marinum*, 301
  against mycobacteria, 302
  against *P. multocida*, 299
  for prevention of Lyme disease, 50
  against *S. maltophilia* and *B.
    Cepacia*, 300
  against *V. vulnificus*, 301
Drake, Lynn, 159
Drug fever, 211
"Drugs for Bugs" list, 312t–313t

Dry mouth, 256
Duricef (cefadroxil), 235
Dye, *Serratia* in marker, 295
Dysgonic Fermenter-2 (DF-2). *See
    Capnocytophaga canimorsus.*
Dystrophic nail. *See* Onychomycosis.

E

Ear disorders. *See* Ototoxicity.
Ecchymosis, 91, 288
Econazole (Spectazole), 156t, 157
Ecthyma, 37–38
Ecthyma gangrenosum, 38
Edema
    in cellulitis, 30
    in clostridial myonecrosis, 44
    in hematoma vs. infection, 129
    in Madura foot, 51
    in mildly infected ulcerations, 117
    in plantar space infections, 123
    in septic arthritis, 76
    from stingray envenomation, 91
    in synergistic necrotizing cellulitis,
        43
Educated guess
    in antibiotic selection, 181
    in diagnosis of lower extremity
        infections, 25–26
Ehrlichia equi, 50
Ehrlichioses, 50
Eikenella corrodens, 81t, 298
Elderly
    and antibiotic selection, 193–194
    and CDAD, 204
    with hematogenous osteomyelitis,
        70, 72
    with osteomyelitis, 56
    with septic arthritis, 78
    with surgical site infections,
        133–134
Electrolytes
    in diagnosis of lower extremity
        infections, 17
    imbalances of, due to penicillin,
        216, 226
Endocarditis
    bacteremia and, 24
    home IV antibiotic therapy for,
        199
    surgical prophylaxis for, 143–145
    viridans streptococci causing, 283

Endogenous pyrogen, 10–11
Enterobacter, 291–292
    beta-lactamase by, 225
    ciprofloxacin against, 264
    in diabetic foot infections, 111
    in moderate to severely infected
        ulcerations, 120
Enterobacter cloacae, 292
Enterobacteriaceae, 290–295
    cefdinir and, 243
    cefepime against, 245
    cefpodoxime proxetil against, 244
    drug resistance of, 191
    ertapenem vs. imipenem against,
        247
    infected vascular gangrene due to,
        46
    nonclostridial cellulitis due to, 41
    ticarcillin against, 222
    in trauma wound infections, 81t
Enterococci, 284–285
    aminoglycosides/beta-lactam
        against, 250, 255
    amoxicillin/clavulanic acid
        against, 226
    ampicillin against, 217, 218
    ampicillin/sulbactam against, 228
    cephalosporins ineffective against,
        232
    clindamycin ineffective against, 257
    erythromycin not against, 271
    imipenem/cilastatin and, 246
    mezlocillin against, 223, 224
    nafcillin ineffective against, 220
    penicillin G and, 217
    tetracyclines not against, 274
    ticarcillin and, 222
    trimethoprim/sulfamethoxazole
        not against, 269
    vancomycin against, 259
    vancomycin/aminoglycoside
        against, 260
Enterococcus
    ampicillin against, 219
    cefoxitin and, 236
    ciprofloxacin and, 265
    in diabetic foot infections, 111
    piperacillin/tazobactam against,
        228
    quinupristin/dalfopristin against,
        261

Enterococcus faecalis, 261, 284–285

Enterococcus faecium, 261, 284–285

Enterococcus, vancomycin-resistant (VRE), 259, 284

  antibiotics for infection with, 285

  quinupristin/dalfopristin against, 260–261

Enzyme-linked immunosorbent assay (ELISA)

  in diagnosis of CDAD, 205

  in diagnosis of lower extremity infections, 16

  and diagnosis of Lyme disease, 49

Eosinophilia, 15, 52

Epidermophyton floccosum, 148, 149

Epstein-Barr infection, 211, 219

Ertapenem (Invanz), 121, 247–248

Erysipelas, 39

Erythema

  in cellulitis, 30

  in hematoma vs. infection, 129

  in mildly infected ulcerations, 117

  in necrotizing fasciitis, 42

  in plantar space infections, 123

  in septic arthritis, 76

  and wound closure, 84

Erythema migrans (EM), 48, 78

Erythrasma, 35, 287

Erythrocyte sedimentation rate (ESR)

  in contiguous focus osteomyelitis, 73–74

  in diagnosis of lower extremity infections, 16

  in hematogenous osteomyelitis, 71

  in moderate to severely infected ulcerations, 119

  in osteomyelitis, 58

  in paronychia, 33

  in plantar space infections, 124

  in puncture wound infections, 88

  in pyomyositis, 47

Erythromycin, 270–271

  against *C. canimorsus*, 298

  against *C. minutissimum*, 287

  vs. dirithromycin, 273

  dosage of, 304t

  for erythrasma, 35

  GI side effects due to, 206

  in hepatic dysfunction, 195

  hepatotoxicity due to, 203

  for impetigo, 37

  for Lyme disease, 49

  ototoxicity due to, 201

  during pregnancy, 195

Escherichia coli, 292

  and ampicillin, 219

  azithromycin against, 272

  cefazolin against, 233

  cephalosporins against, 231, 232

  drug resistance of, 191

  in moderate to severely infected ulcerations, 120

  ticarcillin/clavulanic acid against, 225

  in trauma wound infections, 81t

Eumycetoma, 51

Exelderm (sulconazole), 156t, 158

Exfoliative dermatitis, 209

Exogenous pyrogen, 10–11

Extended spectrum beta-lactamase (ESBL), 191

  amoxicillin/clavulanic acid against organisms with, 226

  cephalosporin resistance and, 231

  Enterobacteriaceae resistance and, 290

  Salmonella resistance and, 295

External fixation devices, 70

Exudate

  absence of, for culture, 23

  absence of, in cellulitis, 30, 31

  in burn wound infections, 94

  in clostridial cellulitis, 40

  in clostridial myonecrosis, 44

  in hematoma vs. infection, 129

  in impetigo, 37

  in infected vascular gangrene, 46

  in mildly infected ulcerations, 117

  in moderate to severely infected ulcerations, 119

  in necrotizing fasciitis, 42

  in nonclostridial cellulitis, 41

  in nonclostridial myonecrosis, 45

  in paronychia, 32

  in plantar space infections, 123, 124

  in pyomyositis, 47

  in synergistic necrotizing cellulitis, 43

  in tinea pedis, 150

  and wound closure, 84

F

Face masks and surgical site
   infections, 135
Facultative bacteria, 41
Fecal contamination, 40, 292
"Fecal fallout", 109
Fetid foot, 110, 123
Fever
   antipyretics and, 12
   body's response of, 10–11
   in diagnosis of lower extremity
      infections, 4
   in ehrlichiosis, 50
   in hematogenous osteomyelitis, 71
   hospitalization for, 26, 50
   in moderate to severely infected
      ulcerations, 119
   in plantar space infections,
      123–124
   in sepsis, 14
   in septic arthritis, 76
   types of, 11–13
Fever curves
   during antipyretic therapy, 12
   in diagnosis of lower extremity
      infections, 11
   during hospitalization, 27
Fever of unknown origin (FUO)
   blood culture in, 24
   determining etiology of, 13
Fish, puncture wounds, 301
Fish tank organisms, 301
Flagyl. See Metronidazole.
Fleming, A, 213
"Flesh-eating bacteria", 282
Florey, HW, 213
Floxin. See Ofloxacin.
Fluconazole (Diflucan), 173–174
Fluid retention, 222, 226
Fluid/electrolyte therapy
   for antabuse reaction, 208
   for CDAD, 205
   for scalded skin syndrome, 37
Flu-like symptoms, 262
Flushing, 259
Folliculitis, 35–36
Food and Drug Administration (FDA)
   approval of antifungals by, 164
   on fluconazole (Diflucan), 173, 174
   on itraconazole (Sporanox), 174
   on oral antifungals, 169

and Pexiganan, 119
   on pulse dosing, 175
   reports of deaths by, 171
   on terbinafine (Lamisil), 176
   on topical antifungals, 167, 168
Food intake
   and amoxicillin serum levels, 220
   and amoxicillin/clavulanic acid,
      227
   and cloxacillin and dicloxacillin,
      221
Foot flora, 293
"Foot infection", 148
Foreign substances/bodies
   in infections following surgery,
      130–131
   in infections following trauma, 80,
      82
   in puncture wound infections, 89
Fortaz (ceftazidime), 242
Fractures, infections of open
   antibiotic therapy for, 97, 100
   debridement for, 97
   fixation for, 100–101
   organisms causing, 81t
Frostbite, osteomyelitis secondary to,
   74
Fruits, contaminated, 299
Fulvicin (griseofulvin)
   history of, 147, 164, 169
   for onychomycosis, 172–173
   for tinea pedis, 155
Fungal cultures
   from bone culture, 60
   contamination of, 160
   in diagnosis of lower extremity
      infections, 22–23
   of erythrasma, 35
   and fungal infections, 152–153
   of onychomycosis, 162, 164
   of tinea pedis, 151
Fungal culture technique of
   dystrophic nail, 163–164
Fungal infections, 147–177. See also
   specific infection.
   cure vs. arrest of, 171
   as diabetic foot infections, 123
   in diagnosis of lower extremity
      infections, 25
   donor-leg cellulitis due to, 32
   erythrasma vs., 35

Fungal infections, (*Continued*)
  predisposing factors for, 149–150
  preventive maintenance and,
    170–171
  septic arthritis due to, 78
  travelers with, 8
Fungal organisms
  classification of pathogenic,
    148–149
  Madura foot due to, 51
  onychomycosis due to, 158–176
  resistance of, 153
  tinea pedis due to, 148–158
Furuncles, 35, 36
Fusobacterium, 290
  in bite wound infections, 92
  in diabetic foot infections, 111
  in trauma wound infections, 81t

G

Gallium scans, 63, 88
Gangrene
  in arterial ulcerations, 122
  infected vascular form of, 45–46
  from *N. meningitidis*, 288
  in secondary osteomyelitis, 75
  in synergistic necrotizing cellulitis,
    43
Garré's sclerosing osteomyelitis, 61
Gas gangrene, 43–44
  due to *C. perfringens*, 286
  infected vascular gangrene vs., 46
  nonclostridial myonecrosis vs.,
    45
Gastroenteritis, *Salmonella*-induced,
    295
Gastrointestinal flora
  Alcaligenes in, 297
  Bacteroides in, 289
  enterococci in, 284
  V. vulnificus in, 301
Gastrointestinal side effects
  due to antibiotic usage, 203–206
  due to macrolides, 271, 272, 273
  due to tetracyclines, 274
Gatifloxacin (Tequin), 268
Gault MH, 17
Generic names of antibiotics,
  305t–309t
Genetic alterations of organisms,
    190–191

Genetic predisposition/
  abnormalities
  to aminoglycoside toxicity, 250
  to fungal infections, 149, 153
  to hemolysis with sulfonamides, 194
Gentamicin (Garamycin), 249
  daily doses of, 252, 254
  for dead-space management, 69
  for noninfected mal perforans, 117
  normal blood levels of, 253
  with other antibiotics, 284
Geophilic organisms, 149
Glossitis, 206
Gloves, surgical, 133
Glucose control, 107
Glucose level, serum
  in diagnosis of lower extremity
    infections, 18
  in mildly infected ulcerations, 118
  in moderate to severely infected
    ulcerations, 119
  in plantar space infections, 124
  in septic arthritis, 78
Glucose-6-phosphate dehydrogenase
    deficiency
  due to antibiotic usage, 194, 207
  sulfonamide side effects in, 270
Glycocalyx
  Bacteroides forming, 112, 289
  clindamycin dissolving, 258
  organisms forming, 134–135
Glycopeptide antibiotic, 258, 263
Gonococcal (GC) arthritis, 77,
    287–288
Gonococcemia, 76
Gonococci
  appearance of, 20t
  ceftriaxone against, 241
  penicillin G and, 217–218
  third-generation cephalosporins
    against, 232
  ticarcillin/clavulanic acid against,
    225
Gonococci, non-penicillinase-
    producing, 217
Gonococci, penicillin-resistant, 288
"Gorillamycin", 245
Gout
  cellulitis vs., 9
  osteomyelitis vs., 62
  septic arthritis vs., 77

Gouty arthritis, acute, 30
Gram stain. *See also* Staining and
    culturing techniques, special.
  anaerobic bacteria in, 21
  of bone culture specimen, 60
  contamination of, 20
  in diagnosis of lower extremity
      infections, 18
  of joint in septic arthritis, 77
  of necrotizing fasciitis, 42
  of nonclostridial myonecrosis, 45
  of plantar space infections, 124
  after puncture wound trauma, 88
Gram stain technique
  collecting specimen for, 181–182
  in diagnosis of lower extremity
      infections, 18–21
Gram-negative cocci, 287–289
Gram-negative organisms
  appearance of, 20t
  in bite wound infections, 92
  in burn wound infections, 96
  in clostridial myonecrosis, 44
  in diabetic foot infections, 109
  in hematogenous osteomyelitis,
      72
  in impetigo, 37
  in infected vascular gangrene, 46
  in Lyme disease, 47
  in moderate to severely infected
      ulcerations, 119–120
  in nonclostridial cellulitis, 41
  in open fracture infections, 100
  in secondary osteomyelitis, 75
  in septic arthritis, 78
  in synergistic necrotizing cellulitis,
      43
  tissue gas due to, 110
Gram-negative organisms (drug
    activity in)
  amikacin for resistant, 249
  aminoglycosides against, 249, 255
  aminopenicillins vs. penicillins
      against, 218
  amoxicillin/clavulanic acid
      against, 226
  ampicillin against community-
      acquired, 219
  ampicillin/sulbactam vs. other
      combinations against, 227
  azithromycin against some, 272

aztreonam against aerobic, 248
aztreonam vs. aminoglycosides
    against, 249
aztreonam with clindamycin
    against, 249
cefazolin against, 233
cefdinir against community-
    acquired, 243
cefepime vs. ceftazidime against,
    245
cefoperazone vs. cefotaxime
    against, 242
cefotaxime against typical, 240
cefotetan vs. cefoxitin against, 236
cefoxitin vs. cefazolin against, 235
ceftazidime similar to cefotaxime
    against, 242
cefuroxime against, 237
cefuroxime axetil against, 238
cephalexin and cephradine against
    some, 235
cephalosporins against, 231, 232
ciprofloxacin against all common,
    264
ciprofloxacin against severe
    infections with, 266
clarithromycin vs. azithromycin
    against, 272
drug resistance of, 191
ertapenem for mixed infections
    with, 248
erythromycin against a few, 271
gatifloxacin against, 268
imipenem/cilastatin against most,
    246
levofloxacin against, 267
mafenide acetate against, 98t
meropenem vs. imipenem against,
    247
metronidazole against anaerobic,
    255
mezlocillin similar to ticarcillin
    against, 223
mupirocin and, 98t
nafcillin ineffective against rods
    of, 220
penicillins' action in, 214
rifampin against some, 262
silver nitrate solution against, 98t
silver sulfadiazine against, 98t
tetracyclines against some, 274

Gram-negative organisms (drug
  activity in) (*Continued*)
 ticarcillin/clavulanic acid against,
  225, 226
 trimethoprim/sulfamethoxazole
  against, 269, 270
 vancomycin ineffective against, 259
Gram-negative rods, aerobic,
  296–301. *See also*
  Enterobacteriaceae.
Gram-negative rods, anaerobic,
  289–290
"Gram-negative tinea", 149
Gram-positive bacilli, 285–287
Gram-positive cocci, 278–285
Gram-positive cocci, anaerobic, 285
Gram-positive organisms
 appearance of, 20t
 in bite wound infections, 92
 in clostridial cellulitis, 40
 in clostridial myonecrosis, 44
 in diabetic foot infections, 109
 in erythrasma, 35
 in impetigo, 37
 in infected vascular gangrene, 46
 in mildly infected ulcerations, 118
 in moderate to severely infected
  ulcerations, 119–120
 in nonclostridial cellulitis, 41
 in pyomyositis, 47
 in secondary osteomyelitis, 75
 in synergistic necrotizing cellulitis,
  43
 tissue gas due to, 110
Gram-positive organisms (drug
  activity in)
 agents against, 258–263
 ampicillin/sulbactam against, 227,
  228
 azithromycin against common, 272
 aztreonam/clindamycin against,
  249
 cefdinir against, 244
 cefepime against, 244
 cefoperazone vs. cefotaxime
  against, 242
 cefotaxime against, 240
 cefotetan vs. cefoxitin against, 236
 cefoxitin vs. cefazolin against, 235
 ceftazidime vs. cefotaxime against,
  242

ceftriaxone vs. cefotaxime against,
  241
 cefuroxime axetil against, 238
 cephalexin or cephradine against
  community acquired, 235
 cephalosporins against, 231
 ciprofloxacin not used for
  osteomyelitis with, 266
 clarithromycin vs. azithromycin
  against, 272
 clindamycin against most, 255, 257
 ertapenem for mixed infections
  with, 248
 ertapenem vs. imipenem against,
  247
 gatifloxacin against, 268
 imipenem/cilastatin against, 246
 levofloxacin against, 267
 linezolid against all, 261
 mafenide acetate against, 98t
 meropenem vs. imipenem against,
  247
 metronidazole against anaerobic,
  255
 moxifloxacin vs. ciprofloxacin
  against, 268
 mupirocin against, 98t
 penicillin G against, 217
 penicillins' action in, 214
 quinupristin/dalfopristin for
  serious infections with, 261
 silver nitrate solution against, 98t
 silver sulfadiazine against, 98t
 ticarcillin/clavulanic acid against,
  226
 vancomycin against all, 258, 259,
  260
Granulocytopenia, 206, 211
Granulomas, 51
Grayson ML, 57
"Greasing the needle", 39, 72
Green-nail syndrome, 299
Griseofulvin (Fulvicin, Gris-Peg,
  Grisactin)
 history of, 147, 164, 169
 for onychomycosis, 172–173
 and peripheral neuropathy, 202
 for tinea pedis, 155
Growth factors for wound healing,
  117
Gustilo RB, 100

H

Haemophilus
  rifampin against, 262
  ticarcillin/clavulanic acid against,
    225
Haemophilus influenzae
  ampicillin and, 219
  cefaclor against, 238
  cefuroxime against, 237
  hematogenous osteomyelitis due
    to, 71–72
  second-generation cephalosporins
    against, 231, 232
  septic arthritis due to, 78
Half-life, drug, 191
Hamburger, contaminated, 292
Headaches due to ciprofloxacin
    usage, 265
Health and Human Services, U.S.
    Department of, 148
Hearing deficit
  due to aminoglycoside, 251
  due to antibiotic usage, 200–201
Heat
  in mildly infected ulcerations, 117
  in plantar space infections, 123
Hematocrit, 44
Hematogenous osteomyelitis
  blood culture differentiation of, 58
  classification of, 54
  differential diagnosis of, 57
Hematogenous osteomyelitis, acute,
    70–73
  bone scan differentiation of, 63
  types of patients with, 70–71, 72
Hematogenous septic arthritis, 76
Hematoma, 129
Hemodialysis, 72
Hemolytic anemia
  due to antibiotic usage, 211
  due to sulfonamide, 207, 270
*Hendersonula. See Scytalidium
    dimidiatum.*
Hepatic dysfunction
  and antibiotic selection, 195
  clindamycin dosage in, 257
  metronidazole and, 256
  nafcillin dosage and, 221
Hepatic failure, 264, 268
Hepatitis B, 81t
Hepatotoxicity, 203, 271

Hexachlorophene, 83
99m Tc-hexamethylpropylene amine
    oxime (HMPAO) scan
  of Charcot's joint, 106
  of osteomyelitis, 64, 65
History. *See* Patient history.
Homans' sign, 32
Home intravenous antibiotics,
    198–200
Homophiles influenza, 298–299
Honey for wound care, 83
Hookworm, 52
Hospital Infectious Program of the
    National Center for Infectious
    Diseases, 128–129
Hospital personnel and surgical site
    infections, 135
Hospitalization, 300
  Acinetobacter infections and, 296
  bacterial culture procedure during,
    181–182
  CDAD and, 204
  Citrobacter infections and, 291
  Enterobacter infections and, 291
  home IV antibiotics for refusal of,
    199
  infection rate related to length of,
    132
  for lower extremity infections,
    26–27
  for osteomyelitis, 67
  for severe diabetic ulcerations, 120
  use of imipenem during, 246, 247
  "Hot tub dermatitis", 35–36
Human bite wound infection
  amoxicillin/clavulanic acid for, 227
  E. corrodens in, 298
  organisms causing, 81t
  variables resulting in, 91–92
Human granulocytic ehrlichiosis
    (HGE), 50
Human immunodeficiency virus
    (HIV) infection
  diagnosis of lower extremity
    infections with, 7
  proximal white onychomycosis in,
    161
  site infections with, 6
Hydrogen peroxide irrigation, 110
Hydroxypyridone antifungal, 158
Hygiene, personnel, 135

Hyperbaric oxygen therapy
  for clostridial myonecrosis, 44
  for infections with *C. perfringens*,
    286
  for necrotizing fasciitis, 43
  for osteomyelitis, 70
Hyperemic flush, 122
Hyperglycemia
  in diabetic immunopathy, 106–107
  in diagnosis of lower extremity
    infections, 18
  in infected vascular gangrene, 46
  in neuropathy, 104
Hyperkeratosis
  in distal subungual
    onychomycosis (DSO), 161
  in noninfected mal perforans, 115
  after toenail removal, 166
Hypernatremia, 222
Hypersensitivity
  to cephalosporins, 233
  immediate vs. delayed, 210
  to penicillins, 216
  to sulfonamides, 269
Hypertension, infection with, 6
Hypokalemia
  due to ticarcillin, 222
  from ticarcillin/clavulanic acid, 226
Hypoprothrombinemia, 206
Hypotension, antibiotic usage and,
  208

I

Imaging, diagnostic, 60–65
Imipenem
  against *Acinetobacter*, 296
  for infections with *C. perfringens*,
    286
  for marine puncture wounds, 90
  for mycobacteria infections, 302
  with other antibiotics, 212
  and seizures, 201
Imipenem and cilastatin (Primaxin),
    245–247
  for clostridial cellulitis, 41
  for clostridial myonecrosis, 44
  for infected vascular gangrene, 46
  for moderate to severely infected
    ulcerations, 121
  for nonclostridial cellulitis, 41
  for nonclostridial myonecrosis, 45

Immune deficit
  in burn wound infections, 94
  in lower extremity trauma, 80
  in proximal white onychomycosis,
    161, 162
  in surgical site infections, 133
Immune status
  antibiotic selection and, 195
  beta-hemolytic streptococci and,
    282
  C. canimorsus and, 298
  Corynebacterium and, 287
  mycobacterium and, 301
  S. maltophilia and *B. Cepacia* and, 300
  surgical prophylaxis and, 139
Immunization. *See* Tetanus
    prophylaxis.
Immunoassay, 25
Immunofluorescence, 25, 49
Immunologic techniques, 25
Immunopathy, diabetic, 106–107
Immunosuppression, 76
Impetigo, 37
Implants, surgical
  antibiotic prophylaxis for,
    139–140
  CNS-infected, 282
  Corynebacterium infecting, 287
  dental procedures after, 144
  infection in, 129, 130–131
  S. epidermidis causing infection
    after, 281
  vancomycin for, 260
Indifference drug interaction, 196
Indium scans, 63
Infants, antibiotic selection for, 194
Infected vascular gangrene, 45–46
Infection, local site
  antibiotics "masking", 5
  classification of diabetic, 112–114
  clinical resolution of, 27
  definition of, 2–3
  hospitalization of patient with,
    26–27
  hyperemic flush vs., 122
  location of, for antibiotic
    selection, 196
  number of bacteria for clinical, 82,
    95
  rules for diagnosis of, 114–115
  systemic infection vs., 2

Infectious Diseases Society of America (IDSA), 114, 311t
Inflammation of site infections, 3
Ingress-egress drainage flush
  after debridement, 69–70
  for septic arthritis, 79
Injection site infection, 38–39, 302
Inoculum effect, 193
Insecticides for prevention of Lyme disease, 50
Instruments, sterilization of surgical, 135
Insulin for wound care, 83
Insurance
  and home IV antibiotic therapy, 200
  and oral antifungal agents, 170
  and topical antifungal agents, 169
Intermittent bacteremia, 24
Intermittent fever, 11
Internet
  alternative products from, 167
  sites about infectious diseases on, 311t
Interstitial nephritis
  due to antibiotic usage, 211
  due to use of cephalosporins, 203
  due to use of penicillins, 203, 216
Intravenous drug abusers
  diagnosis of lower extremity infections in, 7, 8
  with hematogenous osteomyelitis, 70, 72
  home IV therapy contraindicated for, 199
Intravenous route. *See* Parenteral therapy.
Intubation, endocarditis prophylaxis for anesthesia, 144
Invanz (ertapenem), 247–248
Iron supplements and ciprofloxacin usage, 265
Irrigation, wound
  of bite wound, 93
  for infections following trauma, 82–83
  and surgical site infections, 131
  tissue gas due to, 110
Ischemia
  and diabetic neuropathy, 104
  and diabetic ulceration, 113b
  and secondary osteomyelitis, 75

Isoniazid and Griseofulvin, 202
Isopropyl alcohol for surgical scrub, 132
Isoxazolyl penicillins, 221
Itraconazole (Sporanox)
  history of, 147, 169
  for onychomycosis, 174–175
Ivermectin, 52
Ixodid ticks
  ehrlichiosis and, 50
  Lyme disease and, 48

J

Joint dysfunction and diabetic foot infections, 109
Joint implants. *See* Implants, surgical.
Joint infections, 54–79
  ceftazidime for, 242
  P. aeruginosa in, 300
Joint-fluid aspiration
  for diagnosis of Lyme disease, 49
  for septic arthritis, 77, 79
The *Journal of Infectious Diseases*, electronic edition, 311t
"Jungle rot", 8

K

Kaleta JL, 58
Keflex. *See* Cephalexin.
Keftab. *See* Cephalexin.
Kefzol. *See* Cefazolin.
Ketoacidosis in plantar space infections, 124
Ketoconazole (Nizoral)
  dosage of, 156t
  history of, 169
  and onychomycosis, 173
  for tinea pedis, 157
Kidney disorders. *See* Nephrotoxicity; Renal impairment.
Kingella kingae, 288–289
Kirby-Bauer method, 184–185
Klebsiella, 292–293
  appearance of, 20t
  cefazolin against, 233
  cephalosporins against, 232
  drug resistance of, 191
  ticarcillin/clavulanic acid against, 225

L

Laboratory tests
  for determining sensitivity of
    organism, 184–189
  for diagnosis of bone and joint
    infections, 57–59
  for diagnosis of lower extremity
    infections, 14–18
  for identifying organisms,
    182–183
Lacerations, antibiotic prophylaxis
  and, 138
Lamisil AT (terbinafine), 34
  dosage of, 156t
  history of, 169
  for onychomycosis, 175–176
  for tinea pedis, 155
Laser procedures, for paronychia, 34
Lateral subungual onychomycosis,
  161, 162
Left shift index
  in cellulitis, 30
  in diagnosis of lower extremity
    infections, 15
  in pyomyositis, 47
Legionella, 25
Lemont (??), 151
Lethargy and fatigue, 48
Leukocytosis
  in clostridial myonecrosis, 44
  in diagnosis of lower extremity
    infections, 14
  in erysipelas, 39
  in infected vascular gangrene, 46
  in necrotizing fasciitis, 42
  in pyomyositis, 47
  in septic arthritis, 77
Leukopenia, 15, 50
Levofloxacin (Levaquin), 267–268
  for bite wound infections, 93
  for mildly infected ulcerations,
    118
  for moderate to severely infected
    ulcerations, 121
  possibly against *Corynebacterium*,
    287
  for puncture wound infections, 89
  for surgical prophylaxis, 143
Leyden (???), 150
Lichen planus, 163
Limb salvage, 40, 269

Lincomycin, 256
Linezolid (Zyvox), 261–262
  for moderate to severely infected
    ulcerations, 121
  against *S. aureus*, 281
  for VRE, 285
Lipopeptide antibiotic, 263
Lister, J, 126
Liver disorders. *See* Hepatic
    dysfunction; Hepatotoxicity.
Liver function tests (LFTs)
  in diagnosis of lower extremity
    infections, 18
  and penicillins, 216
  prior to antifungal therapy,
    171–172
Loading dose, 252
Long-term care facility, CDAD and,
  204
Loprox (ciclopirox)
  dosage of, 156t
  for onychomycosis, 164
  for tinea pedis, 158
Loracarbef (Lorabid), 239
Lotrimin AF (clotrimazole), 156t,
  157
Lotrisone (clotrimazole and
    betamethasone dipropionate),
  156t, 157
Lyme borreliosis, 47, 241
Lyme disease, 47–50
  doxycycline for, 274
  Internet site for, 311t
  prophylaxis for, 50
  risk of, 50
  septic arthritis due to, 76, 78
  stages of, 48
  transmission of, 48
  travelers with, 8
Lymph angiopathy, 30
Lymphadenitis, 10, 119
Lymphadenopathy, 30
Lymphangitis, 10, 119
Lymphocyte ratio, 15

M

Macrolides, 270–273
  for cellulitis, 31
  vs. clindamycin, 256
  for erythrasma, 35
  against *Kingella kingae*, 289

for marine puncture wounds, 91
against *S. aureus*, 280
for streptococcal infections, 283
Mader, J, 55
Madura foot, 51, 274
Maduromycosis, 51
Mafenide acetate cream, 96, 98t
Magnetic resonance imaging (MRI)
of Charcot's joint, 106
of osteomyelitis, 61, 64–65
of paronychia, 33
of patient with septic arthritis,
76–77
of post-puncture-wound
osteomyelitis, 88
Maintenance doses, 252
Mal perforans ulcerations,
noninfected, 114–117
arterial ulcerations vs., 121
contamination vs. infection in,
114–115
pressure relief for, 116
wound care for, 116–117
Males, Madura foot in, 51
Malignancy
C. minutissimum with, 287
group G streptococci with, 283
onychomycosis vs., 163
Malpractice, medical, 127
Mandol. *See* Cefamandole.
Manual toenail debridement, 164, 165
Marine (water) injuries
A. hydrophilia in, 296
M. marinum in, 301
nonclostridial myonecrosis due to,
45
pedal puncture wounds in, 90–91
V. vulnificus in, 301
"Masked" infection, 5
Matricectomy, 33–34, 166
Maxipime (cefepime), 244–245
Mechanical debridement, 82–83
Medical history in diagnosis of
infection, 6–7
Medicare, 159, 165
Medline Internet site, 311t
Medscape Infectious Disease Page
Internet site, 311t
Mefoxin (cefoxitin), 121, 235
Meningococcemia, 288
Mentax (butenafine), 155, 156t

Meropenem (Merrem), 247
against *Acinetobacter*, 296
for *Kingella kingae* infection, 289
for moderate to severely infected
ulcerations, 121
Metallic taste, 256
Methicillin
history of, 213
vs. nafcillin, 220
nephrotoxicity due to, 203
Methicillin resistance. *See also specific
antibiotic.*
due to beta-lactamase production,
279
in injection site infections, 39
and surgical prophylaxis, 140
Metronidazole (Flagyl), 255–256
against anaerobic gram-positive
cocci, 285
antabuse reaction and, 208
against *Bacteroides*, 290
for CDAD, 205
with ciprofloxacin, 266
vs. clindamycin, 257
for clostridial myonecrosis, 44
dosage of, 304t
E. corrodens resistant to, 298
for ecthyma, 39
for nonclostridial cellulitis, 42
pregnancy and, 195
Mezlocillin (Mezlin), 223–224
with an aminoglycoside, 224, 255
and platelet dysfunction, 207
vs. ticarcillin, 222, 223
Miconazole, 158
Microbiology laboratory, antibiotic
selection procedures by, 181–189
Microsporum audouinii, 148
Migratory arthritis, 48, 49
Mildly infected ulcerations, 117–119
Minimal inhibitory concentration
(MIC)
antibiotic-killing effects and, 192
broth tube dilution technique for,
185–186
drug in vitro activity and, 189–190
inoculum effect and, 193
interpretation and breakpoint of,
186–187
postantibiotic effect (PAE) and, 193
single daily dosing and, 254

Minimum bactericidal concentration
(MBC), 187–188
Minocycline, 273–275
dosage of, 304t
against *M. marinum*, 301
for marine puncture wounds, 91
against *S. aureus*, 280, 281
against *S. maltophilia* and *B.
Cepacia*, 300
Moccasin tinea pedis, 150–151, 175
Molds, 149, 160
Monobactams, 212, 248–249
Morbidity
in arterial ulcerations, 121
in bite wound infections, 91
after fixation of open fracture
infections, 101
in fungal infections, 147
Morganella
beta-lactamase by, 225
ciprofloxacin against, 264
ticarcillin against, 222
Morganella morganii, 293
Mortality
in burn wound infections, 97
in necrotizing fasciitis, 42
in necrotizing infections, 40
in nonclostridial myonecrosis, 45
in synergistic necrotizing cellulitis,
43
Mosby's Drug Consult Internet site,
311t
Motor neuropathy, 105
Moxifloxacin (Avelox), 268
for bite wound infections, 93
for moderate to severely infected
ulcerations, 121
Mucin clot formation, 78
Multiple organ failure, 42
Mupirocin (Bactroban)
for burn wound, 96–97, 98t
for noninfected mal perforans, 117
against staphylococcal folliculitis,
36
Musculoskeletal Infection Society of
N.A., Internet site of, 311t
Myalgias, 261
Mycetoma, 51
Mycobacteria
from bone culture, 60
in marine puncture wounds, 90–91

nontuberculous type of, 301–302
rapid-growing species of, 302
rifampin against, 262, 263
in septic arthritis, 78
Mycobacterium, atypical, 301
Mycobacterium leprae, 8
Mycobacterium marinum, 274,
301–302
Mycobacterium tuberculosis, 72
Mycologic testing, 151–152
Mycoplasma, 25
Mycosel agar, 152
Myocutaneous flap, 69

N

Nafcillin, 220–221
for cellulitis, 31
for pyomyositis, 47
for scalded skin syndrome, 37
Naftifine (Naftin), 155, 156t
Nail debridement, 162
Nail lacquer, 147, 167–168
Nails. *See* Toenail.
Nasal carriage of staphylococci, 132
Nasogastric route for CDAD, 205
National Committee on Clinical
Laboratory Standards (NCCLS)
drug breakpoints established by,
187
sensitivity testing standards by, 152
zone-of-inhibition standards by,
184
National Nosocomial Infections
Surveillance (NNIS) System,
126–127, 128
Nausea and vomiting
due to aminoglycoside, 251
due to antibiotic usage, 205–206,
208
due to ciprofloxacin, 265
due to erythromycin, 271
due to imipenem, 246
Nebcin (tobramycin), 249
Necrotizing fasciitis, 42–43
beta-hemolytic streptococci in, 282
due to *C. perfringens*, 286
due to *V. vulnificus*, 301
imipenem/cilastatin for, 246
in marine puncture wounds, 90
in moderate to severely infected
ulcerations, 119

Necrotizing infections, 39–47
    anaerobic gram-positive cocci in,
        285
    following burn trauma, 94, 95
    following surgical tissue injury, 131
    following trauma, 82
    imipenem/cilastatin for, 246
    in plantar space infections, 124
    in severely infected ulcerations,
        119
    Vibrio vulnificus causing, 300–301
Neisseria, 262
Neisseria gonorrhoeae, 78, 287–288
Neisseria meningitidis, 288
Neosporin, 117
Nephrotoxicity
    and aminoglycoside dosage, 253
    due to aminoglycoside, 250
    due to antibiotic usage, 202–203
    and vancomycin, 259
Neurologic symptoms in Lyme
        disease, 48
Neuromuscular blockade, 201, 251
Neuropathy of diabetes. *See* Diabetic
        neuropathy.
Neurotoxicity
    due to antibiotic usage, 201–202
    due to ciprofloxacin, 265
    due to *C. tetani*, 285–286
Neutropenia
    due to antibiotic usage, 206
    due to cephalosporins, 233
    due to nafcillin, 220
    due to penicillins, 216
    with terbinafine, 176
Neutrophils
    and beta-lactam agents, 206
    in burn wound infections, 94
    in infection following bite wound,
        93
    in infection following trauma, 80
    in septic arthritis, 78
Nizoral (ketoconazole)
    dosage of, 156t
    history of, 169
    and onychomycosis, 173
    for tinea pedis, 157
N-methylthiotetrazole (MTT)
        sidechain, 261–262
    antabuse reaction and, 208
    bleeding disorders due to, 207

    in cefamandole, 237
    in cefoperazone, 242
    in cefotetan, 236
    in cephalosporins, 233
Nocardia brasiliensis, 51
Nonclostridial anaerobic cellulitis,
        41–43
Nonclostridial myonecrosis, 45
Nontuberculous mycobacteria,
        301–302
Nosocomial fever, 10–13
Nosocomial infections, 183
    Alcaligenes in, 297
    cephalosporins for, 231
    ciprofloxacin for, 266
    H. influenza in, 298
    Morganella in, 293
    mycobacterium in, 301
    P. vulgaris in, 294
    Providencia in, 294
    rates of, 127–128
    Serratia in, 295
    surgical prophylaxis and, 140
Nuclear imaging, 61
Nurses and home IV antibiotic
        therapy, 199
Nutrition, patient, 134
Nystagmus, aminoglycoside usage
        and, 251

O

Obesity, infections in, 43, 134
Occupational Safety and Health
        Administration (OSHA)
        Internet site, 311t
Odor, foul
    associated with *Proteus*, 293
    in dermatophytosis complex tinea
        pedis, 151
    in diabetic foot infections, 110
    in moderate to severely infected
        ulcerations, 119
    in plantar space infections, 124
    and wound closure, 84
Office of the Inspector General
        (OIG), 165
Ofloxacin (Floxin)
    levofloxacin vs., 267
    Pexiganan (non-FDA approved)
        vs., 119
Omnicef (cefdinir), 243–244

Onychomycosis, 158–176
  classification of, 160–161
  definition of, 159
  diagnosis of, 162–164
  differential diagnosis of, 163
  facts and figures about, 158–159
  history of therapy for, 147
  microbiology of, 159–160
  monitoring antifungal therapy for,
      171–172
  oral agents for, 172–176
  oral antifungals and, 169–171
  topical antifungals and, 167–169
  treatment for, 161–162, 164–166
Operating room environment and
    surgical site infections, 135
Oral cavity flora, 289
Oropharynx surgery, endocarditis
    prophylaxis and, 144
Osteomyelitis, 54–75
  antibiotic treatment for, 66–67
  bone culture for diagnosis of,
      59–60
  ceftazidime alone for, 242
  Charcot's joint vs., 59, 62, 106
  ciprofloxacin for, 266
  classification of, 54–56
  clindamycin for, 258
  cure vs. arrest of, 65–66
  dead-space management of, 68–70
  diagnostic tests for, 57–59
  fixation devices for, 70
  groups C and G streptococci
      causing, 283
  H. influenza in, 298
  history taking for, 56
  home IV antibiotic therapy for, 199
  host types with, 56, 75
  hyperbaric oxygen therapy for, 70
  imaging for diagnosis of, 60–65
  Kingella kingae in, 288
  P. aeruginosa in, 299
  paronychia and, 32, 33, 34
  penicillin G for, 217
  puncture wounds and, 81t, 88
  S. aureus major cause of, 279
  Salmonella in, 295
  septic arthritis with, 76–79
  surgical treatment for, 67–68
  treatment principles for, 65–66
  types of, 54–55, 70–75

Osteomyelitis secondary to vascular
    insufficiency, 55, 74–75
Ototoxicity
  and aminoglycoside dosage, 253
  due to aminoglycoside, 250–251
  due to antibiotic usage, 200–201
  vancomycin usage and, 259
Over-the-counter products for
    onychomycosis, 167
Oxacillin, 31, 221, 279
Oxazolidinone antibiotic, 261–262
Oxiconazole (Oxistat), 156t, 158
Oxygen therapy, hyperbaric. *See*
    Hyperbaric oxygen therapy.
Oysters, *Vibrio vulnificus* in raw, 301

P

Pain. *See also* Calf tenderness; Skin
    tenderness.
  in arterial ulcerations, 122
  in clostridial myonecrosis, 44
  in dermatophytosis complex tinea
      pedis, 150–151
  in hematogenous osteomyelitis,
      71, 72
  in hematoma vs. infection, 129
  and infected vascular gangrene, 46
  in necrotizing fasciitis, 42
  in nonclostridial myonecrosis, 45
  in onychomycosis, 159
  in osteomyelitis, 57
  in post-op streptococcal
      infections, 282
  in pyomyositis, 47
  in secondary osteomyelitis, 75
  in septic arthritis, 76
  from stingray envenomation, 91
  in synergistic necrotizing cellulitis,
      43
Papineau grafting, 69
Parasitic infections, 51–52
Parenteral therapy and CDAD, 205.
    See also Antibiotic therapy;
    specific antibiotic.
Paronychia, 32–34, 293
Pasteur, Louis, 126
Pasteurella, 92
Pasteurella canis, 81t
Pasteurella multocida, 299
  septic arthritis due to, 78
  in trauma wound infections, 81t

Patient education
  vs. drug promotion, 147
  and home IV antibiotic therapy, 199
Patient history
  and antibiotic resistance, 184
  of bite wound trauma, 93
  in diagnosis of bone and joint infections, 56–57
  in diagnosis of lower extremity infections, 3–8
  of pedal puncture wound trauma, 85
Patient nutrition and infection, 134
Patient preparation for reducing infection, 132
Peak serum levels, 253, 254
Peak specimen, 188
Pedal puncture wound infections, 84–91
  in bone, 89–90
  in marine environment, 45, 90–91, 296, 301
  primary care for, 85–86
  in soft tissue, 89
  statistical data about, 84–85
  tetanus prophylaxis for, 87t
Penems. *See* Carbapenem antibiotics.
Penicillin G, 216–218
  for clostridial myonecrosis, 44
  forms of, 216–217
  history of, 213
  interstitial nephritis due to, 203
  against *S. aureus*, 280
Penicillin, penicillinase-resistant
  E. corrodens resistant to, 298
  P. multocida resistant to, 299
  against *S. aureus*, 280
Penicillin resistance, 214
  and ampicillin, 219
  of anaerobic gram-negative rods, 290
  of *Bacteroides*, 289
  in gonococcal infections, 288
  of group G and viridans streptococci, 283
  and penicillin G, 216–217
  and ticarcillin, 222
Penicillin V, 31, 218
Penicillin-binding protein (PBP), 214, 229

Penicillins, 213–228
  adverse reactions to, 216
  aminoglycosides given with, 198, 253, 283
  aminopenicillins subgroup of, 218–220
  aztreonam for patient allergic to, 249
  beta-lactamase inhibitors with, 224–228
  CDAD due to, 204
  cephalosporin reactions and, 211–212, 232
  classification of, 215b
  for clostridial cellulitis, 41
  for donor-leg cellulitis, 32
  dosages of, 303t
  for endocarditis prophylaxis, 144
  for erysipelas, 39
  for impetigo, 37
  and monobactams, 212
  nephrotoxicity due to, 203
  neutropenia due to, 206
  platelet dysfunction due to, 206, 207
  during pregnancy, 195
  seizures due to, 201
  semisynthetic subgroup of. *See* Penicillins, penicillinase-resistant.
  for tetanus, 286
  ureido- and carboxy- subgroups of. *See* Penicillins, expanded-spectrum.
Penicillins, drug activity of, 214–216
  Aeromonas resistant to, 296
  against anaerobic gram-positive cocci, 285
  Bacteroides resistant to, 289
  against *C. canimorsus*, 298
  against *C. perfringens*, 286
  vs. cefazolin, 233, 234
  vs. cephalexin and cephradine, 235
  vs. cephalosporin activity, 229, 233
  against *E. corrodens*, 298
  against enterococci, 284
  against *Fusobacterium*, 290
  against gonococci, 288
  against group G streptococci, 283
  against *Kingella kingae*, 289
  mechanism of action in, 214

Penicillins, drug activity of, (*Continued*)
against *P. multocida*, 299
vs. piperacillin, 224
S. maltophilia and *B. Cepacia* resistant to, 300
against systemic *N. meningitidis*, 288
vs. ticarcillin, 222
Penicillins, expanded-spectrum, 222–224
against *Citrobacter, Morganella, Serratia*, 291, 293, 295
against *E. coli* and *Klebsiella*, 292, 293
list of agents in, 215b
vs. mezlocillin, 223
spectrum of activity by, 215
Penicillins, natural, 216–218
list of agents in, 215b
nafcillin vs., 220
spectrum of activity by, 214
Penicillins, penicillinase-resistant, 220–221
for cellulitis, 31
vs. ciprofloxacin, 267
for donor-leg cellulitis, 32
list of agents in, 215b
spectrum of activity by, 215
and surgical prophylaxis, 140
Penlac (ciclopirox nail lacquer), 147, 167–168
Peptococcus, 285
cefazolin against, 233
in diabetic foot infections, 111
in moderate to severely infected ulcerations, 120
nonclostridial cellulitis due to, 41
synergistic necrotizing cellulitis due to, 43
Peptostreptococcus, 285
cefazolin against, 233
in diabetic foot infections, 111
in moderate to severely infected ulcerations, 120
nonclostridial cellulitis due to, 41
Periodic acid-Schiff (PAS) preparation, 164
Peripheral neuropathy, 202
Peripheral vascular disease, 6, 46
Pets, infections and, 8
Pexiganan (non-FDA approved), 119
Pharmaceutical industry
drug in vivo activity reported by, 190

promotion of oral antifungals by, 169, 171
promotion vs. education by, 147
Pharmacokinetics, of antibiotics, 191–192
Phenol and alcohol procedure (P&A), 33–34
Phenoxymethyl penicillin, 218
Phlebectomy, cellulitis following, 31–32
Phlebitis
due to cephalosporins, 233
due to IV quinupristin/ dalfopristin, 261
Photosensitivity
due to antibiotic usage, 208–209
due to ciprofloxacin, 265
due to tetracyclines, 274
Physical examination
in diagnosis of bone and joint infections, 56–57
in diagnosis of lower extremity infections, 8–14
in pedal puncture wound trauma, 85
Physicians' Desk Reference
drug renal clearance information in, 195
Internet site of, 311t
Piperacillin (Pipracil), 224
Piperacillin/tazobactam (Zosyn), 228
for bite wound infections, 93
for ecthyma, 39
against enterococci, 284
vs. ertapenem, 248
for infected vascular gangrene, 46
for moderate to severely infected ulcerations, 121
for nonclostridial cellulitis, 42
for post-puncture-wound osteomyelitis, 90
for puncture wound infections, 89
Pityriasis rubra pilaris, 163
Plantar space infections, 123–124
Platelet dysfunction, 206–207, 222
Pneumonia, 12, 270
Podiatric patients, 31
Podiatric physician
manual toenail debridement by, 165
onychomycosis patients of, 158

oral antifungal most ordered by, 175
on oral antifungal therapy, 171
Polymerase chain reaction (PCR), 49,
77
Polymorphonuclear leukocytes
(PMNs), 14–15, 20
Porphyromonas, 81t, 92
Porphyromonas asaccharolytica, 290
Postantibiotic effect (PAE), 193, 254
Postoperative infections. *See also*
Surgical site infections.
beta-hemolytic streptococci in, 282
cellulitis in, 9–10
clostridial myonecrosis in, 44
contiguous focus osteomyelitis as,
73
costs of, 127
etiologies of, 4
necrotizing fasciitis as, 42
septic arthritis as, 76
tissue gas in, 110
Potassium hydroxide (KOH)
preparation, diagnostic
in diagnosis of lower extremity
infections, 22–23
for onychomycosis, 162, 163, 164
for tinea pedis, 151
Potassium level, 17
Povidone iodine (Betadine)
for infections following trauma, 83
for noninfected mal perforans, 117
for puncture wound infections, 86
Pregnancy
antibiotic selection during, 195
and tetracycline, 203, 274
Preoperative preparation for
reducing infection, 132–133
Pressure relief for noninfected mal
perforans, 116
Prevotella melaninogenica, 290
Primaxin. *See* Imipenem and cilastatin.
Probenecid
amoxicillin with, 220
ampicillin with, 219
cefazolin and, 234
cephalexin and cephradine and, 234
cloxacillin and dicloxacillin with,
221
mezlocillin and, 223
nafcillin with, 220
penicillin G with, 217

ticarcillin with, 222
Procaine penicillin, 216, 217
Proctoscopy, for diagnosis of CDAD,
204
Prostaglandin production, drugs
inhibiting, 11
Prosthetic joint implants. *See*
Implants, surgical.
Protein binding of drug, 192
cefoperazone and, 242
ceftriaxone and, 241
Proteus, 292–294
azithromycin against, 272
in moderate to severely infected
ulcerations, 120
second-generation cephalosporins
against, 231, 232
ticarcillin against, 222
in trauma wound infections, 81t
Proteus mirabilis
and ampicillin, 219
cefazolin against, 233
cephalosporins against, 231
in diabetic foot infections, 111
foot flora with, 293
noninfected mal perforans and,
116
paronychia due to, 33
tinea pedis and, 149
*Proteus morganii. See Morganella
morganii.*
Proteus vulgaris, 294
Prothrombin time, 207
Providencia, 264
Proximal white onychomycosis, 161,
162
Pruritus
in cutaneous larva migrans (CLM),
52
due to antibiotic usage, 211
due to vancomycin, 259
in erythrasma, 35
in vesicular tinea pedis, 150
Pseudomembranous colitis,
205–206, 256
*Pseudomonas. See also Burkholderia
cepacia; Stenotrophomonas
maltophilia.*
appearance of, 20t
beta-lactamase by, 225
cefepime against, 244

Pseudomonas. (*Continued*)
  cefoperazone dosage in infections
    with, 243
  ciprofloxacin against, 264
  color of infection with, 95
  ecthyma due to, 38
  glycocalyx formation by, 134
Pseudomonas aeruginosa, 299–300
  in burn wound infections, 96
  diabetic foot infections and, 111
  ecthyma due to, 38, 39
  folliculitis due to, 35
  hematogenous osteomyelitis due
    to, 72
  infections caused by, 4
  in IV drug users, 7
  in marine puncture wounds, 90
  noninfected mal perforans and, 116
  onychomycosis vs., 160
  osteomyelitis due to, 26
  paronychia with, 34
  septic arthritis due to, 78
  tinea pedis and, 149
  in trauma wound infections, 81t, 88
Pseudomonas aeruginosa (drug activity
    in)
  aminoglycosides against, 249
  aztreonam against, 248
  beta-lactamase inhibitor
    combinations against, 225
  cefdinir ineffective against, 243
  cefepime against, 245
  cefixime and ceftibuten ineffective
    against, 244
  cefoperazone against, 242
  cefotaxime ineffective against, 240
  ceftazidime most active for, 242
  cephalosporins against, 231, 232
  ciprofloxacin against, 264, 266
  drug combinations against, 249
  ertapenem ineffective against, 247
  imipenem/cilastatin and, 246
  levofloxacin less active against, 267
  levofloxacin vs. ciprofloxacin
    against, 268
  list of antibiotics against, 310t
  meropenem against, 247
  mezlocillin against, 223
  mupirocin poor against, 98t
  piperacillin against, 224
  ticarcillin against, 222

  tobramycin against, 249
Psoriasis vs. other infections, 161, 163
Pulmonary emboli, nosocomial fever
    with, 12
Pulse dosing
  drug interactions and, 170
  pros and cons of antifungal,
    174–175
Pulse volume recordings, 122
Puncture wound infection. *See also*
    Pedal puncture wound
    infections.
  antibiotic prophylaxis preventing,
    138
  bone scan differentiation of, 63
  contiguous focus osteomyelitis
    secondary to, 73
  organisms causing, 81t
  septic arthritis from, 76, 78
  V. vulnificus causing, 301
Pus, skeletal muscle, 46–47
Pyomyositis, 46–47
Pyridoxine, 202
Pyrogens, 10–11

Q

QT interval changes, 264
Quality of life, 159
Quantitative bacteriology, 22
Quinine, 50
Quinolone resistance in non-U.S.
    gonococcal infections, 288
Quinolones, 264–269
  for bite wound infections, 93
  vs. cefoperazone, 243
  vs. cefotaxime, 240
  dosages of, 304t
  drug combinations using, 224, 257
  for infected vascular gangrene, 46
  for marine puncture wounds, 90
  for moderate to severely infected
    ulcerations, 121
  for nonclostridial cellulitis, 42
  for open fracture infections, 100
Quinolones, drug activity of
  against *Acinetobacter*, 296
  against *Aeromonas*, 297
  against *B. henselae*, 297
  against *C. canimorsus*, 298
  against *Citrobacter, Morganella,
    Serratia*, 291, 293, 295

against *E. coli* and *Klebsiella*, 292, 293
against *E. corrodens*, 298
against *H. influenza*, 299
against *Kingella kingae*, 289
against *P. mirabilis*, 294
against *P. multocida*, 299
against *P. vulgaris* and *Providencia*, 294
against *Salmonella*, 295
Quinupristin/dalfopristin (Synercid), 260–261, 285

R

Radiography
of bite wound, 93
of Charcot's joint, 106
of clostridial cellulitis, 40
of clostridial myonecrosis, 44
of contiguous focus osteomyelitis, 73
of hematogenous osteomyelitis, 71
of infected vascular gangrene, 46
of nonclostridial myonecrosis, 45
of osteomyelitis, 60, 61, 65
of paronychia, 33
after pedal puncture wound trauma, 85
of plantar space infections, 124
of puncture wound infections, 88
of septic arthritis, 76
Rash
due to ampicillin, 219
due to antibiotic usage, 208–209, 210
due to cephalosporins, 233
due to rifampin, 262
due to sulfonamide, 269
due to tetracyclines, 274
Red man (Red neck) syndrome, 208, 259
Renal failure
amoxicillin dosage in, 220
amoxicillin/clavulanic acid dosage in, 227
ampicillin/sulbactam dosage in, 227
cefazolin dosage in, 234
cefotaxime dosage in, 240
cephalexin and cephradine dosage in, 234
clindamycin dosage in, 257

due to quinolones, 264
nafcillin dosage and, 221
single daily dosing and, 254
ticarcillin/clavulanic acid dosage in, 226
Renal function
antibiotic dosages and, 17
metronidazole usage and, 256
normal, defined, 252–253
vancomycin usage and, 259
Renal impairment. *See also* Creatinine levels, serum.
aminoglycosides toxicities and, 255
antibiotic selection in, 194–195
aztreonam dosage in, 248
cefotetan dosage in, 236
cefoxitin dosage in, 236
ceftazidime dosage in, 242
ceftizoxime dosage in, 240
ceftriaxone and, 241
cefuroxime dosage in, 237
ciprofloxacin dosage in, 266
cloxacillin and dicloxacillin dosage in, 221
diabetic foot infections and, 109
imipenem/cilastatin dosage in, 246
nephrotoxicity and, 202–203
ototoxicity and, 200, 202
penicillin G dosage in, 217
penicillin V dosage in, 218
Respiratory tract infections
cefdinir for, 243
cefixime and ceftibuten for, 244
clarithromycin for, 272
Klebsiella in, 293
viridans streptococci causing, 283
Rheumatoid arthritis
septic arthritis vs., 77
septic arthritis with, 76
surgical prophylaxis for, 139
Richmond-Sykes I beta-lactamase, chromosomal
beta-lactamase combinations and, 225
carbapenem agents resistant to, 245
cefotaxime and organisms with, 240
cephalosporins inactivated by, 229

Rifampin, 262–263
with ciprofloxacin, 265
with ethambutol, 91, 301
with minocycline, 274, 281
possibly against *Corynebacterium*,
287
with trimethoprim/
sulfamethoxazole, 281
with vancomycin, 197, 263
with vancomycin, and an
aminoglycoside, 281

S

Sabouraud's agar, 152
Safety
of aminoglycosides, 249, 250, 254
in antibiotic selection, 181
of azithromycin vs. erythromycin,
271
of aztreonam, 248
of cephalosporins, 232
of cloxacillin and dicloxacillin, 221
of linezolid, 262
of oral antifungals, 169
of penicillins, 216
of quinupristin/dalfopristin, 261
of "T&T" combination, 223
of tetracyclines vs. other
antibiotics, 273
of vancomycin, 259
Saliva, injection site infections and,
39
Salmonella, 295
ampicillin and, 219
cephalosporins against, 231
hematogenous osteomyelitis due
to, 72
ticarcillin/clavulanic acid against,
225
Salt water organisms, 301
Saphenous vein graft, cellulitis
following harvesting of, 31
Saprophytic molds, 149, 160
Sardinia, 228
Scalded skin syndrome,
staphylococcal, 36–37
Scarring, osteomyelitis and, 57
Schlicter test, 188–189
Scintigraphy
of osteomyelitis, 61
paronychia and, 33, 34

Scopulariopsis brevicaulis, 160
Scytalidium dimidiatum, 149, 160
Scytalidium hyalinum, 149
Seizures
due to antibiotic usage, 201–202
due to imipenem, 246
due to metronidazole, 256
myoclonic, from penicillins, 216
Sensory neuropathy, 105
Sepsis, 13–14
aminoglycosides for, 255
in burn wound infections, 94, 97
criteria for diagnosis of, 14
CRP indicator of, 58
differential diagnosis of, 8
hospitalization for, 26
in moderate to severely infected
ulcerations, 119
in necrotizing fasciitis, 42
P. aeruginosa causing, 299
in plantar space infections, 124
Vibrio vulnificus causing, 300–301
Septic arthritis (SA), 76–79
bacterial etiology of, 78
bite wound infections causing, 92
ceftriaxone for, 241
differential diagnosis of, 77
gonococcal infection and, 287–288
gout vs., 77
groups C and G streptococci
causing, 283
H. influenza causing, 298
Kingella kingae causing, 288
laboratory findings of, 77–78
osteomyelitis secondary to, 73
penicillin G and, 217–218
rapid-growing mycobacteria in,
302
types of, 76
Septicemia. *See also* Bacteremia;
Toxemia.
in clostridial myonecrosis, 44
in marine puncture wounds, 90
in pyomyositis, 47
in scalded skin syndrome, 36
Septra, 269–270
Serrati S, 295
Serratia, 295
beta-lactamase by, 225
ciprofloxacin against, 264
in diabetic foot infections, 111

gentamicin against, 249
trimethoprim/sulfamethoxazole
    and, 269
Serum bactericidal titer (SBT),
    188–189
Serum sickness, 211
Shaving and infections, 132
Shigella, 219, 231
Shoes
    and noninfected mal perforans, 116
    and onychomycosis, 159
    and tinea pedis, 153
    "Shotgun therapy", 197
Sickle cell disease, osteomyelitis in,
    72, 295
Sigmoidoscopy for diagnosis of
    CDAD, 204
Signs and symptoms in diagnosis of
    lower extremity infections, 4–5,
    8–14
Silvadene (silver sulfadiazine), 117
Silver nitrate solution, 96, 98t
Silver sulfadiazine (Silvadene)
    for burn wound, 96, 98t
    for noninfected mal perforans, 117
    and wound care, 83
Sinus tract, in osteomyelitis, 57
Skeletal muscle, pyomyositis of, 46
Skin and soft tissue infections,
    30–53. *See also* Fungal
    infections.
    Acinetobacter in, 296
    amoxicillin/clavulanic acid for, 227
    azithromycin for, 272
    beta-hemolytic streptococci in, 282
    cefdinir for, 243, 244
    cefpodoxime proxetil for, 244
    ceftazidime for, 242
    groups C and G streptococci in, 283
    levofloxacin for, 267
    moxifloxacin for, 268
    P. aeruginosa in, 300
    Vibrio vulnificus in, 300–301
Skin changes with
    infections/trauma, 94, 109
Skin flora, 286
Skin graft, 69, 96
"Skin popped", 38
Skin tenderness, 36
Smoking in diagnosis of lower
    extremity infections, 7

"Sneaker osteomyelitis", 88
Soaks, foot. *See also* Compresses,
    warm.
    and paronychia, 33
    for puncture wound trauma, 86
    for stingray envenomation, 91
Social history in diagnosis of lower
    extremity infections, 7
Society of Critical Care Medicine,
    13–14
Sodium hypochlorite (Dakin's
    solution), 117
Sodium level, serum
    in diagnosis of lower extremity
        infections, 17
    and mezlocillin usage, 223
    and penicillin usage, 216
    and ticarcillin/clavulanic acid
        usage, 226
Southern U.S.
    cutaneous larva migrans (CLM) in,
        52
    Madura foot in, 51
Spectazole (econazole), 156t, 157
Spleen, *C. canimorsus* in patients
    without, 298
Spondyloarthropathies,
    seronegative, 77
Sporanox (itraconazole)
    history of, 147, 169
    for onychomycosis, 174–175
Staining and culturing techniques,
    special
    for Lyme disease, 49
    for Madura foot, 51
    for onychomycosis, 164
Staphylococcal scalded skin
    syndrome, 36–37
Staphylococci
    in bite wound infections, 92
    in burn wound infections, 96
    carried by surgeon, 133
    furuncle and carbuncle due to,
        36
    indications for use of clindamycin
        against, 257
    infected vascular gangrene due to,
        46
    nonclostridial cellulitis due to, 41
    in osteomyelitis, 58
    paronychia due to, 33

Staphylococci (drug activity in)
aminoglycosides in drug
combinations against, 250
amoxicillin/clavulanic acid
against, 226
ampicillin/sulbactam against, 228
azithromycin against, 272
cefamandole against resistant, 238
cefazolin against, 234
cefdinir against, 243
cefepime against, 244
cefpodoxime proxetil vs. cefdinir
against, 244
ceftriaxone against, 242
cefuroxime against, 237
cefuroxime axetil against, 239
cephalexin/cephradine vs.
penicillins against, 235
cephalosporins against, 232
cloxacillin and dicloxacillin
against, 221
erythromycin against, 271
levofloxacin vs. ciprofloxacin
against, 267
mezlocillin not against most, 223
nafcillin against, 221
piperacillin ineffective against,
224
quinupristin/dalfopristin against,
261
resistance to ciprofloxacin of, 265
rifampin against, 262
tetracyclines against, 274, 275
ticarcillin and, 222
ticarcillin/clavulanic acid against,
225
trimethoprim/sulfamethoxazole
against, 269, 270
Staphylococci, coagulase-negative
(CNS), 111, 281–282
Staphylococci, non-penicillinase-
producing. See *Staphylococcus
aureus*, penicillin-sensitive.
Staphylococci, penicillinase-
producing. See *Staphylococcus
aureus*, methicillin-sensitive.
Staphylococcus
appearance of, 20t
glycocalyx formation by, 134
susceptibility of, 140
Staphylococcus aureus, 278–281
antibiotics for infection with,
280–281
cefazolin against non-resistant, 233
cefepime against, 245
ceftriaxone against, 242
cellulitis due to, 31
cephalosporins against, 229
clindamycin against, 257
diabetic foot infections due to, 111
endocarditis prophylaxis against,
144
folliculitis due to, 35
hematogenous osteomyelitis due
to, 71
impetigo due to, 37
injection site infections due to,
38–39
mildly infected ulcerations due to,
118
moderate to severely infected
ulcerations due to, 120
noninfected mal perforans and, 116
notoriety and virulence of, 134
open fracture infections due to,
100
post operative infections due to, 4
puncture wound infections due to,
88
pyomyositis due to, 47
resistance patterns of, 279–280
scalded skin syndrome due to, 37
septic arthritis due to, 78
surgical prophylaxis against, 140
in trauma wound infections, 81t
Staphylococcus aureus, methicillin-
resistant (MRSA), 279
antibiotics for infection with, 281
in burn wound infections, 96, 97
in community setting, 183
in hematogenous osteomyelitis, 72
in hospital and community
settings, 140
imipenem against some strains of,
246
in IV drug users, 7
laboratory reporting of, 280
minocycline against, 274
mupirocin against, 98t
in open fracture infections, 100
quinupristin/dalfopristin against,
261

significant resistance to
ciprofloxacin of, 265
in surgical setting, 4
as "therapeutic hole", 197
trimethoprim/sulfamethoxazole
against, 269, 270
vancomycin against, 259
Staphylococcus aureus, methicillin-
sensitive, 279
antibiotics for infection with, 280
first-generation cephalosporins
against, 231
nafcillin against, 220, 279
Staphylococcus aureus, penicillin-
sensitive, 279
antibiotics against, 280
first-generation cephalosporins
against, 231
and penicillin G, 217
Staphylococcus aureus, vancomycin-
intermediate (VISA), 259,
279–280
antibiotics against, 281
in hospital and community
settings, 140
prevention best treatment for, 281
Staphylococcus epidermidis, 281–282
contamination by, 25
hematogenous osteomyelitis due
to, 72
infections caused by, 4, 5
in joint implant infections, 140
latent infections due to, 134
noninfected mal perforans and, 116
in prosthetic joint implants, 129
in trauma wound infections, 81t
wound closure and, 84
Staphylococcus epidermidis,
methicillin-resistant (MRSE),
282
in implant infections, 140
in surgical site infections, 4, 134
vancomycin against, 259, 260
Staphylococcus epidermidis,
vancomycin-resistant (VRE),
261, 282
Stenotrophomonas maltophilia, 300
resistant to aztreonam, 248
resistant to ciprofloxacin, 265
resistant to imipenem/cilastatin,
246

trimethoprim/sulfamethoxazole
against, 269, 270
Sterilization, surgical instrument, 135
Steroids, septic arthritis and, 76, 78
Stevens-Johnson syndrome, 209, 269
Stingray envenomation, 91
Stomatitis due to antibiotic usage, 206
Streptococcal fasciitis, 42–43
Streptococci
in bite wound infections, 92
in burn wound infections, 96
ecthyma due to, 38
endocarditis prophylaxis for, 144
nonclostridial cellulitis due to, 41
paronychia due to, 33
in puncture wound infections, 88
Streptococci, alpha-hemolytic, 81t
Streptococci (drug activity in)
aminoglycosides/beta-lactam
against, 250, 255
amoxicillin/clavulanic acid
against, 226
ampicillin against, 218, 224
azithromycin against, 272
cefazolin vs. penicillin against,
233, 234
cefdinir vs. cephalexin against, 243
cefepime against, 244
cefpodoxime proxetil vs. cefdinir
against, 244
cephalosporins against, 231, 232
ciprofloxacin unreliable against,
265
clindamycin against, 257
erythromycin against, 271
levofloxacin vs. ciprofloxacin
against, 267
nafcillin vs. other penicillins
against, 220
penicillin G against, 216, 217
piperacillin and other penicillins
against, 224
rifampin against, 262
tetracyclines against, 274, 275
ticarcillin vs. penicillin against,
222
ticarcillin/clavulanic acid against,
225
trimethoprim/sulfamethoxazole
against some, 269
vancomycin against, 259

Streptococci, group A beta-hemolytic, 282–283. *See also Streptococcus pyogenes.*
  cellulitis caused by, 31
  donor-leg cellulitis due to, 32
  erysipelas due to, 39
  impetigo due to, 37
  injection site infections due to, 39
  limb necrosis due to, 129
  necrotizing fasciitis due to, 42
  in trauma wound infections, 81t
Streptococci, group B beta-hemolytic, 282–283. *See also Streptococcus agalactiae.*
  common infections with, 4
  infected vascular gangrene due to, 46
  in moderate to severely infected ulcerations, 120
  septic arthritis due to, 78
  in trauma wound infections, 81t
Streptococci, group D. *See* Enterococci.
Streptococci, groups C and G beta-hemolytic, 283–284
Streptococci, viridans, 283–284
Streptococcus
  appearance of, 20t
  myonecrosis due to, 45
  in trauma wound infections, 81t
Streptococcus agalactiae, 282–283. *See also* Streptococci, group B beta-hemolytic.
  in diabetic foot infections, 111
  mildly infected ulcerations due to, 118
Streptococcus pyogenes, 111, 282–283. *See also* Streptococci, group A beta-hemolytic.
Subacute bacterial endocarditis (SBE), 8
Subcutaneous infections, 39–47
Sugar for wound care, 83
"Suicide agent", 225
Sulconazole (Exelderm), 156t, 158
Sulfonamides, 269–270
  agranulocytosis due to, 206
  hemolytic anemia with, 194, 207
  hypoglycemia with, 194
  "Superbug", 284
Superficial infections, 30–39

Superinfection, 145, 206, 274
Suprax (cefixime), 244
Surgeon preparation for reducing infection, 132–133
Surgery, endocarditis prophylaxis and elective, 144
Surgery length
  antibiotic prophylaxis and, 139
  infection rate related to, 131
Surgical apparel and surgical site infections, 135
Surgical debridement
  of bite wound, 93
  of burn wound, 96
  for clostridial cellulitis, 40, 41
  for clostridial myonecrosis, 44
  for contiguous focus osteomyelitis, 74
  to diagnosis necrotizing fasciitis, 42
  and dorsal space infections, 125
  followed by dead-space management, 68–70
  followed by home IV antibiotic therapy, 199
  during hospitalization, 27
  for infections following trauma, 82
  for infections with *C. perfringens*, 286
  for marine puncture wounds, 90
  for mildly infected ulcerations, 118
  for mycobacteria-infected sites, 302
  for necrotizing fasciitis, 43
  for nonclostridial cellulitis, 41
  for nonclostridial myonecrosis, 45
  for noninfected mal perforans, 116
  for post-puncture-wound osteomyelitis, 89
  for secondary osteomyelitis, 75
  for synergistic necrotizing cellulitis, 43
Surgical drains, infection in, 130
Surgical incision and drainage
  of bite wound, 93
  endocarditis prophylaxis for, 144
  of furuncles and carbuncles, 36
  of infected puncture wounds, 89
  of *M. marinum*-infected lesion, 301
  of marine puncture wounds, 90, 91

of moderate to severely infected
ulcerations, 120
of mycobacteria-infected sites, 302
of plantar space infected abscess,
124
of pyomyositis pus, 47
of septic arthritic joints, 79
of *V. vulnificus*-infected wounds,
301
Surgical prophylaxis, 138–140
adverse effects and failures of, 145
antibiotic agents for, 141–143
antibiotic selection and
administration for, 140–141
cefamandole for, 237
cefazolin for, 234
cefuroxime for, 237
cephalexin/cephradine for
outpatient, 235
for risk of endocarditis, 143–145
vancomycin for, 260
Surgical scrubs for reducing
infection, 132–133
Surgical site infections (SSIs),
126–135. *See also* Postoperative
infections.
history and incidence of, 126–127
operating room factors in, 135
pathogen factors of, 134
patient factors of, 133–134
rapid-growing mycobacteria in,
302
risk factors of, 127–128, 127f
surgical factors of, 128–133
Surgical technique, breaches of,
129–133
Survival rate for leg amputees, 104
Sutures and sutures technique,
infections caused by, 130
"Swarming" organism, 294
Swimming pools
fungal infections and, 153
puncture wounds and, 90–91
Synercid (quinupristin/dalfopristin),
260–261
Synergistic necrotizing cellulitis, 43
Synergistic nonclostridial anaerobic
myonecrosis, 45
Synergy drug interaction, 196–197
Synovial fluid analysis, 77–78
Systemic lupus erythematosus, 209

T

Tachycardia, 208
Taste disturbances
due to clarithromycin, 273
due to metronidazole, 256
with terbinafine (Lamisil) usage,
175, 176
Taylor GJ, 136
Tazicef/Tazidime (ceftazidime), 242
Tea tree oil (*Melaleuca alternifolia*),
155, 167
Technetium 99 MDP bone scans
for diagnosis of osteomyelitis,
62–63, 65
in post-puncture-wound
osteomyelitis, 88
Teeth, staining of, 274
Teichoic acid antibodies, 16–17, 58
Teicoplanin (non-FDA approved),
143, 263
Tendonopathies, 265
Tequin. *See* Gatifloxacin.
Teratogenicity, 195
Terbinafine (Lamisil AT)
dosage of, 156t
history of, 147, 169
for onychomycosis, 175–176
for tinea pedis, 155
Tetanus prophylaxis, 285–286
after bite wound trauma, 93
indications for, 87t
after puncture wound trauma, 86
Tetracycline, 273–275
children and, 194
dermatologic reactions due to,
208–209
dosage of, 304t
GI side effects due to, 206
hepatotoxicity due to, 203
against *Kingella kingae*, 289
for marine puncture wounds, 90,
91
pregnancy and, 195
for tetanus, 286
Tetracyclines, 273–275
vs. macrolides, 273
against *S. aureus*, 280
Theophylline, 265
"Therapeutic holes", 197
Thermoregulation, 10, 13
Thiabendazole, 52

Thienamycin, 245
Thrombocytopenia
    due to linezolid, 262
    due to penicillins, 216
    in ehrlichiosis, 50
Thrombophlebitis. *See also* Deep vein
    thrombophlebitis (DVT).
    vs. donor-leg cellulitis, 32
    due to erythromycin, 271
    due to tetracyclines, 274
    nosocomial fever with, 12
Thrombosis, 124
Ticarcillin, 222-223
    platelet dysfunction due to, 207
    pregnancy and, 195
Ticarcillin/clavulanic acid
    (Timentin), 225-226
    for bite wound infections, 93
    for infected vascular gangrene, 46
    for moderate to severely infected
        ulcerations, 121
    for nonclostridial cellulitis, 41
    vs. piperacillin/tazobactam, 226,
        228
    against *S. maltophilia* and *B.
        Cepacia*, 300
    vs. ticarcillin alone, 225
Tick-borne zoonosis, 50
Timentin. *See* Ticarcillin/clavulanic
    acid.
"Tinea incognito", 151
Tinea pedis, 148-158
    cellulitis due to, 32
    definition of, 148
    diagnosis of, 151-152
    erythrasma vs., 35
    microbiology of, 149
    oral agents for, 155, 170, 172
    topical agents for, 154-158
    treatment for, 153-154
    types of, 150-151
    variants of, 148
Tinea unguium, 159
Tinnitus, 200, 251
Tioconazole (non-FDA approved), 167
Tissue gas
    in clostridial cellulitis, 40
    in clostridial myonecrosis, 44
    CT scan to locate, 65
    in diabetic foot infections, 110
    in infected vascular gangrene, 46

    in moderate to severely infected
        ulcerations, 119
    in necrotizing fasciitis, 42
    in nonclostridial myonecrosis, 45
    in plantar space infections, 124
    in synergistic necrotizing cellulitis,
        43
Tissue infections. *See* Skin and soft
    tissue infections.
Tissue penetration of drug, 191-192
Tissue transplant, 69
Tobramycin (Nebcin), 249
    for dead-space management, 69
    normal blood levels of, 253
    with ticarcillin, 223
Toenail
    avulsion of, 33-34
    debridement of, 165
    discoloration of, 160
    DSO in stratum corneum of, 161
    fungal infection of, 159
    infected ingrown, 32
    proximal white onychomycosis in,
        161
    surgical removal of, 166
    treatment of fungal infections in,
        161-162
    white superficial onychomycosis
        (WSO) in, 161
Total dystrophic onychomycosis,
    161, 162
Toxemia. *See also* Bacteremia;
    Septicemia.
    in clostridial cellulitis, 40
    in clostridial myonecrosis, 44
    in impetigo, 37
    in moderate to severely infected
        ulcerations, 119
    in necrotizing fasciitis, 42
    in nonclostridial cellulitis, 41
    in synergistic necrotizing cellulitis,
        43
Toxic epidermal necrolysis (TEN),
    36, 209
Toxic megacolon, 205
Toxic shock syndrome, 282
Toxicities. *See* Antibiotic usage.
Toxin titers and diagnosis of CDAD,
    204
Toxins
    from *Bacteroides*, 289

from *C. perfringens*, 286
from *C. tetani*, 285
Trade names of antibiotics, 305t–309t
Transcutaneous oxygen, 122
Transient bacteremia, 24
Trauma
  cellulitis due to, 9, 30
  clostridial myonecrosis after, 44
  Madura foot after, 51
  myonecrosis from marine, 45
  necrotizing fasciitis from, 42
  onychomycosis vs. changes from, 163
  puncture wound in marine, 90–91, 296, 301
  pyomyositis and, 47
  septic arthritis from, 76, 77
  surgery as, 133
Trauma, infections following, 80–102
  Acinetobacter in, 296
  antibiotic prophylaxis for, 138
  bite wounds and, 91–94
  burn wounds and, 94–97
  factors leading to, 80–82
  open fractures in, 97–101
  organisms causing, 81t
  pedal puncture wounds and, 84–91
  surgical prophylaxis for, 139
  tissue gas due to, 110
  wound care for, 82–84
Travel history
  cutaneous larva migrans (CLM) and, 8, 52
  in diagnosis of lower extremity infections, 7–8
  Madura foot and, 51
  pyomyositis and, 46
Treponema, 25
Treponema pallidum, 81t
Trichomonas vaginalis, 255
Trichophyton mentagrophytes
  fungal infections due to, 148
  tinea pedis due to, 149
  vesicular tinea pedis due to, 150
  white superficial onychomycosis (WSO) due to, 161
Trichophyton rubrum
  distal subungual onychomycosis (DSO) due to, 161

fungal infections due to, 148
  moccasin tinea pedis due to, 150
  proximal white onychomycosis due to, 161
  tinea pedis due to, 149
Trichophyton tonsurans, 148
Trimethoprim/sulfamethoxazole (Bactrim, Septra), 269–270
  against *Aeromonas*, 297
  against *B. henselae*, 297
  against *Citrobacter, Morganella, Serratia*, 291, 293, 295
  dosage of, 304t
  against *E. coli* and *Klebsiella*, 292, 293
  against *E. corrodens*, 298
  against *H. influenza*, 299
  against *M. marinum*, 301
  for marine puncture wounds, 90
  for mycobacteria infections, 302
  against *P. mirabilis*, 294
  against *P. multocida*, 299
  against *S. aureus*, 280, 281
  against *S. maltophilia* and *B. Cepacia*, 300
Tropical regions, infections in, 46, 51
Trough serum levels, 253, 254
Trovafloxacin (Trovan), 268–269
Tuberculosis (TB), osteomyelitis with extra-pulmonary, 72
Type I reaction, 210

U

Ulcerations. *See also* Mal perforans ulcerations.
  anaerobic gram-negative rods in, 290
  in arterial insufficiency, 121–122
  classification of, 112–114
  of injection site, 38–39
  in osteomyelitis, 73, 75
  risk of, 104
Ulcerations, mildly infected, 117–119
Ulcerations, moderate to severely infected, 119–121
Unasyn. *See* Ampicillin/sulbactam.
"Unholy triad", 104
University of Texas, San Antonio, 113b

Ureidopenicillins, 215t, 223, 224
Urinary tract infection (UTI)
  bacteremia due to, 24
  carbenicillin for, 222
  hematogenous osteomyelitis due
    to, 72
  nosocomial fever with, 12
  trimethoprim/sulfamethoxazole
    for, 269
Urine, alternative therapy using, 83,
  167
Urosepsis, 8
Urticaria, 211
U.S. Army, 213

V

Vancomycin (Vancocin), 258–260
  and beta-lactam, 281
  for CDAD, 205
  for cellulitis, 31
  against *Corynebacterium*, 287
  for dead-space management, 69
  for ecthyma, 39
  against enterococci, 284
  to fill "therapeutic holes", 197
  monitoring blood levels of, 209,
    260
  nephrotoxicity and, 203, 250
  neutropenia due to, 206
  for open fracture infections, 100
  ototoxicity due to, 201
  for pyomyositis, 47
  red man syndrome due to, 208
  resistance to, 259, 279
  and rifampin, 197
  against *S. aureus*, 280, 281
  for scalded skin syndrome, 37
  for streptococcal infections, 283
  for surgical prophylaxis, 142
Vantin (cefpodoxime proxetil), 244
Vascular insufficiency, osteomyelitis
  and, 55, 74–75
Vascular studies, 32, 75
Vegetables, contamination of, 299
Velocef (cephradine), 234–235
Venography, 32
Venous occlusions, acute, 9, 30
Vertigo, 201, 251
Vesicles
  in impetigo, 37
  in vesicular tinea pedis, 150

Vestibular impairment/toxicity,
  200–201, 251
Vibrio
  vs. *A. hydrophilia*, 296
  in marine puncture wounds, 90
  myonecrosis due to, 45
Vibrio vulnificus, 300–301
Viral infections
  and ampicillin, 219
  with bacterial infections, 211
  in diagnosis of lower extremity
    infections, 25
  septic arthritis from, 78
Vision and diabetic foot infections,
  108
Vitamin K, 207
Vitamin K metabolism disorders,
  206, 207

W

Wagner classification system of
  ulceration, 112–113, 114
Waldvogel, F, 55
Warts, 148
"Water-loving" organisms, 90–91,
  296
Western blot techniques, 49
Wet mount, 152
White blood cell count (WBC)
  and antibiotic usage, 206
  in cellulitis, 30
  and contiguous focus
    osteomyelitis, 73
  in diagnosis of lower extremity
    infections, 14–15
  in hematogenous osteomyelitis,
    71
  hospitalization for elevated, 26, 27
  in mildly infected ulcerations, 118
  in moderate to severely infected
    ulcerations, 119
  in plantar space infections, 124
  prior to antifungal therapy, 171
  in puncture wound infections, 86
  in sepsis, 14
  in septic arthritis, 78
White blood cells in site infections, 3
White superficial onychomycosis
  (WSO), 161, 162
Wood's lamp examination, 35, 287
World War II, 213

Wound care
    following burn trauma, 97,
        98t-99t
    following pedal trauma, 85–86
    for infections following trauma,
        82–84
    for puncture wound infections, 89
Wound care, passive, 116–117
Wound closure
    of burn wound, 96
    infections caused by surgical, 131
    for infections following trauma,
        83–84
    of noninfected bite wound, 93
Wound healing
    cellulitis with, 9
    dead-space infection in, 129
    dead-space management for, 68
    growth factors for active, 117
Wound prophylaxis, 138

X

Xanthomonas. See Stenotrophomonas
    maltophilia.
X-ray. *See* Radiography.

Y

Yeast infection. *See also Candida.*
    due to antibiotic usage, 206
    mafenide acetate and, 98t
    silver nitrate solution for, 98t
    silver sulfadiazine for, 98t

Z

Zaias N, 149, 160
Zinacef (cefuroxime), 237
Zithromax. *See* Azithromycin.
"Zone of inhibition", 184
Zoonosis, 8, 50
Zoophilic organisms, 149
Zyvox (linezolid), 261–262